(*continued on back*)

THE PRACTICE OF HYPNOTISM

The Practice of Hypnotism

Volume 2: Applications of Traditional and Semi-Traditional Hypnotism. Non-Traditional Hypnotism

André M. Weitzenhoffer

WILEY

A WILEY-INTERSCIENCE PUBLICATION

JOHN WILEY & SONS

New York • Chichester • Brisbane • Toronto • Singapore

Library of Congress Cataloging in Publication Data:

Weitzenhoffer, André M. (André Muller), 1921–
    The practice of hypnotism / André Weitzenhoffer.
        p.   cm.—(Wiley series on personality processes)
    Includes bibliographies and indexes.
    Contents: v. 1. Traditional and semi-traditional techniques and
    phenomenology—v. 2. Applications of traditional and semi-
    traditional hypnotism ; Non-traditional hypnotism.
    ISBN 0-471-62167-6 (v. 1).   ISBN 0-471-62168-4 (v. 2)
    ISBN 0-471-62199-4 (2-vol. set)
    1. Hypnotism.   2. Hypnotism—Therapeutic use.   I. Title.
II. Series.
    RC495.W43   1989
    615.8′512—dc19   88-20902
                                                              CIP
ISBN 0-471-62167-6 (v. 1)
ISBN 0-471-62168-4 (v. 2)

Printed in the United States of America

10 9 8 7 6 5 4 3 2 1

This volume is dedicated to
Janet and Mark,
my daughter and son,
and to
Michelle, David, and Wesley,
my grandchildren

Series Preface

This series of books is addressed to behavioral scientists interested in the nature of human personality. Its scope should prove pertinent to personality theorists and researchers as well as to clinicians concerned with applying an understanding of personality processes to the amelioration of emotional difficulties in living. To this end, the series provides a scholarly integration of theoretical formulations, empirical data, and practical recommendations.

Six major aspects of studying and learning about human personality can be designated: personality theory, personality structure and dynamics, personality development, personality assessment, personality change, and personality adjustment. In exploring these aspects of personality, the books in the series discuss a number of distinct but related subject areas: the nature and implications of various theories of personality; personality characteristics that account for consistencies and variations in human behavior; the emergence of personality processes in children and adolescents; the use of interviewing and testing procedures to evaluate individual differences in personality; efforts to modify personality styles through psychotherapy, counseling, behavior therapy, and other methods of influence; and patterns of abnormal personality functioning that impair individual competence.

IRVING B. WEINER

Fairleigh Dickinson University
Rutherford, New Jersey

Acknowledgments

I wish to acknowledge the cooperation of the following publishing houses and journals:

The American Journal of Clinical Hypnosis for permission to reproduce text and tables from the 1958, 1959, 1974, 1975, and 1976 volumes, copyright 1958, 1959, 1975, and 1976 by the American Society of Clinical Hypnosis; J. B. Lippincott and Company for permission to reproduce text from W.S. Kroger, *Clinical and Experimental Hypnosis,* copyright 1963; Grune & Stratton, Inc. for permission to reproduce text from L. R. Wolberg, *The Techniques of Psychotherapy, Part I,* copyright 1967; The Psychological Corporation for permission to reproduce text from L. R. Wolberg, *Medical Hypnosis, Volume I,* copyright 1948; Brunner/Mazel, Publishers, for permission to reproduce text from J. K. Zeig, *A Teaching Seminar with Milton H. Erickson, M.D.,* copyright 1980; W.W. Norton and Company, Inc., for permission to reproduce text from J. Haley, *Uncommon Therapy,* copyright 1973; *The Medical Clinics of North America* for permission to reproduce text from M. H. Erickson, Hypnotic Psychotherapy, New York issue, pp. 572, 573, 574, 575, copyright 1948 by W. B. Saunders Company, Publishers; *Behavioral Science* for permission to reproduce text from the 1956 volume, copyright 1956 by the Society for General System Research; Real People Press for permission to reproduce text from R. Bandler and J. Grinder, *Frogs into Princes,* copyright 1979; Irvington Publishers for permission to reproduce text from M. H. Erickson, E. L. Rossi, and S. I. Rossi, *Hypnotic Realities,* copyright 1976 and from M. H. Erickson and E. L. Rossi, *Hypnotherapy. An Exploratory Casebook,* copyright 1979.

Contents

Contents for Volume 1

1

Introduction

Volume 1 focused on techniques of induction that are of general applicability and devotes considerable space to the production of the many possible hypnotic phenomena, without concern about how they can be put to practical use. In this volume, the focus shifts to specific applications. These have mostly been in the health sciences, but we shall also look at other types of applications.

Volume 1 also focused on *semi-traditional* hypnotism, an approach to the production and utilization of hypnotic phenomena that is rooted in the traditional use of direct suggestions. It also approaches this production and utilization with greater flexibility and attention to ongoing events and gives special attention to the personal contributions the subject can make to the overall process. It has a relationship to *non-traditional* hypnotism, an approach first used by Milton H. Erickson and now practiced by his students and followers. This approach will also be discussed.

The domain of clinical applications is extremely broad; there are probably as many ways of applying hypnotism in a given situation as there are clinicians. This is particularly true in the area of psychotherapy. No single volume can cover in detail all the many ways of applying hypnotism in a clinical setting, nor is this necessary. A reasonable sampling of applications, accompanied by a discussion of such general principles as may be involved, can suffice. Many procedures used in one situation can often, with a few modifications, be readily carried over to other similar situations. In any case, the many variations in the use of hypnotism in a given type of problem are partly determined by the kind of person the patient is and the surrounding circumstances. These are highly variable factors and essentially unpredictable; the clinician must be left to improvise in ways that one cannot fully cover in any single book. Other elements of the determination of procedures, especially with psychotherapy, are the therapist's interpretations of the symptomatology, the role of contextual factors, and the particular school of therapy he belongs to. If a clinician is adequately trained in the fundamentals of his specialty, he does not need to be explicitly told how to adapt the various procedures that were discussed in Volume 1 or that will be discussed presently. I take this position partly on the basis of my own experience in using hypnotism in clinical settings and also on the basis of experience accrued from conducting workshops for professionals. The writing of this volume was very much guided by the latter experience.

As was pointed out in Volume 1, hypnotism is as much, and possibly more, of an art than a science, and this is even more the case in the applied areas. It is especially true in the area of psychotherapy because we have to cope with the inadequacies of our knowledge about hypnotism which are compounded with the inadequacies of our knowledge about the nature of psychotherapy.

It may seem that I have allocated a disproportionate amount of space to the traditional, and especially the semi-traditional, approach to clinical hypnotism. One keeps hearing how superior the Ericksonian type of approach to clinical hypnotism is. Why, then, bother with any other approach? First, this superiority has by no means been clearly demonstrated. The claims of superiority come mainly from individuals who have never known or used any other approach. In my experience, if used with understanding, traditional, and especially semi-traditional, procedures (these contain elements found in the Ericksonian approach) can be just as effective. Furthermore, there are many medical applications for which these are particularly well-suited, much better than the Ericksonian approach. One advantage is that with the traditional approach easy, straight-forward, logical steps are taken making it easier to follow the therapeutic process. The Ericksonian approach can be rather circuitous and involved, and is appreciably more difficult to use when properly done. It has been held against the traditional approach to clinical hypnotism—and this holds true for the semi-traditional approach, as well—that it is hypnotist-centered; that is, that the therapist plans and directs the way the cure or amelioration will take place. This is in contrast to the non-traditional approach that is said to be client-centered and that works from the position that the patient can find his own cure from within himself and should be allowed and encouraged to do so. However, no one has, as yet, clearly shown that patients really do this. Furthermore, there are no necessarily negative aspects involved in planning the therapeutic steps and, indeed, this should be effective in many situations. This objection seems to be more of a philosophical issue than of one based on facts.

Erickson's writings show considerable evidence that he was often quite directive, and that, most of the time, he had a great deal of input into and control of the therapeutic process. I also seriously question that every individual knows, deep down, how to cure himself or solve his problems. Lastly, Fromm (1987) has made the excellent observation that the Ericksonian and Neo-Ericksonian movement may be a fad that will pass. Erickson did make some valuable contributions, but their correct place may be in the further evolution of semi-traditional hypnotism. For these reasons, the time has not yet come to discard traditional and semi-traditional approaches.

The relative amount of space I have devoted to the two main approaches that are taken up in this volume has largely to do with the highly individualized approach Ericksonian therapy takes. It is difficult to give general models because no two like problems are ever approached the same way. Erickson's followers see this as an essential feature. The best one can do, short of presenting extensive case descriptions (in which the literature on Ericksonian and strategic therapies abounds), is to try to abstract the essential features. One can find a small number of such features that can be discussed in relatively little space. Much of what is found in the literature concerning Erickson's approach is an adulterated version of what he said and did, and as such does not belong in this volume. (I say this having had the good fortune of knowing Erickson personally and of spending many hours with him over the years.) This adulteration has partially come about because an increasing amount of the relevant literature has originated from individuals who have had no personal contact with Erickson. As Fromm (1987) aptly states it, today we are speaking of a Neo-Ericksonian rather than of a pure Ericksonian approach. I have tried to present a view of Erickson's thoughts and *modus operandi* that is as free as possible from my personal elaborations and distortions, but I am quite certain that I have only partially succeeded in doing this.

As in the first volume, I have tried to separate fact from fiction. Hypnotism may not yet be a science, but one can still approach it with a scientific spirit and with a critical mind, whether one discusses suggestions, techniques of induction, its phenomena, or its applications.

The format followed in Volume 1 is not fully applicable here. Nevertheless, I have continued, in a selective manner, to give detailed examples of procedures as models to guide the reader and student. Here, *even more* than in the case of the models given in Volume 1, the reader should keep in mind *the need to modify these models to meet the needs of the patient and of the situations encountered.*

The present volume assumes that the reader has a background of knowledge equivalent to the contents of Volume 1. As an aid in the study of the

present volume, the glossary included in the first volume has been duplicated and follows the last chapter.

Reading a book is only the beginning in learning to work with hypnotism.
Before embarking on any specific project using it, whether research or therapy, one should get first-hand experience with hypnotic phenomena and
their production in an informal setting, with no other goal than to try things
out. This should be a preliminary period of free exploration. If at all possible, every student of hypnotism should experience being a subject. There is
an invaluable, unique, subjective knowledge to be obtained in this manner
that cannot be obtained in any other way.

2

General Overview and Principles of Traditional and Semi-Traditional Clinical Hypnotism

INTRODUCTION

As explained in Volume 1, Chapter 1, I prefer to speak of *clinical hypnotism* rather than *clinical hypnosis,* as has been so widely done for at least the last 30 years. As pointed out, *hypnosis* is a state, or condition, of mind and being. *Hypnotism* is the use of suggestion with or without hypnosis being present, although for many individuals, hypnosis is always implied when this term is used. There are also those who deny that hypnosis exists. For those who do not, it is meaningful and useful to distinguish between *intra-hypnotic* and *extra-hypnotic* suggestions, according to whether or not a suggestion is given in the presence of hypnosis. However, it must always be kept in mind that a suggestion is a suggestion whether or not given during hypnosis. This is at least true concerning its ideational content and the ideodynamic action it brings about. Because traditional and semi-traditional hypnotism view suggestion as the essential agent and instrument in the production and use of hypnosis, it seems reasonable to speak more specifically, in this case, also of *hypnosuggestion* and *hypnosuggestive* phenomena when we want to emphasize that hypnosis is presumed to be involved. We will keep the expressions *suggestion* and *suggestion phenomena* to designate cases of the use of suggestion in which the absence or presence of hypnosis is not of concern. It is also particularly important to recognize that hypnosis per se not only has a limited phenomenology of its own, but, for the most part, also has very little therapeutic value by itself when viewed in the framework of traditional hypnotism. Such limited therapeutic effects as have been ascribed to it have been poorly documented. Its main value in clinical work seems to lie in its ability to enhance suggestibility. Because the therapeutic effects of implicit suggestions were not well-recognized by classical hypnotism, it did seem, to the very early workers in the field, that hypnosis was, indeed, the therapeutic agent even when it was not. They may have ascribed the term in far more cases than were warranted. For post-traditional hypnotism, best exemplified by Ericksonian hypnotism, suggestion effects and hypnosis are inseparable. In this case, the ascribing of therapeutic value to hypnosis per se has a somewhat better foundation.

There is no reason to think that applying hypnosis and suggestion effects alters their basic nature, nor that the domain of application is itself basically changed. The problems may differ, but the same general phenomenology of hypnotism applies in a selective manner. It is for this reason that I prefer to think in terms of clinical hypnotism rather than in terms of medical, dental, psychological, or psychiatric hypnotism. These seem to dangerously and subtly imply an essential difference. Briefly stated, *clinical hypnotism is the explicit planned use of hypnotism for purposes of furthering the physical and mental health of individuals, whether it be in the treatment of an existing condition or a prophylactic utilization of hypnotism.* The prophylactic use has been greatly overlooked in the past by health practitioners. Many features of the preoperative preparation of surgical patients with hypnotism are good examples of such a prophylactic use.

The problem of distinguishing intended from effective therapeutic suggestions is appreciably greater in the clinical situation than in other situations because an intended suggestion acted on at a strictly voluntary level, as an instruction, may nevertheless be therapeutic. For example, an intended posthypnotic suggestion might be given to a patient to insure that he will religiously follow a prescribed procedure (such as taking a pill every other day). Obviously, if the suggestion does not take as such, but the patient faithfully carries out what is now only an instruction, the desired therapeutic step will still occur. Spiegel's (1970) hypnosuggestive treatment of tobaccomania (nicotinism) provides us with a good example. At one point, the patient is given the intended posthypnotic suggestion that he will go through a brief specified ritual whenever he feels the urge to light a cigarette. This step may simply work because the response constitutes a positively reinforced inhibiting act. It is clear from the literature on behavior therapy that a similar act done as a voluntary response to appropriate effective instructions would be expected to have a similar effect. This being the case, it becomes immaterial whether or not the intended suggestion ever becomes effective.

Clinical uses of hypnotism fall into two main classes. There are those in which hypnotism is used as the *principal* mode of treatment. Other nonhypnotic procedures and agents may be used, but the use of hypnotism is the *core* of the overall treatment. In such cases, it is legitimate to speak in general of *hypnotherapy.* There are times when one wishes to emphasize that psychotherapy with hypnotism is the subject matter. The term *hypnopsychotherapy* can then be used. Likewise, if it is important to make it clear that the therapy using hypnotism is not psychotherapy, the term *hypnosomatotherapy* denotes this situation. This term covers all strictly somatically oriented applications in medicine, dentistry, and related fields. The use of the qualificatives *hypnotherapeutic, hypnopsychotherapeutic,* and *hypnosomatotherapeutic* is the same. I realize that there are applications in which a combination of somatic and psychic therapeutic steps have to be undertaken jointly as, for example, in the treatment of severe gastric ulcers or when the patient has a severe emotional reaction to his illness or its treatment. Sometimes such situations involve somatic treatment by a medical specialist with conjoint psychotherapy by a psychiatrist or psychologist. Sometimes it consists of joint interventions, in the sense to be defined, by the same health professional, usually a physician or dentist. There are many situations, however, in which hypnosuggestive methods are employed in a limited, peripheral manner and, therefore, in which hypnotism is no longer the core of treatment. It is now an *adjunct,* rather than the principal, agent. In such instances, it is much more appropriate to speak of a hypnotherapeutic and a hypnosuggestive *intervention.* These are not quite the same. In the first usage, there is a goal of a defined, limited direct therapeutic action. In the second, there is *no* direct therapeutic goal in itself. An example taken from my own practice was the use of hypnotism to treat tension headaches in a patient whose primary therapy, conducted by another therapist, was for the abusive use of alcohol. Consider also the hypnotic treatment of a wrist drop in an individual who was in treatment with another therapist for a major personality disorder. Neither of these examples used hypnosis to treat the primary problem, but a limited therapy of an associated problem was performed with it; these are therefore hypnotherapeutic interventions.

A good example of hypnosuggestive intervention is the use of hypnotically induced analgesias or anesthesias for dental, surgical, and obstetrical work. Consider also my incidental use of hypnoanalgesia to relieve the pain of a sprained shoulder that one of my patients had suffered in an accident while she was in psychotherapy with me. In this particular instance, I was also using hypnotism extensively in a central way in her psychotherapy. This is a good example of a double use of hypnotism, in a clinical setting, for hypnotherapy and for intervention.

Going back a moment to the tension headache case, the treatment was purely ancillary. In this case, if a hypnopsychotherapeutic approach had been used for the patient's dominant problem, this could have been made an integral part of the total treatment because the abusive use of alcohol centered around his attempts to handle stress. His primary therapist chose to proceed otherwise, presumably with good reasons.

I have found, over the years, that one of the more effective ways of approaching the clinical use of hypnotism is by thinking of it as the *methodical* application of hypnosuggestive phenomena to the solution and resolution of clinical problems. In such an approach, every proposed clinical use of hypnotism should begin, as much as possible, with the following seven basic questions being considered:

1. What is the exact clinical problem to be solved?
2. What does hypnotism offer in its phenomenology that can be used to solve the problem?
3. What is the patient capable of producing in the line of hypnosuggestive effects?
4. What are the patient's assets and liabilities, particularly, but not exclusively, of a psychodynamic nature?
5. What is practical, feasible, and desirable for the patient in terms of his everyday life?
6. What is clinically sound and appropriate for a given case?
7. How will the chosen or available use of hypnotism fit into the overall therapeutic framework in which it will be employed?

This is mostly a common-sense approach that has its parallel in other applied fields. In many instances, some of these questions have to be answered by hypotheses, which are then tested. If they are rejected, new ones are made. Answering these questions for each patient may appear to be time consuming. It frequently is. I have rarely had a patient with whom I undertook hypnotic treatment on the first, or even second, session. There is a need for preliminary fact gathering and much thinking, followed by planning a preliminary course of action and implementation. Then, with luck, and/or because one has done an exceptional job of this groundwork, one might occasionally hold a single hypnotherapeutic session and effect a seemingly miraculous "cure." Most of the time, this does not happen. Many of the remarkable therapies reported by Milton H. Erickson were, by his own accounts, actually the result of much groundwork of the kind just outlined. In brief, a comprehensive treatment plan is as much advocated here as it is in other clinical applications.

Prospective users of clinical hypnotism should be aware that even though there appears to have been more miraculously "brief" therapies reported with the use of hypnotism than with other forms of psychotherapies, this, in actuality, may be more the exception than the rule. Many psychotherapies in which hypnotism is used can still last several years and require multiple weekly sessions. There is no question that there have been and can be some spectacular results obtained with psychotherapy using hypnotism, and that it has been a powerful ingredient in some reported cases of "briefer" psychotherapy. Still, the qualification "briefer" is relative, and usually spells out, in the best of cases, a dozen and more therapy hours, rather than the couple of hours that seems to be the popular perception and expectation. Then, too, are "brief" therapies, in general, really briefer? Briefer than what? Unfortunately, once patients have been cured with a so-called brief therapy, there is no way to go back and find out what other therapies would have done for them. Other approaches might have been just as effective. Even if a patient has gone unsuccessfully through one or more "long-term" therapies previous to undertaking a successful brief therapy, there is a problem in drawing conclusions about the true effectiveness of the presumably briefer therapy. Who knows how near success the previous therapy had come before the brief therapy was instituted? Did the latter capitalize on this? Even if the prior therapy was nowhere near reaching success, how much may it, nevertheless, have contributed to the success of the brief therapy? Did the shift to the new therapy itself serve as a catalyst? A formal statistical approach comparing groups of patients going through the two types of therapies seems to be the only way of settling the question. This has never been done and for good reasons. It would be a horrendous enterprise! Semi-formal statistical comparisons are much more feasible; in spite of certain weaknesses, they would be useful. To my knowledge, none have been done. Thus, the relative effectiveness of clinical hypnotism, particularly in the area of psychotherapy, is not a clearly established matter.

We will now look more closely at the above questions. Some of the examples used briefly will subsequently be covered in greater detail in later chapters.

The Problems

It is not necessarily the total syndrome the patient presents or the particular symptom he complains of that the actual clinical problem to be solved with hypnotism is concerned with. There are reasons for this. First, hypnotism has its limitations, even under ideal conditions, although more with some individuals than with others. Second, a symptom may only be one element in a long causative chain of events, and the preferred treatment may be to deal with only one or more of the other elements in the chain. There are also many situations in which it is feasible, or even indicated, to be concerned only with one or several aspects of a syndrome, but not with the latter *in toto.* For example, chronic tension headaches are often more easily treated symptomatically by attacking the associated muscular tension rather than the pain. In a case of diaphragmatic myoclonus that I once treated, the most effective way of helping the patient was by focusing treatment on the control of the associated abdominal myoclonus. Finally, in the treatment of a case of chronic painful head jerking that had resulted from a neck injury, effective treatment consisted of focusing on decreasing the pain experience, on the patient's awareness of the head movements, and on reducing her emotional reaction to having the movements. Very little was done to reduce the movements; this was not necessary.

Although the patient initially stated that she had sought help to stop the jerking of her head, she was really seeking relief from her embarrassment over this. This information was revealed in the course of the initial session and also several times as therapy aimed at controlling the movements went on. She felt that the problem would be solved if the movements stopped, and this was her goal. True, the pain was also a motivation, but it was a secondary one. Initially, I accepted her request at face value and, indeed, this was a perfectly reasonable solution. Unfortunately, while the associated pain easily came under control, the head movements would not. On the other hand, they were not so severe as to physically interfere with her carrying out her daily activities. Because this was the case, and because pain was no longer a factor, I focused on the more basic problem of her embarrassment. Had I listened more carefully in the initial session, I might have saved the patient a number of possibly unnecessary sessions and saved myself much work.

It must also be recognized that the manifestations of many ailments are multiple, and treatment often needs to be multifaceted. More often than not, hypnotism can be used for more than one purpose in dealing with an ailment. The case of the woman with the head jerk is an example, too, of a double use of hypnotism. In the case of severe body burns, hypnotism has been found useful in relieving the patient not only of the attending pain during healing, but also of the pain caused by debridement, the changing of surgical dressings, and skin grafting. In addition, hypnotism has also been found helpful in promoting adequate food intake, facilitating physical therapy, and improving the patient's morale. All of this can usually be accomplished with simple direct suggestions of the desired effects.

Sometimes in the course of treating a patient for a problem, one may identify other possible problems. Tempted as one may be to also deal with these, unless treating them is essential to the treatment of the initial problem, it is advisable to stay with the main problem. Later, one can discuss with the patient the option of treating the other problems. Even when this additional treatment is necessary, the patient's consent is still desirable. In my early days of practice, I lost a patient by allowing her, without her consent, to have a spontaneous cathartic experience with regard to an incident that was not clearly related to the problem for which I was treating her.

Sometimes, there may be no reason to treat, or it may be inadvisable to treat, the perceived additional problems. Once a psychiatry resident at a hospital where I worked asked me to treat, with hypnotism, one of his patients who had a back pain. The pain seemed to be primarily somatogenic, since it was related to a back injury and to scar tissue that was caused by earlier surgery of the back. Two sessions were required to relieve the pain. At least two years later, the man was still pain free. However, in the course of treatment, the man was found to have some paranoid ideations. The resident, who had been much impressed by the pain alleviation, was very eager to move on to a treatment of the paranoia. I refused because I would not have used hypnotism for this and because the man had come to us with the complaint of a somatogenic chronic back pain and nothing more. Equally important, there were no indications that his paranoid thoughts were creating any problems. I advised against further work with the patient. The two-year follow-up showed no indications that such problems had developed.

Hypnotic Possibilities

In theory, hypnotism offers a multitude of effects that one can utilize in treatment. Of course, not all are suitable in every case. Suitability will usually be determined by a great many factors. One is that there are usually limitations regarding what can actually be evoked in any given patient. While most of these are a function of the patient, there are some limitations inherent in the nature of some of the effects that one may propose to induce.

For example, it is very doubtful that one can *directly* affect reflexes by suggestion, even in the most suggestible persons. Tissue and organ changes induced by *direct* suggestion are more the exception than the rule. Whether this is a constitutional matter or a matter of requiring an unusually great suggestibility is not clear. The recovery of forgotten material through suggested hyperamnesia and age regressions is greatly subject to confabulation. Deciding what specific effects might be used is also dependent upon an understanding of the nature of the problem to be treated and upon a good knowledge of what can be produced with suggestions. The treatment of Reynaud's disease, a progressive circulatory disorder, by suggestion is a case in question. One might, at first, consider this to be an impossibility, because direct suggestions are generally unable to affect the vascular system directly to the degree that would be required to re-establish proper blood circulation in the patient's extremities. Instead, one could use an indirect method, such as having the patient hallucinate that his hands and/or feet are immersed in warm water. Might not this lead to a conditioned reflex dilation of blood vessels in just the right place? This was, indeed, tried once by Milton H. Erickson as part of a very successful hypnotherapy in a similar case.

Quite some years after Erickson had told me about his case, I had the opportunity to similarly treat a young man who had been greatly handicapped by Reynaud's disease. The treatment was fully successful; the patient recovered full use of his hands and now, some 20 years later, he is still free of symptoms.

The full implementation of the treatment in these two cases was somewhat more complex than just described, but the extra details are not needed to make the desired point. Deciding just what can be done may call for a study of the pertinent literature, especially if the problem is an unfamiliar one, as it was for me in the case of the diaphragmatic myoclonus. Other factors that might be considered will be better discussed in the context of some of the material which follows.

Patient Potentials

Although the patient's ability or inability to produce suggested effects can justifiably be viewed as part of his total assets and liabilities, this matter is better considered separately from others. In general, hypnotism offers a much wider variety of potentially usable effects than the individual to be treated can produce, because most persons have a limited suggestibility. Reason tell us that every person must possess physical and mental limitations that cannot be transcended by suggestions. Also, it is doubtful that one can create, by suggestion, a new ability or capacity unless the ground for it already pre-exists. Thus, a tone-deaf individual will most likely remain tone-deaf when hypnotized. Someone who has never had an exposure to calculus is not likely to suddenly develop the ability to solve calculus problems under hypnosis. An individual born with a limited intellect will generally continue to have a limited intellect under hypnosis. Such limitations must be taken into account in doing clinical hypnotism. Clinical hypnotism is no different than clinical work without hypnotism. On the other hand, failure on the part of a patient to produce a suggested effect does not necessarily preclude his producing a related phenomenon that can be put to good use instead. For example, a patient who is unable to produce suggested dreams may be able to produce equally useful vivid guided fantasies when hypnotized. A woman unable to produce a suggested saddle block for delivery may still be able to produce a satisfactory suggested analgesia and even anesthesia. One may not be able to lift an amnesia directly, yet the desired material may be recovered by means of a regression or, failing this, through automatic writing or, possibly, dreams. When a direct suggestion of analgesia or anesthesia fails, it may be possible to get the desired result by means of a suggested dissociation of the part of the body which is to be involved. In some cases, the use of age regression is another way out. A simple separation of affect from the pain experience could also be the solution. A good knowledge of the phenomenology of hypnotism, a flexible treatment plan, and a readiness *to utilize whatever the patient has to offer* in the line of responses to suggestions all help in reducing many limitations inherent in the use of hypnotism. Utilization is one of the key words and concepts of Ericksonian psychotherapy and is possibly the most important one.

Assets and Liabilities

Basically, any factor that can hinder therapeutic effectiveness is a liability, and, conversely, any facilitating factor is an asset. Anything that can be used is an asset, whereas that which cannot be used is a liability. Low suggestibility is a liability, but high suggestibility is an asset. For hypnopsychotherapy, as well as for other psychotherapies, a strong ego is an asset; a weak one is a liability. Cooperation or lack of cooperation from the patient's family is respectively an asset and a liability. Husbands will sabotage their wives' therapy and conversely, and parents will sabotage their children's therapy. I once had a woman patient whose husband insisted that after each session, she go over with him in detail what had transpired in my office. Not only did she strongly resent this invasion of her privacy, but she was placed in a quandary because the husband was a frequent topic of conversation. Another husband decided to learn the rudiments of hypnotism and placed pressure upon his wife to let him hypnotize her instead of her continuing to see me. Such situations are usually an indication that the spouse or parent is also in need of psychotherapy, or that marital or family counseling (therapy) are also indicated. I have encountered cases in which one or both parents wanted me to use hypnotism with a child to deal with what they considered to be behavior problems, when actually the indicated simple solution lay in a quite different direction.

In two cases that I have in mind, the use of hypnosis would have constituted a contraindicated coercive action. On the other hand, Erickson (1963) has reported, in great detail, a most ingenious use of a patient's family to bring about, in one of his patients, planned therapeutic frustration over a long period of time. Having a patient with whom one cannot communicate verbally is a liability, but the former's ability to respond to non-verbal suggestions is an asset that can make up for the liability. This was nicely demonstrated by Erickson (1964), who could not speak Spanish, in the case of a Mexican subject who did not understand English.

Feasibility

Practicality, feasibility, and advisability of suggested effects in regard to the patient's everyday life situation is an important issue that should not be overlooked. Suggestions, the effects of which are to carry over into his or her daily activities, should take the potential problems that they might cause into consideration. One of the first clinical applications of hypnotism, frequently done during the nineteenth century, was in the treatment of alcoholism. The patient was given the very simple posthypnotic suggestion that any time he tried to drink an alcoholic beverage, he would be unable to do so. The trouble with this suggestion was that it often created a very embarrassing, and even distressing, situation because the patient's hand refused to bring the glass to his mouth. As he persisted in trying, he developed tremors and jerky, convulsive movements resulting in liquid being sloshed over the glass. In a case I witnessed, the suggestion to the subject that cigarettes would have a "vile" taste resulted in the subject becoming violently ill upon placing a cigarette to her mouth.

These two examples show the importance of choosing one's words carefully when constructing suggestions. Thus, "become unable" is too broad an expression. Likewise, "vile" is too unspecific and strong. Usually, satisfactory modifications can be found that allow one to proceed with, essentially, the planned suggestion. An individual who has sustained a painful injury and whose pain has been relieved will often carry out activities that are contraindicated. This is often the case with past back injuries that may become associated with chronic pain and must be prevented.

One of the first patients I treated for chronic pain was a woman who had suffered a back injury in a fall from a horse. She felt "so good" after I had removed the pain that she started to ride a horse again. Fortunately, this resulted in a new attack of pain before she had done any new damage. Removing the new pain was not particularly difficult, and having done this, I carefully explained to her that horse riding was no longer an option. I also discussed the inadvisability of carrying out certain other potentially stressful acts. Her next visit, shortly thereafter, was prompted by a recurrence of pain. She assured me that she had been very careful not to put undue stress on her back. However, in thoroughly discussing her activities, it became clear that she had been overly active because she felt so good again. She had cleaned her large two-story home from top to bottom; thus, she had effectively put stress on her back in a different, less obvious way. As I will discuss in more detail later, it is quite feasible to give, in such a treatment, additional broad posthypnotic suggestions that are very effective countermeasures against such occurrences. However, when one does this, it is also advisable to make provisions for the possible occurrence of situations in which there may be no other alternative but for the patient to put strain on his or her body.

Consider, for example, the case of one of my patients who had a weak back that prohibited her from lifting her small grandchildren, whom she often babysat. One can easily conceive of life-threatening situations that might make it imperative for this woman to lift and carry such a child. Dramatic as it may sound, fires, accidents, tornados, and other unpredictable events do occur that call for this very type of action. Injunctions such as "always" and "never," and the stipulation of highly specific times and places in connection with therapeutic posthypnotic suggestions, should be used with the utmost care and as little as possible.

Finally, it is important in clinical hypnotism, as in any other clinical practice, to consider how the therapy may affect the family stability or some specific family member. This is especially true when psychotherapy is involved. A physician once approached me regarding a woman patient who suffered from a *tic douloureux*. Could I decrease or remove the pain? The first interview with the patient evinced an association between attacks, exacerbation of her symptoms, and certain interactions with her husband. Further inquiry gave indications that the husband might become psychotic if her symptoms were totally removed. In this case, a compromise had to be made that was satisfactory to both the patient *and* her spouse. Such compromises are not always possible.

Clinical Soundness

Hypnosuggestive interventions and certain forms of hypnotherapy that may otherwise be effective and satisfy the above criteria may still not be clinically sound. This issue probably appears most often in the case of symptom removal, which was the goal of therapeutic traditional hypnotism in its early days. It should be clear that there is no problem with symptoms that have a purely somatic origin. Symptoms that are psychogenic or have a psychogenic component are another matter. Opinions have greatly varied, ranging from "never remove symptoms" to "removing symptoms is always permissible." As is usually the case in this type of situation, the truth seems to lie somewhere in the middle. There are now clinical data that show direct symptom removal can be quite successful. But it is also clear that it can be deleterious. Seitz (1953) has shown this in an experimental study done in a clinical setting with an actual patient. This study also provides important information regarding the nature and mechanism of symptom substitution.

The issue of clinical soundness has many ramifications. We have already seen how patients relieved from pain may then overtax their body unless steps other than the removal of pain are taken. Another example from my case files is that of a patient whom I treated for mild obesity. In her particular case, and under other circumstances, I would have given her suggestions severely limiting her sugar intake. Because she was a diabetic taking insulin and subject to hypoglycemia, such a step could have led to hypoglycemic complications. Special provisions had to be incorporated to obviate such occurrences. This case also shows the importance of obtaining a complete medical history and the importance for clinical psychologists of having some understanding of medical problems that may arise as a consequence of the use of a therapeutic suggestion or treatment. Consulting with the patient's personal physician is a good alternative to studying the medical literature.

Appropriateness and soundness are closely related. Quite some years ago, a man contacted me who wanted me to see his wife, whom he described as having what seemed, at the time, to be psychotic homicidal episodes. I did not feel that this was a case I should handle, and advised him to consult a psychiatrist. Time passed, then one day a pediatrician contacted me asking me to see the mother of one of his young patients. From his description, I very quickly identified this woman as being the one whom I had previously been asked to see. I explained to the pediatrician my reasons for not wanting to take this case and my feelings that a psychiatrist should see her. He replied that she had been unable to get an appointment with any of the local psychiatrists. As a favor to him, he wanted me to see the woman just to make a diagnosis. I agreed to do so. She came, and I could detect no indication of psychosis in her. It seemed that, intermittently, she found herself becoming increasingly tense. This tension would often culminate in her getting a kitchen knife and threatening her family while screaming at them. She had, thus far, never actually hurt anyone. There did not seem to be any regularity about these attacks. I chose a tentative diagnosis of episodic hysteria and agreed to continue to see her. During the second session, it was revealed that she had very irregular menses. She could not say whether or not there was a coincidence between her attacks and her menses. I thought that there might be, and consulting some relevant textbooks reaffirmed this. I also found that she had not consulted a gynecologist, or any other physician, in the last two years, so I contacted one. I presented the case to him, as well as my suspicion that I was dealing with a case of premenstrual syndrome. He agreed that this was a likely diagnosis and indicated that there was a simple medical treatment for this problem. I referred my patient to him. There were no further homicidal episodes. I never used hypnotism with this woman. I had considered doing so in my third session with her. This would have been the next step, and a way of further exploring the nature of her symptoms. Using the alternative somatic approach seemed more appropriate at that point. Had this failed, I most likely would have gone on with the use of hypnotism.

On another occasion, I was contacted by the parents of a young boy. They stated that their son, who had, not long ago, been a top student, was now doing poorly in school and had become withdrawn and apathetic. The boy's IQ was well above average, and I agreed he should have been able to do much better. They wanted me to hypnotize their son and change him back to what he had been. A further session with the parents elucidated that the father was an engineer with aspirations to move upward socially and economically. To further this goal, he had moved his family into a new housing development where many of his more successful colleagues, as well as many other professionals, lived. The boy had entered a new school where it seemed that each grade consisted of two groups of children who were taught separately. One group consisted of only Caucasian children who were primarily children of professional people. The other was made up of children from a lesser socioeconomic level, including many Hispanics. Unfortunately for the boy, the average IQ of his class was appreciably above his. He had been able to produce an above average performance with ease, but now was unable to do so even with some effort. Neither his teachers nor his parents were particularly sensitive to his situation. This case hardly seemed to be one that could or should be solved with hypnotism. I thought that a better first-step solution would be to transfer the boy to the other class, where he would again become one of the brighter students. This recommendation was poorly taken by his parents. "What would our neighbors and friends think!" was the father's immediate response. This simple solution was quite unacceptable to the parents. Why could I not hypnotize their son and make him perform as he should? That was the last I saw of the parents and their child. I am not saying that the child did not need some kind of supportive therapy, but neither this nor hypnotism, if the latter were to have been used in other ways, could have been effective without a situational change first being made.

My last example is a case of a child being brought to me because he was becoming a juvenile delinquent. Currently, his behavior was making him a problem-child in his school. The parents were divorced; the boy's father had custody. In the first two sessions, I heard, from both the boy and the father, a rather horrible story. My one reaction was to wonder why the boy was not worse. Psychotherapy, with or without hypnotism, definitely seemed indicated. Then, during the third session, I discovered that the boy's problems in school had started about the time he had been held back a grade because of reading difficulties, and that he continued to have great problems with reading. I wanted to get an idea of just what kind of difficulties he had, so I asked him to read some material. At this point, I discovered that the child had a visual problem. I told the father this, and that his son probably simply needed to be fitted with glasses. I recommended that he contact an ophthalmologist. The father followed my advice, the boy was given glasses, and the behavior problems soon ceased without any further intervention on my part. Would the boy have benefited from therapy? Certainly he had gone through a great deal of psychological trauma by the time I saw him, and I cannot say that it did not lead to later problems. However, the problem I had been consulted about was caused by the need for glasses, and there was no actual evidence that anything more needed to be done. There is such a thing as unnecessarily opening a can of worms.

These last three examples are evidence that hypnotism is not always the most appropriate answer.

This seems a good place to consider the use of taped suggestions and inductions for clinical work, especially when done on a large scale. A number of commercial enterprises (usually not accredited health-providing agencies) have, for many years, sold cassettes to the public for eating and smoking problems, for improving study habits, and for other highly questionable purposes. A now-deceased physician, who became well-known in the fifties for his workshops in clinical hypnotism, strongly advocated the mass treatment of patients by having them listen to individualized tapes. The idea was that a half-dozen patients or more could come to his office and be simultaneously treated in the same hour. I know one physician who, in more recent times, started a "medical hypnosis clinic," in which he had a half-dozen cubicles where six patients could sit or recline at one time and listen to a generalized or a personalized tape. He did not supervise these sessions; he left that to so-called technicians who presumably watched each patient by means of closed circuit TV monitors. At best, tapes lend themselves to situations where a set formula can be expected to be effective. *Within limits,* this includes the preparation of patients for surgery and dental work, testing for suggestibility and hypnotizability, inducing deep relaxation, and also hypnosis. The main problem with the use of taped material is that effective hypnotherapy and, especially, hypnopsychotherapy, is built upon a moment-to-moment interaction between therapist and patient and upon events occurring between sessions. Good therapy of any kind, in which feedback plays an important part, is dynamic rather than static. Two-way, not one-way, communication is a crucial element. Additionally, non-verbal communications frequently constitute an important element. The effective utilization of the patient's behavior is eliminated by the use of tapes. In the best of applications, taped material will fail to give maximum benefit. A last objectionable feature of the use of tapes is that even seemingly innocuous suggestions and instructions sometimes have unexpected, undesirable effects. In a face-to-face situation, the therapist can often catch such occurrences and remedy these before any real harm has been done. Relying on video monitoring and inadequately trained human monitors is hardly better than no monitoring.

Therapeutic Framework

We now come to the final question. The clinical uses of hypnotism, when they are not the entire therapy—that is, when they constitute interventions —are most effective when they are carefully fit within a framework of overall therapy. Hypnosuggestive interventions need to be coordinated with whatever else one is doing with the patient. The selection of effects to be used should take into account all of the factors that have already been discussed and, also, how best the therapy can be implemented. One of the few exceptions to this rule may be found in some crisis interventions where there is very little time or opportunity to do much more than act as the situation indicates.

The importance of the above consideration is, perhaps, most evident in the case of psychotherapy, which is potentially the richest field for the applications of hypnotism. Different kinds of psychotherapies call for the use of different kinds of suggested effects. For example, hypnotically induced dreams and fantasies can be used with appropriate modifications with all three main traditional types of psychotherapies: supportive, re-educative, and reconstructive. On the other hand, age regressions can be advantageously used with reconstructive therapies, but have no place in supportive therapies, and, at best, have only limited value for re-educative therapy. In further contrast, suggested attitude changes can effectively be used with both supportive and reeducative therapies, but are of limited value for reconstructive therapies. Shifting focus momentarily from the traditional to non-traditional Ericksonian-type therapy, there seems to be no limitation to what can be effectively used.

One should not confuse the use of hypnotism as an adjunctive tool within the framework of a general, non-hypnotic therapeutic approach with the creation of a *new* form of therapy, hypnotic or otherwise. For example, a client-centered therapy remains *the same* client-centered therapy when one uses hypnotism *properly* within it. Likewise, the use of a client-centered approach in the production of hypnotic phenomena should not be expected to create a new state of hypnosis or change the basic nature and character of the associated phenomena. It is proper to speak of an Ericksonian *approach to* hypnotism and to hypnotherapy, but much less so to speak of an Ericksonian *hypnotism* (or hypnotherapy) without further qualification.

Group Therapy

Bernheim, as well as a number of other nineteenth-century practitioner-hypnotists, frequently did group treatment of a very simple kind. As a precursor of hypnotism, early mesmerism might be mentioned, too. Unlike using taped material, group hypnotism does permit face-to-face contact and interaction between therapist and patients at all times. But with large groups (over four persons), such contact is so diluted as to be of little value. A further problem peculiar to group situations is that all group members are exposed to the same suggestions and instructions. To some extent, this problem can be circumscribed by appropriate procedures aimed at creating selectiveness at appropriate times. In general, the larger the group is, the less each member can be given individual attention. I find that it is generally a far more exhausting form of therapy for the therapist than other group therapies, particularly since this form of group treatment frequently does not lend itself well to the participation of a co-therapist.

We are now finished with the examination of the seven questions listed earlier. One conclusion that can be derived from this material is that the clinical uses of hypnotism must generally be tailored to each patient, each problem, and each type of therapy. *There are no set rules* for the treatment of most problems. Given a patient capable of producing certain specific, suitable, suggested effects, the therapist selects one or more of these effects, brings them about, and shapes and controls them in the context of solving the problem as dictated in part by the overall therapeutic plan and, in the case of psychotherapy, by his psychotherapeutic orientation and training. This is anything but a cut-and-dried procedure. Effective use of hypnotism calls for ingenuity, creativity, and flexibility. The ability to shift in midstream and to improvise is an important asset. The extent of the therapist's knowledge regarding hypnosuggestive phenomena is obviously very important. No less important is his clinical knowledge and acumen in the area of normal and abnormal human behavior and functioning. In the remainder of this chapter, a few other basic issues will be examined which did not easily fit under previous headings.

FACTORS FOR SUCCESS

It would be a delightful situation if one could determine under exactly what conditions hypnotism will be successfully used in any given therapy. This simply cannot be done as yet. It is clear that being a good hypnotic subject is not necessarily an indication that an individual is a good candidate for hypnotherapy and hypnopsychotherapy. On the other hand, some poor hypnotic subjects can, nevertheless, sometimes greatly benefit from hypnotic intervention. Persons who seek a miraculous cure for behavioral problems are frequently poor prospects for traditional and semi-traditional hypnotic therapy. Persons who look to hypnotism as a magical source from or through which they will acquire the will-power or the power of concentration, which they claim is all they need to solve their problems in life, are also poor prospects. Individuals with weight and smoking problems, with poor study and work habits, and, more generally, poor self-discipline, also frequently fall in the above group of poor prospects. Unless their thinking can be reoriented, they usually drop out of therapy after two or three sessions.

Success with clinical hypnotism is also dependent upon the therapist's personality. Not everyone should undertake this kind of work. For reasons not altogether clear, some therapists using hypnotism seem to do better with one type of problem than with others. This, of course, is not a unique characteristic of clinical hypnotism. In any event, personality differences among therapists, especially psychotherapists, can probably account for differences in success with clinical hypnotism. Unresolved conflicts and prejudices can cause difficulties and lack of success. Also, for reasons not always clear, some therapists do much better with a certain approach than others. In particular, many practitioners feel very uncomfortable with an authoritarian approach. As a consequence, they are not able to use effectively certain forms of hypnotherapy that lend themselves better to such an approach. There is nothing wrong with acting selectively in some of these respects. Some of the more successful users, who are enthusiastic supporters of clinical hypnotism, do tend to specialize with regard to both types of patients and of methods they use. In many of these instances, this seems to be an intuitive choice.

Claims have been made by past therapists that they have had close to, and even 100% success with this or that method. If there had ever been a method that gave that kind of results, we would all be using it by now! Gross exaggerations of the facts, overenthusiasm, premature reports, or poor controls and statistics, and especially lack of proper follow-ups, are generally behind such reports. Criteria for success are relative; make them sufficiently lax and you can have great success. One physician, who was a well-known authority on clinical hypnotism, once assured me that he had never failed to induce hypnosis, and he stated his puzzlement over laboratory reports that invariably spoke of a certain percentage of failures. His criterion for the presence of hypnosis, as it turned out, was obtaining a general muscular relaxation that he tested by raising a hand and arm or a foot and leg a few inches and letting them go. Back in the mid 1950s, when the use of ideomotor signaling was at its highest, one highly respected teacher and worker in the field reported, at a scientific meeting, having had 100% success in predicting the sex of unborn children by having the pregnant patient hold the Chevreul pendulum. After I questioned him, he admitted that he was reporting on a few cases only and that much of his data were second hand that had come from physicians who had done the testing and had reported their results to him.

The approach one takes to the patient is probably an important element in determining the success of a therapy. There is much to be said in favor of the use of a client-centered approach, thus, in some cases, of non-traditional hypnotism. Contrary to the opinion held by those who favor this, I do not think it is necessarily a suitable approach in all instances. There is also a place for strong, persuasive, authoritarian maneuvers. By virtue of his training, the therapist generally knows more than the patient, or at least knows things that the patient does not know; thus knowledge can be used advantageously by the therapist to help the patient in a planned therapy.

I also have a firm belief in the reality of psychodynamics and in Stekel's "psychic scotoma" (blind spots). Because of these, a therapist is able to perceive and understand things about a patient and his life that the patient can neither know nor understand. The therapist is in a position to view matters and present them back to the patient in a different, helpful light. There are situations in which the therapist must formulate a series of steps leading to a therapeutic change and must take a strong directing role.

In the absence of indications to the contrary, it seems reasonable to start treatment with fairly direct steps aimed at eliminating or improving a patient's difficulties. If it works, it is the quickest way. If it fails, one can then go on to less direct means. The concern that failure of the direct approach might have adverse effects upon further progress with a different approach does not appear to be supported by facts.

THE ISSUE OF HYPNOTIZABILITY

Many therapists worry considerably about the hypnotizability of their patients. They should actually be more concerned about their suggestibility. I have a basic rule: *If a patient can produce what I need in hypnosuggestive effects, he is sufficiently suggestible and hypnotized, if indeed he is hypnotized.* Since suggestibility is really what is important, it is actually not material whether or not hypnosis is also present. Note, too, that the patient may not be able to produce many other effects; obviously, this is also immaterial. For this reason alone, there is usually little point in using one of the accepted scales of hypnotic susceptibility and hypnotic depth to pretest potential candidates for clinical hypnotism, and there is no particular reason to test their suggestibility once presumably hypnotized. The administration of such scales is time-consuming, requiring as much as an hour. The time can be better devoted to actual therapy. Tests such as the Postural Sway Test and the Chevreul Pendulum Test tend to take on a bizarre quality in a practitioner's office. They should be used only if they have an educational value for the patient in his preparation or if they are needed to facilitate the induction of hypnosis. Alternative scales and, in particular, clinical scales, have been published, but as indicated in Volume 1, they are of doubtful validity and utility. In general, if one wants some measure of a subject's suggestibility or depth of hypnosis, a fair estimate can frequently be obtained from the subject's responses and overall behavior during a hypnotherapeutic session. Such estimates are probably more meaningful because they represent the therapeutically utilizable suggestibility of the patient. In any case, it is surprising *how far a little suggestibility,* as measured on an accepted scale, *can really go in a therapeutic setting* (Weitzenhoffer, 1962).

Nevertheless, it does stand to reason that the production of certain effects by suggestion will not be possible, and that this will impose limitations on what can be therapeutically accomplished by suggestions alone, be they direct or indirect. Frankel (1987) has reported pertinent interesting statistics concerning this.

Let us now discuss the so-called "refractory" and "difficult" patient. Some patients can be placed in this category because of resistance, a topic that was considered in Volume 1 and to which we shall come back later. Others are categorized as such for other reasons. In any case, every patient that seeks or agrees to be hypnotized and to undergo various hypnotic interventions may or may not respond to all suggestions, or may respond poorly to any number of them. This is not cause to reject the use of hypnotism in an absolute manner, and one should not let the patient do so. In cases of patients who are unable to become sufficiently hypnotized, I will initially say something like, "Well, possibly you are not quite *ready* for this. There are a number of other things we can do until you become ready. In fact, they may work so well that we will not need to come back to the use of hypnotism." There are, of course, two indirect suggestions deliberately introduced in this statement. One is to become ready. The other is that different interventions will be effective. In any event, I do go on to non-hypnotic interventions for at least awhile. A similar approach can be taken with a patient who, although hypnotizable, is unable to produce a certain desired effect, or cannot do so to the degree required. Obviously, this kind of maneuver is not always practical. It works best in the context of psychotherapy and least well in an emergency medical situation.

I must emphasize that *one should not expect that sooner or later one will always succeed in getting the desired hypnotic responses in all cases and that it is only a matter of using the right approach.* There are going to be failures, possibly because of one's inability to come up with the right approach, but *possibly because there is none to be found.* This must be said because the Ericksonian schools of hypnotism have given the opposite impression. Listening to or reading Erickson's accounts of brief hypnotherapy cases, one receives the impression that his approach never failed him. Indeed, it may be true that he never knew failure; however, it is more likely that he never reported his failures. This is unfortunate, because there is much to be learned from failures. I think, too, that Erickson had a way of presenting what may have been unique, one-time successes in such a way that one cannot help but think that they were reflective of all his cases. Also, many of Erickson's accounts of cases in seminars and workshops were often greatly abbreviated; important details that may have shown them in a rather different light were left out. I consider myself, perhaps incorrectly so, as a good clinician; one who is quite adept at working with hypnosis. I will readily admit that I have had some great successes, but also an appreciable number of failures. I have been told that Erickson did report some cases of failures, but I have been unable to obtain specific references to where this had been published, if, indeed, it was.

DANGERS

There are dangers in the use of hypnotism. Some are quite obvious, and I think it is absurd to deny their existence, as certain well-known clinicians have done in the past, even when faced with actual evidence to the contrary. To argue that the use of hypnotism does not carry with it more dangers than any other clinical approach to health problems does not do away with its dangers, some of which are specific to it. Nor does the correct assertion that "hypnosis" is not dangerous; *per se,* it is not. *Such dangers as do exist lie primarily in its misuses or, more correctly, in the misuse of suggestions.* From a clinical standpoint, this is a matter of mismanagement of therapy cases. In all documented cases that I have been able to examine in which untoward effects had resulted, these effects had originated from overall poor therapeutic, particularly psychotherapeutic, practices and management, specific procedural errors, and improperly worded suggestions and instructions. A striking example of procedural error reported in the literature was that of a young woman treated for bruxism (teeth grinding) by a practicing lay hypnotist, one of the many individuals who hold no recognized academic professional credentials and who offer their services as hypnotists, hypnotherapists, and, in more recent times, as hypnotechnicians. Not uncommonly, they hold questionable degrees of "doctor of hypnotherapy" and variations on this theme, and/or are members of questionable organizations and unions, and/or certified or licensed by questionable boards. One such person I know of created his own association, named himself president of it, and certified himself! Of course, he made much use of these "credentials" with considerable success. Many such individuals have had years of experience as hypnotists, but little else in the line of clinical education or experience. Such hypnotists may have been brought into a case, as in the above example, by a legitimate health provider, but this does not compensate for their lack of essential knowledge or their clinical incompetence. The hypnotist mentioned above decided that if his client would sleep with her tongue between her teeth, she would naturally be awakened by the pain that she would experience in her tongue as soon as she began to clench her jaws and attempt grinding movements. Thus, the bruxism would be prevented from taking place. Accordingly, he implanted appropriate posthypnotic suggestions in his client. Had this succeeded, one cannot help but wonder how much sleep the woman would have had, and the possible consequences of greatly curtailed sleep on her overall health and life. Obviously, the hypnotist did not consider this issue. As it happened, his client slept on while chewing up her tongue! She did wake up, luckily, before she had completely severed her tongue! This happened with a lay hypnotist, but it could also easily happen with some licensed practitioners. I know of a physician who, faced with a patient he had diagnosed as having a streptococcus infection of the throat, chose to ignore the generally accepted and very effective use of antibiotics. Instead, he limited himself to suggesting to the hypnotized patient that his unconscious would effect a cure!

Symptom removal can be quite successful, and without side effects. On the other hand, this is not always the case. Seitz (1953) has clearly shown how it can also lead to severe decompensation, thus supporting other less clear evidence of this that is found in the literature. I have a simple rule for symptom removal: *If a symptom is refractory to treatment or repeatedly reappears after removal, it is best to let the symptom alone until further therapy of a different type has been done.* Unless the specific technique of symptom substitution is being used for the therapy, it is also a good idea not to attempt a new symptom removal of one that has been spontaneously substituted.

There is little question that with hypnotism, one can breach a patient's psychological defenses; he may even give these up prematurely. This kind of action courts disaster. Repressed material can frequently be uncovered through hypnotic techniques. Subsequently confronting a patient with such material, even though the repression has been allowed to remain, can have serious repercussion and even cause decompensation. In the case of individuals with weak defenses, such uncovering can weaken the repressive mechanism to the point of allowing threatening material to seep prematurely through the defensive barriers. A pertinent case is that of a 19-year-old girl referred to me by a physician who said that she had been diagnosed as a pseudoschizophrenic, although the diagnosis is not important for our purposes. I was not particularly certain what I could do for her, but as a favor to this physician I did go ahead and see her. She had one main complaint: she insisted that day by day her mind was being gradually drained of memories by "something." Presently I found out that, according to her, this draining was being done by magnetic tapes that she was regularly listening to. Further inquiry elicited the following information: this young woman had previously been in treatment in a clinic where tapes had been made of her verbalizations when under the influence of LSD. When released from her hospitalization, she had been sent home with these tapes, and had been instructed to listen to them over and over on a regular basis. She had no clear idea of the actual contents of the tapes. The foundation of her delusion should be obvious. Much, perhaps all, of the material on the tapes had been repressed material released by the influence of the LSD. As she listened to the tapes, she would transiently become aware of this material, which then soon became repressed again. This experience became distorted into her delusion. Admittedly, this case has no connection with hypnotism beyond that the patient was referred to me for hypnopsychotherapeutic work. It is, however, quite clear that what had been done with LSD could just as easily have been done with hypnotism. This example demonstrates the dangers of premature exposure to uncovered repressed material. Because the patient's defenses were still strong enough to repress the material presented to her, the harm done was much less than it could have been otherwise.

Improperly worded suggestions and instructions can be a source of potential trouble. The following incident exemplifies this. The case is that of a woman described by her obstetrician as a "deep" hypnotic subject. In preparing her for painless childbirth, he had told her under hypnosis that the onset of the very first labor contraction would be a signal for her to become totally unaware of further sensations in her abdominal and pelvic regions. When the time came, this is exactly what happened. The result was that the patient, who was then at home, did not become aware that she had entered labor until she felt fluid from the broken amniotic sac streaming down her legs! She did get to the hospital, but barely in time to deliver the baby. After detailing the above to me, this obstetrician commented "I just don't understand it . . . she is such a good subject!" The implication was that if she was such a good subject, somehow there would not have been a near miss.

Indeed, she was such a good subject that she carried out his suggestion perfectly!

Finally, I would also remind the reader that, as I have shown (1974), what is intended *as an instruction* when given during hypnosis *may actually function as an effective suggestion.* This may also happen with instructions given immediately after dehypnotization. In fact, anything said at such a time may have unexpected effects because of the residual hypnosis which can be present.

CONTRAINDICATIONS

Some writers, mostly those not favoring the use of hypnosis, frequently point to the possibility of creating or exacerbating dependency by such a use as a reason for hypnotism to be contraindicated, especially in cases already having a dependency problem. Even if this was always the case, I would not call this a danger, although it certainly would be of concern. It has never been demonstrated that the use of hypnotism per se does facilitate dependency. Dependency problems that develop during hypnotherapy and hypnopsychotherapy are usually a function of the therapist and his way of conducting the therapy. If dependency problems are going to arise with a given case, they most likely will do so whether or not hypnotism is used. In general, dependency needs should be handled in the clinical hypnotism situation in the same manner as they would be handled in any other therapeutic situation. They certainly should not be used as a major contraindication for the use of hypnotism.

There is little evidence to show that the use of hypnotism is contraindicated in any particular situation in which its use is *appropriate.* We have already seen examples of uses that were inappropriate. Assertions found in the literature that there are contraindications seem to be largely based on speculation and theory. For example, orthodox psychoanalysts insist that hypnotism is incompatible with psychoanalysis. This, they feel, is inherent in the first rule of psychoanalysis: that of free association. They wonder how one can freely associate if one's mind is controlled by someone else. I question whether this argument is truly valid. There are some research data available that indicate, on the contrary, that hypnosis facilitates free association. Contemporary orthodox psychoanalysts reject hypnotism in emulation of Freud's rejection, with no true understanding of why he did so. Still, if one is working within the framework of a certain school of psychotherapy, of a personality or behavioral theory, or of a theory of psychopathology, it is certainly viable to allow one's framework to be a guide with regard to what is indicated or contraindicated. By doing so, the therapist will at least feel more comfortable about what he is doing. I would, however, caution all therapists, whatever their persuasion, to keep in mind the seven points I have made earlier; they are generally applicable. When in doubt, clinical intuition is often a good guide. If there is doubt about the use of a proposed hypnosuggestive intervention, it is frequently possible to test it safely in a modified, miniature form. It is quite generally agreed that hypnotism should not be used with paranoid psychotics, or only with extreme care. I agree with this.

While there are probably few, if any, contraindications regarding the use of hypnotism, it should, at the same time, not be overused. Some therapists are oversold on its use. With some clinicians, hypnotism has acquired an uncalled for and an unhealthy mystical and evangelical quality; they are tempted to use it for everything, often disregarding the true treatment of choice. Such excesses are, of course, not unique to hypnotism. We have seen psychiatrists using electroshock therapy for each and every condition, and there was a short period when lobotomies and lobectomies were being used rather indiscriminately.

INDICATIONS

As for specific indications, the use of hypnotism is certainly to be considered when everything else has failed or before embarking upon risky last-resort procedures. The case of diaphragmatic myoclonus I referred to earlier was such a case. Everything else in the line of medical intervention had been tried except surgery. Not only were there no guarantees that surgery would work, but it was likely to leave the patient seriously incapacitated in other ways. One should not, however, consider the use of hypnotism *only as a last resort*. Too often this is what happens, to the detriment of the patient. In medicine and dentistry there are, of course, clear first-choice procedures for most disorders. In psychotherapy, the situation is very different, and hypnotism should be considered as a potential tool *from the very beginning* of the planning of any treatment. Keep in mind, however, that there are conditions, such as process schizophrenia and all the depressions except psychoneurotic (aka reactive) depression, for which, while not contraindicated, hypnotism has not been found particularly effective. Hypnotism has been found particularly useful in psychoanalytically-oriented therapies and behavior modification therapy. It can be quite useful in crisis intervention, but this is not for the beginner or the faint-hearted. In contrast to the psychoses and character disorders, the psychoneuroses are usually quite amenable to hypnotherapeutic interventions.

The conclusion is that there are no fixed rules regarding how or when to use hypnotism in therapy or how much or how little of it to use. This must be determined for each case. In some instances, one will use it early, perhaps even at the start; in others, only when well along in the therapy. In some cases, it will be used sparingly or on occasion, but in other cases, it will be used frequently and extensively. In some cases, it will never be used, either because it is not needed or for other reasons. Most persons seeking help through hypnotism have unrealistic expectations, and in all fairness to both patient and therapist, the patient's expectations should be corrected from the beginning. The prospective patient needs to be made aware that the most effective way of using hypnotism is usually in combination with other therapeutic steps that may even come first or be equally used. The patient should also be made aware that the therapist can most effectively use hypnotism if he is not pressured into doing so prematurely and, especially, if he is not expected to produce immediate results with it. The therapist needs to be free to conduct therapy in a flexible manner and in the most profitable way for the patient. He must be able to use his own discernment in using or not using hypnotism. The contract made by the therapist with the patient should always provide for this freedom. One should certainly never contract to use hypnotism as the only method of treatment.

Is there a *best* method for hypnotizing? A *best way* to use it? A sure fire method? Where traditional and semi-traditional hypnotism are concerned, there are none. Ericksonian-type hypnotists, of course, view the Ericksonian approach as superior in every way. There seems to be a general tendency among them to view the approach as infallible. But even within it, there are choices to be made as to what one does, and there are certainly no set rules to follow. Again, the situation and the hypnotist's perception and understanding of it are strong determinants of what is to be done within the framework of Ericksonian hypnotism. Nor does it demonstrably offer briefer therapy than traditional and semi-traditional hypnotism, at least not very clearly; if it does, this has been poorly documented.

The general overview presented in this chapter is now complete. The remainder of this volume is devoted to expanding and detailing this material.

3

Specific Procedures in Traditional and Semi-Traditional Clinical Hypnotism: Preparation of the Patient

INTRODUCTION

There have been extensive uses of hypnotism with respect to the maintenance of health. Mesmerism, out of which hypnotism grew, originated in
the context of healing. It may be useful to have a tabulation of some of the
uses of modern hypnotism in the health field. The list that follows is by no
means exhaustive; it is mostly a list of medical applications. This should not
be interpreted as indicating that physicians have used hypnotism more extensively than other health care professionals. Physicians using hypnotism
have been, and continue to be, relatively few. The list does not give a true
picture of how extensively hypnotism is actually used in medicine, but
primarily shows the variety of medical applications. The list partly reflects
that hypnotism was first used by physicians who, for a long time, were
mental health as well as physical health care professionals. It also partly
reflects the nature of physical ailments and that medical nosology readily
provides this kind of a list. Even with the classification offered by the
DSM-III-R, nothing quite comparable is possible in the area of mental
health. This list does not reflect that psychosomatic and somatopsychic
problems fall under the province of both physical and mental health. In
particular, psychosomatic problems are likely to be first seen by physicians
who may or may not refer the cases to mental health professionals. Either
way, these cases must be viewed as physical problems. Even in the field of
medicine, it is unclear whether psychosomatic medicine should stand as an
entity on its own or fall under the more inclusive heading of internal
medicine. I think that a gastric ulcer caused by stress justifiably comes
under the heading of internal medicine or of gastroenterology, even if effectively treated by psychotherapy.

Under what headings should alcoholism, drug addiction, and the tobacco habit fall? On the basis of five years spent treating alcoholics on an
inpatient unit, I think that at some stage of development alcoholism does
become associated with serious physical changes and problems and can
hardly be viewed as just a deleterious habit. Some drug addictions most
likely present similar features. What of the so-called tobacco or nicotine
habit? There is most likely a physiological addiction involved in the case of
the majority, but not at all comparable to the one involved with other
addictive substances. However, because medicine has still not recognized
excessive smoking as a true medical problem, one can probably justifiably
continue to treat it as a habit problem with medical consequences, although it would be more appropriately placed under the heading of a
psychophysiological problem.

As specialization in medicine progressed, mental health eventually became the province of psychiatry. Today it is a domain shared with clinical

psychologists and social workers. Because the ways of using hypnotism in psychotherapy are the same for these specialties, there is need for only one entry. My choosing to list the psychotherapeutic uses of hypnotism under psychiatry is in no way intended to indicate that psychotherapy more legitimately belongs to medicine than to other disciplines. There is no basic reason why much of hypnopsychotherapy should not be discussed independently, or under a non-medical specialty. On the other hand, psychiatry, as the more comprehensive of the disciplines concerned with mental health, seems a reasonable choice.

The following is a list of major specialties, with examples of areas of applications, in which hypnotism has been used. It should be understood that this list is only a sampling. It is largely based on reports in the relevant literature and, in some instances, there have been only a few patients involved. For example, only a small number of cases of Reynaud's disease have been treated with hypnotism. Also, no attempt has been made to distinguish disorders or problems with a strong psychogenic component, such as anorexia nervosa, obesity, or nail biting, from those that are purely organic. One reason is that they usually first come to the attention of a physician in one of the listed specialties and, not infrequently, they have been treated by this same physician. The other reason is that many of these disorders and problems have traditionally been thus categorized. There is a certain amount of inevitable overlap because a specific disease entity is likely to be encountered in more than one specialty and to be treated by more than one specialist. For example, an internist, a pediatrician, and an allergist will all treat asthma cases. This has not always been made clear in this listing. Also, some obvious uses will not be found listed under a given specialty because they are included under another heading. For example, the use of hypnoanesthesia and hypnoanalgesia in obstetrics is covered under labor.

1. *Hypnotism in Internal Medicine*
   Cardiovascular disorders
   Gastrointestinal disorders
   Metabolic diseases
   Obesity
   Enteritis
   Constipation
   Hyperthyroidism
   Asthma
   Anorexia nervosa
   Bulimia

      Allergies
      Reynaud's disease
      Headaches
      Insomnia

2. *Hypnotism in Surgery and Anesthesiology*
      Anesthesia and analgesia
      Preoperative and postoperative care

3. *Hypnotism in Obstetrics*
      Labor
      Postpartum period
      Pregnancy
      Spontaneous abortion
      Lactation
      Toxemia

4. *Hypnotism in Gynecology*
      Pelvic examinations
      Amenorrhea
      Dysmenorrhea
      Pseudocyesis
      Uterine bleeding
      Infertility
      Frigidity
      Low back pain
      Pelvic pain
      Premenstrual syndrome
      Menopause
      Intersexuality

5. *Hypnotism in Dermatology*
      Warts
      Urticaria
      Pruritus
      Ichthyosis
      Alopecia
      Herpes
      Neurodermatitis
      Hyperhidrosis

    Psoriasis

    Skin allergies

6. *Hypnotism in Ophthalmology, Otolaryngology, and Rhinology*

    Glaucoma

    Squint

    Amblyopia

    Tunnel vision

    Blepharospasms

    Myopia

    Contact lenses

    Tinnitus

    Globus hystericus

    Aphonia

    Dysphonia

    Rhinitis

    Epitaxis

    Analgesia

    Anesthesia

    Gag and salivary reflex

7. *Hypnotism in Genitourinary Conditions*

    Postoperative urinary retention

    Chronic bladder irritability

    Premature ejaculation

    Impotence

    Cytoscopy

    Vasectomy

    Infertility

8. *Hypnotism in Oncology*

    Facilitating chemotherapy and radiation therapy

    Pain in terminal cases

    General management

9. *Hypnotism in Pediatrics*

    Enuresis

    Tics and habit spasms

    Stuttering

    Mental retardation

12. *Hypnotism in Psychiatry*
    Alcoholism
    Excessive smoking
    Substance abuse
    Sleep disturbances
    Phobias
    Compulsions
    Neuroses in general
    Psychoses in general
    Reactive depressions
    Psychosomatic disorders
13. *Hypnotism in Physical Rehabilitation*
    Amputees
    Poliomyelitis
    Parkinsonism
    Multiple sclerosis
    Hemiplegia and quadriplegia
    Paraplegia
14. *Hypnotism in Dentistry*
    Gag reflex
    Salivation
    Analgesia
    Oral surgery
    Prophylaxis
    Periodontics
    Tongue thrust
    Thumb sucking
    Bruxism
    Postoperative and preoperative treatment
    Dental hygiene

Readers will find journal references for many of these applications in Crasilneck and Hall (1975).

The rest of this chapter as well as the next three will be devoted to the applications of traditional and semi-traditional hypnotism only. Ericksonian hypnotherapy will be discussed in Chapter 7. Neurolinguistic programming as it is related to hypnotism will be the subject of Chapter 8.

It is assumed throughout this book that the reader will be familiar with Volume 1 and will be well acquainted with the contents of Chapters 2, 3, and 5. These chapters serve as a foundation for the material that follows.

INITIAL PROCEDURES

Potential candidates for the clinical use of hypnotism fall into two groups: those who come to the therapist asking to be hypnotized and those who have not, but for whom, at some point, the therapist decides that the use of hypnotism is indicated. These two groups must be approached differently. In contrast to the first group, the second must be introduced to the use of hypnotism. This may be done in a number of ways, depending on the nature of the problem to be treated, the kind of person the patient is, and other factors. In addition, practitioners have personal preferences as to how this is done. Finally, ethical and professional standards may be factors. In this section, I will discuss certain features of the process of introducing and initiating the use of hypnotism which are of general applicability. It should be understood that they are open to individual modifications.

When the Patient Asks for the Use of Hypnotism: Indications and Contraindications

A patient may request the use of hypnotism, but that does not necessarily mean he is well-informed about it. Before agreeing to his request, it is important to find out what he knows and what his expectations are. Having this information, the therapist can go on to the next step, which may be that of correcting false ideas that the patient has. The use of hypnotism may or may not be indicated—then or at any future time. In that case, the patient needs to be therapeutically apprised of this. Timing, rather than absolute contraindication, is usually the issue. With a patient who has never been seen before, but who comes to the office asking to be hypnotized, first obtain a personal history. In some cases, a short one will do; in others, more extensive data may be needed. This may require several more sessions. There will be times when the therapist will want to contact the patient's personal physician or access hospital records. A physician may first want to do a physical examination and even some laboratory work. Doing these things involves a delay before using hypnotism, or even before agreeing to do so. Absolute contraindications are rare. Those that exist are usually a function of the case and may only be temporary. Many contraindications have their basis in the patient's attitude and expectations. Sometimes it is simply a matter of feasibility or practicality. The following examples will help to clarify this important aspect.

A prospective patient came to me saying, as he sat down, "Doc, hypnotize me and tell me to stop drinking." A quick inquiry showed this person expected that this could be easily done in one short session. He would accept nothing else in the form of treatment and was not even willing for me to obtain a personal history from him. I had little choice than to refuse to proceed as requested. In my experience and opinion, alcoholics are, in the first place, poor prospects for hypnotherapy under the best of conditions. With one who appears to have a hidden agenda and is unwilling to cooperate to the extent of giving a history, the chances of success are nil. In this case, the induction of hypnosis would probably have failed. Had this patient been willing to provide a history, I would have felt obligated to inform him that a one-session cure bordered on the miraculous, and that there would not be much point in initiating treatment unless he was willing to enter a longer term treatment. Unrealistic expectations of extremely brief hypnotherapy are a common occurrence, and the therapist owes it to the patient and himself to educate the prospective patient.

My next case is that of a young woman who came to my office requesting that I use hypnotism to enlarge her breasts that, by most standards, were quite adequate, especially for her body build. This was before surgical techniques for doing this had been developed. She had heard of the possibility of this being done. There, indeed, had been some poorly documented and overpublicized reports of this having been accomplished. Although skeptical about the matter, I could not completely discard the possibility of some success in a few cases. I was frank with the patient. I gave her my opinion that the matter was highly controversial and, at the risk of creating a negative set, added that the likelihood of success was quite low, but that if she wanted to chance it, I would be willing to work with her. However, I first asked whether she would be willing to tell me why she felt she needed bigger breasts. My patient informed me that her husband seemed to be obsessed with large-breasted females. He collected all kinds of girlie magazines and was openly enthused over the well-endowed women that were pictured. She felt that he had repeatedly given her clear hints that he wished she was more like them. This information placed the whole matter in a totally different light, suggesting that issues of self-image and self-worth were at stake and that the marital situation needed to be explored.

This case has a parallel in women seeking plastic surgery in order to improve a poor marital relationship. Wise and ethical plastic surgeons are unwilling to perform surgery under these conditions. Without altogether refusing to accede to the original request, I was able to focus the patient upon the more relevant issue, and therapy proceeded accordingly. Had the patient insisted that I work *only* on enlarging her breasts, I doubt that I would have accepted her as a patient.

One question the above case raises is that of the professional ethics involved in a psychologist getting involved with something like breast development. I do not feel that this is an issue because the treatment is non-intrusive, does not call for a physical examination or for manipulations, and is unlikely to cause any deleterious physiological changes if successful.

A patient from the inpatient psychiatric unit at a VA Hospital where I was employed approached me, wanting to be hypnotized. He was a member of a therapy group I met with biweekly, and he had been diagnosed as a paranoid schizophrenic. In general, there are no indications for using hypnotism with this kind of pathology, but quite apart from that there is considerable danger with such patients that the hypnotic experience will become incorporated in their delusional systems. Still, every case must be decided on its own merit. To my inquiry as to how I could help him with hypnotism, all that this normally well-articulated man could or would cryptically say was, "You have the key!" He would not or could not elaborate on this answer and was unwilling to work with me on any other individual basis than that I hypnotize him. Under these circumstances, I felt it would be unwise to accede to the request.

I have encountered two cases of paranoid schizophrenia, both of whom were women who believed that they were in a permanent state of hypnosis induced by some other person. Both were ambulatory and had jobs. They both sought to be hypnotized as a way of removing this hypnosis. The first of these cases came to my attention while I was briefly visiting in a city near the town where the woman lived. My main reasons for not attempting such removal were that there would be no opportunity to do a satisfactory anamnesis and for therapeutic follow-up sessions. Also I was not licensed to practice in the state where she lived.

The second of these cases came to my attention at the time I was working on my doctoral dissertation. Not only did I not have proper professional accreditations, but my research and studies did not allow appropriate time for such an undertaking. This last was actually more of an issue because, while one session might have succeeded, the likelihood of a need for follow-up sessions was quite high, and my schedule did not allow for this. Added to this, the woman, who was not in therapy, lived in another city that was an appreciable distance from where I lived. For these reasons, I also had to decline this case. Had the situations been otherwise than as I have described, would it have been wise to use hypnotism on either of these women? Altering that which was most likely a delusion was a possibility, but what then? In such an instance, one must assume that the delusion of being in a permanent state of hypnosis (supposedly induced by a man in each case) served a definite purpose. To alter it without proper understanding of what this purpose was would carry serious risks.

Sometimes, interference with a delusion is the only way one can find out what its function is. In this case, one must be prepared for the possibility that the patient may react catastrophically and have to be hospitalized. Had

I been in a position to take these cases on, I might have done so, but only with the clear understanding that I would decide when the time was right to use hypnotism to remove the alleged hypnosis. I would also make it clear that this might be some indefinite time in the future, and that in the meantime therapy would be instituted and approached differently.

The next case is that of a man who lived on the West Coast, about 1500 miles from where I resided and who, some years ago, requested an appointment with me without saying why. Flattering as this was, I felt that before this man undertook the long and expensive trip, it would be wise if he would first tell me his reasons for wanting to consult me on a face-to-face basis. While I did not know for certain that this was a potential therapy case, I suspected that it was. There were a number of well-established hypnotherapists close to where he lived; why had he not consulted one of them? What did I have to offer him that they could not? Thinking that perhaps he was ignorant of the availability of closer aid, I felt an appropriate referral would be in order. (I firmly believe that it is part of a therapist's professional obligation to make referrals when so indicated. It has also been my experience that there is a percentage of patients seeking hypnotherapy that can be better served by such referrals. Examples of such cases have been briefly described in Chapter 2.) There was also a puzzling aspect to this man's request. I was not particularly well-known as a therapist; the name I had made for myself was in research. Why, then, had he selected me? The man was not willing to divulge any information. Over a period of several years, he contacted me a number of times by telegrams and letters, and once by telephone. He was willing to travel and would stay in the city where I lived, as long as necessary. On several occasions, he made vague appeals to my research interests. Except for this obsession that I become his therapist, and his insistence on secrecy, the man sounded normal. I suppose I could have given him an appointment. After all, if he wanted to travel this far with no idea of what the outcome of his visit would be, it was his business. Part of my reason for not giving in was, I suspect, my own need for knowing ahead of time what I might be getting into. Also, I was aware that he might settle down indefinitely in Oklahoma City if I agreed, even this once, to see him. He could become a very real problem. Therefore, I held firm, insisting that I must have at least a modicum of information regarding his purpose in seeing me. He finally divulged that he wanted to see me so that I would age regress him. He wanted this to be his main treatment for an unstated problem. Based on his reading of my published writings, he believed that I was the only one who could do this successfully. This added a new puzzle, because age regressions had not been an area in which I had done any research. There seemed to be an unfounded expectation. Additionally, there happened to be a well-known researcher and psychotherapist, with an office in the city the man lived in, who had done considerable recognized work with age regressions. It seemed unlikely that this man was ignorant of this, but I went ahead and recommended that he first see my colleague. His reply was that he had already consulted this expert; he then made some highly uncomplimentary remarks about him. Then he divulged that he had seen a great number of hypnotherapists and psychotherapists without getting the results he sought. Next, he enumerated the procedures he wanted me to follow and told me, at last, what the manifested problem was. He also pointed out that no one had ever been able to hypnotize him, even with the aid of drugs. Finally, possibly thinking that my reluctance at accepting him as a patient could thus be overcome, he proposed that I take him on as an experimental subject. Perhaps his own reluctance to divulge any details until now was his accurate realization that I would probably not be willing to work with him once I heard his story, and his partially accurate perception that once I did see him, I would feel an obligation to continue to do so. At this point, I firmly refused to consider him any further as a potential patient. In retrospect, I believe that to have acted differently in this situation would have been unwise, and not in the best interests of either this man or myself.

Finally, there is the case of a patient who originally came to me because he was suffering from a rare form of leukemia. He had heard of the Simonton method of treating cancer and wanted me to give him hypnotic suggestions that would facilitate and reinforce the application of this technique. I did not have much faith in Simonton's ideas and little reason to believe that any kind of hypnotic suggestion could reverse the course of the disease. Still, there was a small probability that a positive result might follow. I made it clear to the patient that since I had not previously worked in this area, I would have to proceed on a purely experimental basis. This being agreeable to him, the course of treatment was instituted. The patient died within a year, with no indication that any kind of improvement or positive change had taken place. Some readers may take the position that my attitude and beliefs may have adversely affected the course of the treatment. I was aware of this possibility. But I was also aware that I did not altogether disbelieve. For me, the production of blisters by suggestion and psychosomatic effects are very much of a reality. Also, I felt that placing the therapy within the framework of an exploratory experiment would help to eliminate negative influences of this type. Had I thought otherwise, I would have felt obligated to refer the patient to a more appropriate hypnotherapist.

The issue of when to treat and not to treat with hypnotism is anything but a clear matter. A safe position would probably be never to use hypnotism with psychotics. I say this in spite of reports of this being done successfully. For the most part, these are poorly documented reports and, in some instances, one must question the accuracy of the diagnoses. In at least one detailed case reported by Wolberg (1945), he raises the possibility that the patient had been wrongly diagnosed as being a hebephrenic schizophrenic. Also, on the basis of personal experience, I do not recommend using hypnotism with alcoholics, at least not as the main treatment modality. I would take the same position on theoretical grounds with regard to the hypnotic treatment of chemical dependency in general. I have not found homosexuality, as such, to be particularly treatable with hypnotism. On the other hand, emotional problems centering around a person's homosexuality can be treated effectively. Sociopathy is no more amenable to hypnotic treatment than it is to other forms of treatment. Nor is hypnotism particularly useful in treating character disorders.

In general, it is advisable when doing hypnopsychotherapy that the therapist be sure the patient clearly understands and agrees that the therapist will have the last word as to when and how hypnotism will be used. I always make this a part of my initial contract with the patient. I explain to the patient that I most likely will not solely use hypnotism in treating him, and that there will be sessions when I will make no use of it. Generally, when doing psychotherapy, I use no hypnotism in the first two or three sessions, which are my initial fact-gathering sessions. When psychotherapy is not involved, such as when training an individual to develop anesthesia for childbirth, only the first session will usually be free of the use of hypnotism, and in many cases, I will do the first induction in the latter part of this first session. Crisis intervention is also another exception to the rule.

When the Therapist Proposes Hypnotism Be Used

When it is the therapist who wishes to institute hypnotic treatment, the situation differs from the above in a number of ways. Although this is an increasingly less frequent occurrence, some patients have no idea what hypnotism is about. More often, they have some knowledge, but it is not necessarily accurate. In either case, some education is indicated as the starting point. Even when this is done, patients may retain certain archaic ideas, faulty beliefs, and misperceptions about hypnotism, and they may reject its use. There is not much one can do about this. The best approach, in this case, is to proceed as well as possible in an acceptable therapeutic manner, with the hope that in time the patient will change his mind.

In the past, some practitioners, especially dentists, were reluctant to use the terms hypnosis and hypnotism. Instead, they would propose to use "relaxation" techniques with the patient. If, indeed, relaxation is all that is being sought, there is little more to be said about the matter. However, if the aim is to induce a state of heightened suggestibility and to produce various hypnotic effects, or even just one, such as anesthesia, then a deception is being perpetrated upon the patient. To recommend the use of hypnotism as part of a treatment is no different than recommending other kinds of interventions. One should be forthright about the matter. Whatever fears and misconceptions the patient may have should be dealt with. If a practitioner feels uncomfortable about informing his patient of his intent, or if he is concerned about what his colleagues might think of his using hypnotism, then he should refrain from using it. Fortunately, this situation is becoming much less frequent as the professional world becomes better informed about and more willing to accept hypnotism.

If hypnotism seems to be the best approach to use, from the very start of therapy I usually introduce the possibility of using it by merely saying to the patient something like, "I believe the use of hypnotism would be the best way to handle your (this) problem," or "Hypnotism has been used successfully for this kind of problem. Would you like to go that route?" On the other hand, having begun therapy along some other line, I may, at some point, come to the conclusion that hypnotism is now indicated. In this case, I might say, "I think we ought to consider using some hypnotism in your treatment." If it is to be used for some specific purpose, such as getting through a mental block or clarifying a dream, I will usually refer to these in proposing hypnotism.

Significance of Hypnotic Depth, Hypnotic Susceptibility, and Hypnotizability; Problem of Simulation

Many practitioners, especially those starting out in the use of hypnotism, tend to be overly concerned with two questions: "How do I know (when) my patient is hypnotized?" and "How can I be sure (tell) that my patient is not pretending?" A third question that comes up, but less often, is "How can I tell how deeply my patient is hypnotized?"

As explained in Volume 1, scales of hypnotic depth are *at best* measures of suggestibility. None, by themselves, can tell us whether or not a patient is hypnotized in any other sense, and how deeply, except by fiat. Furthermore, the use of lengthy test batteries, such as the Stanford Scales of Hypnotic Susceptibility, Forms A and B (Weitzenhoffer & Hilgard, 1959), seems rather out of place in the office of a therapist. Clinical scales are more suitable, but many are of questionable validity and reliability. This is particularly true for Spiegel's popular eye-roll test described in Volume 1. One problem with many of these scales is that the items on them rarely have direct relevance to therapeutic effects. Keeping in mind what has already been said regarding hypnotic scales in general, Table 3.1 offers a clinical scale that is a modification I have made of one proposed earlier by Wolberg (1948). No reliability or validity has been established for it, nor has it been formally standardized. It is merely one that was empirically put together. It obviously closely models other, better established scales and to this extent probably has a validity and reliability of the same magnitude as they have. It can be a useful instrument for gauging suggestibility for clinical purposes and obtaining an index of the kinds of hypnotherapeutic steps one might undertake with a patient if one wishes to go to the trouble of pretesting. Going from top to bottom, it is a Guttman-type scale (see Volume 1). Having established the limiting suggestibility, the therapist knows that any item below this limit can probably be

TABLE 3.1. Stages (Depth) of Hypnosis in Relation to Clinical Applications[a]

Criteria	Degree
Eyes smart and/or water Eyelids heavy Eyelids flutter	Waking
Feeling of heaviness in the extremities Drowsiness *Psychobiologic therapy (reassurance, persuasion, reeducation, confession, and ventilation) *Hypnoanalysis (free association, induced fantasies) *Pain threshold raised through relaxation *Reduction of general muscular tension	Hypnoidal state
Eye closure Overall physical relaxation Eyelid catalepsy (paralysis) Limb catalepsy (waxy flexibility) Induced limb rigidity Induced paralysis Induced automatisms *Psychobiologic therapy (guidance) *Light analgesia (tension headaches, labor and some deliveries, simple dental work)	Light hypnosis
Suggested partial posthypnotic amnesia Suggested alterations of the various cutaneous senses Glove anesthesia Partial posthypnotic analgesia Generalized automatism Suggested superficial personality alterations *Hypnoanalysis (induction of dreams, role playing) *Facilitation of physical therapy *Analgesia for labor and deliveries, dental work and minor surgery	Medium hypnosis
Simple posthypnotic suggestions Extensive suggested posthypnotic amnesias General anesthesia Induced emotional effects Suggested deep alterations of the personality Hallucinations Alterations of the sense of time Age regressions and progressions *Psychobiologic therapy (certain desensitizations) *Hypnoanalysis (automatic writing, painting, use of modeling clay) *Symptom removal *Semi-general use of suggestions as adjunct to medical interventions. Anesthesia for major surgery.	Deep hypnosis

TABLE 3.1. *(Continued)*

Criteria	Degree
Total spontaneous posthypnotic amnesia	
Ability to open the eyes in hypnosis	
Suggested profound alterations of the personality	Profound
All posthypnotic suggestions including posthypnotic	hypnosis
hallucinations possible	(somnam-
*Psychobiologic therapy (reconditioning)	bulism)
*Hypnoanalysis (crystal gazing, psychodrama, induced artificial conflicts, revivifications)	
*General use of suggestions as adjunct to medical treatment.	

Source: Modified from Wolberg, 1948. With permission of The Psychological Corporation.
[a] This scale is a modification of one first presented by Wolberg (1948). An asterisk indicates the kinds of suggestibility most suitable for various hypnotherapeutic interventions (*).

successfully used. The kinds of therapeutic interventions that are possible at various levels have been marked with an asterisk.

To establish whether the patient is hypnotized, clinicians may use one or more of the clinical signs of hypnosis described in Chapter 3 of Volume 1.

How important is it in therapy *to predict* a patient's ability to respond to suggestions, or to develop a hypnotic state? It is rarely important. Apart from considerations taken up in the last chapter, the other reason is that the use of accepted scales is usually for the purpose of establishing whether or not the patient can be hypnotized and whether or not he produces a satisfactory response to given test suggestions. The theory, partly supported by experience, is that if he responds positively to a test suggestion, he will then respond positively at any other time the suggestion is given. Conversely, failure leads to the prediction that he will always fail. All other things being equal, one can simply wait until a certain effect is needed to suggest it. Nothing is gained by doing this ahead of time. Also keep in mind that available scales do not actually tell us whether or not a patient can enter a hypnotic state.

One reason that one might want to establish ahead of time what the patient is capable of doing would be in order to plan a complex course of hypnotherapy before instituting it. Certainly, knowing that it is likely that the patient will be unable to produce certain classes of phenomena can be useful. One can employ the above scale for this purpose.

Another reason for using such devices as the Stanford Scales is that they can be conceived as useful both for training, (preparing the patient for future uses of hypnotism) and as methods of induction combined with a deepening procedure. As discussed in Volume 1, this deepening effect is not well documented, but is widely believed to exist.

Finally, for the novice, such scales offer ready-made inductions and deepening procedures.

When I started doing hypnotherapy, I would invariably proceed through a series of the traditional test suggestions described in Chapter 2 of Volume 1 before I attempted to induce hypnosis. This included the Postural Sway Suggestion, the Finger Lock (Hand Clasping) Suggestion, the Arm Rigidity Suggestion, and sometimes the Eye Catalepsy Suggestion, given in this order. Over the years, I found that most of this was unnecessary. It was much better simply to induce hypnosis and go on from there, testing only as needed for the purposes of the therapy as it progresses. Most of what one needs to know about the patient's suggestibility and hypnotic depth can be learned in the course of therapeutically working with him.

Having just said the above tests are *usually* not called for, I now must add that occasionally there is a place for one or the other. For example, producing an arm rigidity is a good way of introducing the patient to the possibility of producing muscular rigidity in some other part of his body, as was required in the case of diaphragmatic myoclonus mentioned earlier. It was also a way for me to ascertain whether this approach was at all feasible. Other instances of a use of induced arm rigidity can be found in the medical literature in connection with the transfer of skin grafts from a forearm to the face. A standard way of inducing anesthesia in other parts of the patient's body has been by first inducing a glove anesthesia in one of the patient's hands.

I continue to use one non-hypnotic test of suggestibility—the Hands Together Test—but much less as a way of ascertaining the patient's suggestibility than as a way of introducing him to suggestion effects and to the kind of mental set that he needs to have. At the same time, information is obtained regarding his ability to respond to suggestions. This is useful, but not essential. As discussed in Volume 1, "hypnotic depth" is mainly a reference to suggestibility, the latter being used as its measure.

Finally, a word or two about simulation. This issue originates in two ways: from the therapist and from the patient. The concern may be whether or not the patient is really hypnotized. Or, there may be no question about hypnosis being present, but there may still be a concern about the genuineness of the presumably induced behaviors and experiences. Validating or, as Milton H. Erickson preferred to say, ratifying, the hypnotic state, behaviors, and experiences can be a big issue for some therapists, especially when they first begin working with hypnotism. Some subjects may also make an issue of it. One of the appeals of Ericksonian hypnotism is that it eliminates much of this concern by allowing almost any response to be a valid hypnotic response. Traditional and semi-traditional hypnotism are not quite that lenient.

This is not as big an issue as it may seem to be when doing therapy. From a therapeutic standpoint, if the desired result is obtained, it does not make much difference what the true nature of the response was. For example, the authenticity of many age regressions can be questioned. In many cases, one has reasons to suspect that they are largely fantasies. As such, they can still have a powerful therapeutic effect. What conclusions one can draw from them regarding the patient's past is the only concern one should have. Regressions into past lives have been a popular therapeutic tool in recent times. I do not question their efficacy at times, but I seriously question their veridicality.

The Initial Induction; Preparation of the Patient Before, During, and Following the Induction

There are any number of ways one can initially induce hypnosis. Volume 1 describes traditional and semi-traditional procedures that can be used in the context of therapy as well as outside of it. While it cannot be said that any one method is superior to the others, except in respect to certain features, there are reasons for choosing a passive as against an active form of induction. Generally, one will use active forms if one wants the patient to be able to function very actively within the hypnotic state. Otherwise, passive forms are probably to be preferred. Sometimes, in order to obtain a high degree of active suggestibility, it is necessary to use a passive form first. All of this has been fully discussed in Chapter 3 of Volume 1. You may wish to review the pertinent material before proceeding.

In general, I like my therapy room to be arranged so that the patient sits in a comfortable armchair, frequently a recliner. I sit on his left, somewhat diagonally from him, so that I can at least have an oblique view of his face. I am close enough, in most cases, so that by partly rising and leaning forward I can touch his left hand or arm when it is on the arm rest. Directly across from the patient, 9 to 12 feet away, near the ceiling, is a small metal disk (button, very large thumbtack, etc.) that is used as a visual fixation target. One or more small folding tables (TV-tray type) nearby are useful for holding a cassette recorder and other paraphenalia. It is always a good idea to have available, in addition, at least one straight-back chair, and even an adjustable stool (piano type). Adjustable lighting can be useful. Figure 3.1 is a diagram of this arrangement.

A therapy room thus arranged is not always available. One may have to use an office with a desk, files, and bookcases. In this case, the best one can do is to approximate the above as closely as possible for routine hypnotherapy. In situations such as crisis intervention, one usually has to forego all of these niceties.

Some of the information that I give to the patient regarding hypnosis and its induction may take place in a session prior to the one in which I attempt the first induction. This will usually be an explanation that hypnotism is

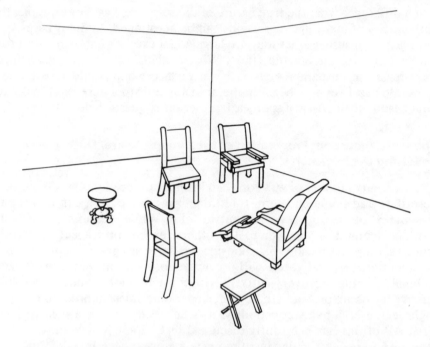

Figure 3.1 Suggested furniture arrangement for a therapy room.

simply the use of suggestion. Suggestion, I explain, consists of ideas that I present in such a way that they can have a special, direct action upon him. Such effects, I add, take place without the patient doing anything to make them happen. I further explain that the best way the patient can help this to happen is to just let happen whatever seems to want to take place, and that he should neither hinder nor help the process. I tell him that hypnosis is merely a state of mind that the patient will probably be able to attain and that will facilitate this process; it is not, however, essential that it occur. I also explain that although some hypnotized persons feel like they are asleep when hypnotized, or, when it is over, that they have been asleep, hypnosis is not sleep or unconsciousness. If I do not plan to follow up these explanations immediately with an induction of hypnosis, I may or may not go on with the use of the Hands Together Suggestion. Generally, I prefer to make it a part of the induction. In any case, the way I present the use of this suggestion is by telling the patient that I will now give him an opportunity to experience what a suggestion is like. Having said this, I go on to use the Hands Together Suggestion as described in Chapter 2 of Volume 1. I always follow it up with the test for non-voluntariness.

There are a number of reasons for using this suggestion at this time. It gives the patient an opportunity to experience a mild, non-threatening, and interesting suggested effect, and it is good preparation for the induction to follow. By its nature, the suggestion is neither aided nor hindered by factors other than the subject's suggestibility and mental set. If the subject has any difficulty with it, the nature of the problem is usually, but not always, easy to pin down and correct. A strong response to this suggestion is usually a good indictor that the Hand Levitation Induction can be successfully performed. On the other hand, the absence of any response is a clear indication that the patient is relatively or totally refractory and that the prognosis for an easy induction is poor. An eye-fixation technique with suggestions of relaxation is indicated in this case. It should be kept in mind that even when no movement of the hands is observed, the patient may nevertheless experience unusual sensations when the Hands Together Suggestion is used. This can be acknowledged as a sign of some responsiveness. In an effort both to pace and to lead, a new attempt should now be made in which references to the sensations are incorporated into the suggestion. Compounding of these sensations with the suggested movement can be quite effective.

In the therapy situation, one is not concerned with obtaining measures of suggestibility under standardized conditions, but, instead, with eliciting and using whatever suggestibility is available. Because of this, weak and incomplete responses to the Hand Movement Suggestion are just as acceptable as a strong movement. The injection in the suggestion of additional ideas, such as those of a force acting on the hands, or of instruction to the patient to visualize his hands moving together, or of anything else the therapist may think will aid or reinforce the suggestion, is permissible. This can be done while initially giving the suggestion or on a subsequent trial. When a second attempt is made, one should, of course, also be guided by such information as the patient may have provided regarding his experience on the first trial.

Occasionally, the patient will be frightened by the experience of his hands moving or even by the precursor sensation of impending movement. This is not too common, but it does happen, and one should always be on the lookout for signs of anxiety, as the patient will frequently not say or do anything more. In such instances, one should stop the suggestion, inquire about what is going on, and act accordingly. On the other hand, patients may state that they do not want to go any further with the test. Such a response should always be accepted and preferably followed up with some inquiry and discussion. Surprisingly, some of these patients will have no difficulty with a passive induction. One can surmise that for such individuals, loss of control is too threatening. Clearly, at this stage, they are not candidates for a hand levitation induction or active induction in general. However, it may be possible to use these methods later.

With patients in psychotherapy, any untoward or unexpected responses should always be considered as possibly meaningful with respect to their problems, and therefore of psychotherapeutic value. This is particularly true with patients' reactions to the induction and/or the experience of hypnosis. From this standpoint, an induction can be viewed as a potential diagnostic tool.

Eliciting non-hypnotic suggestibility is by no means a necessity. The existing situation often dictates what one will do. There are also personal preferences. When several attempts with the above test suggestion have failed, one can always try the Chevreul Pendulum Test. This is probably the test that requires the least suggestibility. If any kind of positive response is obtained, one can often then use it to develop the subject's suggestibility further, and even use it to induce a hypnotic state, as explained in Volume 1. If no response is obtained with this test, one should, for the time being, abandon the idea of using hypnotism.

The first induction of hypnosis is the next step. It may be done immediately following the use of the Hands Together Suggestion, or delayed until the next session. Of course, the induction does not depend upon doing this test first. That is, one can directly proceed to an induction of hypnosis. Sometimes this is necessary, as, for example, when working with a quadriplegic. Another example is in crisis intervention, where time is of the essence and the situation frequently is not suitable for such testing. With regard to choice of induction method, one should use a method which feels comfortable. Using an eye fixation technique is a good general approach that fits most situations. All other things being equal, when I have a good reason to expect that a hand levitation procedure will work, I give it preference. I cannot say exactly why, beyond my feeling that it induces a deeper hypnosis and does so more rapidly. Whichever method I use, I always follow it up with the modified fractionation method described in Volume 1, in which I use a count of 1 to 20. Also at this time, I introduce the various safeguards and special posthypnotic instructions that I also described in Volume 1. Of course, this may also be the time to introduce preliminary suggestions relevant to the problem under treatment. After the patient has returned to his normal state, one should ask him to give a brief account of his experience. This material is useful in several ways. First, it gives the therapist some information regarding the extent to which the patient was hypnotized. Also, as will be seen shortly, the material is useful for subsequent inductions. Usually the combination of preinduction testing, induction, and the above mentioned intrahypnotic work takes up a one-hour session.

I have not found the 60-minute session to be the most feasible way of doing hypnopsychotherapy, although this is the traditional length for psychotherapy sessions. Usually, I allow for an hour-and-a-half to two hours, while at the same time aiming to keep the session within a 60-minute limit. My patients are told from the beginning that if I feel it will be useful, I may extend the session beyond an hour and that, if on some occasions they cannot stay longer, they should let me know at the beginning of the session so that I can plan the work accordingly. On occasions, I have extended sessions beyond several hours because, when using hypnotic methods in psychotherapy, there is more of a possibility of the occurrence of unexpected, unplanned happenings that need to be immediately followed up and that may require the expenditure of extra time. There have been times, too, when I have deliberately planned ahead to hold special, long sessions, such as when a patient has travelled several hundred miles in order to receive treatment. This has been especially true when the patient could not make weekly trips and needed continued therapy. The case of diaphragmatic myoclonus was one requiring extra-long sessions, as was the case of a certain quadriplegic. It is an old cliche, partly substantiated by fact, that some patients in psychotherapy will attempt to extend the therapy session beyond its allotted time, and therapists are warned against falling into this trap. The classical example of this is the patient who, at the last minute, suddenly declares that there is something that absolutely must be talked about before ending the session. With the use of hypnotism, this does not seem to be as great of a problem. Manipulations by the patient to gain extra time are not altogether eliminated, but they are minimized.

Long sessions are not limited to hypnopsychotherapy, and they can be viable for somatic problems. However, with somatic problems (with the exception of the initial induction), sessions can often be limited to 30 minutes or less and, generally, will be limited in number and/or spread over time. Most hypnosomatic treatments have a clear end point, which is in contrast to hypnopsychotherapy, which rarely does.

There is one last point to make regarding long sessions in hypnosis: one needs to make an allowance for the possibility that the patient may need to relieve himself. Characteristically, unless otherwise instructed, hypnotized patients will not volunteer information regarding discomfort or act independently in this regard. For this reason, I always incorporate instructions in the initial induction to insure that the patient will speak up if need be. I simply say to him something like, "If at any time something bothers you, such as needing to go to the bathroom, or you feel uncomfortable in some other way, you will let me know."

Beyond the Initial Induction

What follows the initial induction will vary from case to case. The therapist may decide to develop a deeper hypnosis by devoting several more sessions to this process. Hartland (1971) recommends doing this routinely and devoting up to four sessions to this part of the preparation of the patient.

As discussed in Volume 1, the concept of hypnotic depth is equivocal. In brief review, there is no satisfactory foundation for thinking that hypnosis is a state with depth or degree. The impression of depth on the part of subject and hypnotist is largely subjective. Suggestibility is the only feature that can be objectively measured, and its relation to a postulated depth remains to be established in a definite manner. Any "deepening" procedure can be better viewed as increasing suggestibility and/or increasing the extent of participation by the patient at a non-voluntary level. Some patients show an ability to develop greater suggestibility. Why they do is not at all clear. Part of it may be because the patient becomes more comfortable with relinquishing control and more willing to do so; part may be because the patient learns the best way to give up control and then allows the suggestion effects to take place. There may also be a build-up of one kind or another and a generalization (spread) of the fundamental processes underlying suggestibility proper, whether this be ideodynamic action or something else. (I spoke of this aspect of homoaction and heteroaction in Volume 1.) Finally, at some point in the induction or deepening process, there may be an actual state change that may or may not affect suggestibility proper, but that gives hypnosis its trance-like character. I will continue to refer to the "depth of hypnosis" and to "deepening" hypnosis, but with the above understanding.

Unless one is seeking to produce a highly specific effect by suggestion (this being most often the case when working with somatic problems), I do not feel that one should usually devote more than one session to developing the patient's ability to become hypnotized. As I perceive it, hypnotherapy and, especially hypnopsychotherapy, are not so much the art of developing deep hypnosis in the patient and then utilizing it as the art of utilizing *whatever* degree of hypnosis one can obtain at any moment. How this is done will be seen in some of the specific examples which will be discussed as we go along. Frequently, as therapy progresses and hypnotism is repeatedly induced and used, the patient's suggestibility will, if at all possible, increase. That this may not be possible must be recognized, because it is probable that everyone has a suggestibility ceiling.

It is true that the more suggestible a patient is, the more hypnotic phenomena can be produced. On the other hand, it is most important to recognize that, in most cases, one does not have to produce the entirety of hypnotic phenomena. Most novices in the use of clinical hypnotism become overly concerned with the production of this or that phenomenon, when actually they have no need to be. What does it matter if a patient can or cannot have a vivid visual hallucination if the goal is merely to bring about an attitude change toward life? The ability to age regress is irrelevant if all one seeks to produce is an analgesia. The capacity for developing an anesthesia is of no relevance to the ability to have dreams. Many beginners are particularly vexed by the many patients who seem to be unable to develop an amnesia for their hypnotic experiences. Why is that so important? In many cases, it is not. This is not to say that for some applications it is not desirable, perhaps even essential, to obtain a posthypnotic amnesia, whether spontaneously or by suggestion. The strong appeal that amnesia has for many hypnotists is that, if it is observed, it is a dramatic ratification of hypnosis having been present. Braid made amnesia the *sine qua non* of the presence of hypnosis, and traditional hypnotism followed him, but this probably is not the main reason for the view of today's hypnotists. However, it is rather historically significant to me that, in his writings, Braid reported that a fair percentage of the patients he attempted to hypnotize showed ameliorations and even cures, in spite of the fact that he did not consider them to have been hypnotized because amnesia was absent. They did present other symptoms he associated with the hypnotic state, but none so crucial as amnesia. Braid failed to recognize the significance of the above observation and left it to Liébeault and Bernheim to do this. As pointed out in Volume 1, I believe, along with Bernheim, that there is a form taken by hypnosis which is associated with spontaneous amnesia; this form is the true artificial somnambulism of traditional hypnotism. One may think of it as a phase of hypnotism, or one of several forms that constitute a complex to which the generic term hypnosis has been and can be applied. Somnambulism is unquestionably the ideal form of hypnosis to work with, but its incidence appears to be quite low and, in practice, one can do most of what is required with patients in its absence. In any case, the failure to obtain posthypnotic amnesia, even with suggestions, should not be considered a stumbling block.

Deepening Techniques and Routines

Whatever the plans for the utilization of the session following the initial induction, it is my practice, and one I recommend, to perform the second induction by repeating the original one with a slight variation. Suppose the Visual Fixation Method was used. The patient is now told that it is again time for him to be hypnotized. He is asked to look at the target, but now, rather than suggesting what is going to take place, he is asked to recall the events of the previous session, with the therapist guiding, pacing, and leading while he does so. It is particularly advantageous to use the very words the patient had previously used in describing his experience after the first hypnotization. For example, the patient might be told, "As you look at the

target, you remember how last time it seemed to get much brighter . . .
then how it seemed to scintillate . . . and then how it became blurry . . .
just as it is doing now . . . and, one, your eyelids have become heavy, just
like last time . . . two, so heavy that it is hard for your eyes to stay open
. . . three, four . . . you have become quite relaxed . . . five . . . and
getting more relaxed . . . [assuming the eyes have closed at this point]
that's right, you can close your eyes and keep them closed while I continue to
count toward twenty and you let yourself go farther and deeper into the
hypnotic state that you have now entered . . ."

In this example, "brighter," "scintillate," and "blurry," were words used
by the subject in describing his first experience in becoming hypnotized.
Notice how the posthypnotic suggestion that was then given regarding the
count of 1 to 20 as an inducing procedure is injected in the new induction.

This second induction is also terminated somewhat differently than the
first, because this time the Modified Fractionation Technique is not used.
However, the suggestion regarding the effects of forward and backward
counting is reiterated for reinforcement, and backward counting is used to
dehypnotize the patient.

Some readers may wonder why, when one asks the patient to describe his
experience after the initial induction, he does not re-enter a hypnotic state
by reintegration, as he does in the above. This can happen, and the wise
therapist will not only watch for signs of this occurrence and act accordingly, but he will, as a matter of course, reassert to the patient that he is fully
back in his normal state before going on to other matters. If one suspects
that hypnosis has been reinstated, but is not sure about this, one can ask the
patient whether he feels fully normal (awake). If he indicates that this is not
the case, he can be told to close his eyes, to take a deep breath, and, as he
exhales, that now he is no longer hypnotized (he is now wide awake). Most of
the time, hypnosis does not become reinstated during this recall. What
makes the difference has not been established. One reason is probably because, the therapist having just terminated the hypnotic state, there is an
implied message to the patient that whatever follows next will be associated
with the normal state. On the other hand, when recall is used for reinduction, this is generally done in the context that hypnosis is to be induced. The
therapist may have just announced this, as above, or the patient will have an
expectation that this will be done during the session.

In general, anything associated with going into hypnosis or being in it
may serve as a reintegration cue. With this in mind, when a patient seems to
have difficulty in coming out of hypnosis, having him change chairs will
often resolve the problem. Presumably, the chair in which he is sitting when
he is dehypnotized acts as a cue to be in hypnosis since it is the one he was

sitting in when hypnosis was induced. Milton H. Erickson used to go a step further by asking the patient to trade chairs with him.

An interesting and effective way of applying this is to have two chairs available: one for the induction of and work with hypnosis, and one for non-hypnotic interactions. With the patient initially in the non-hypnosis chair, when it is time for the induction, he is asked to change chairs. He is then asked again to do this after he is dehypnotized. When this is done routinely, other factors may become operative. For one thing, sitting in the hypnosis chair may become a posthypnotic cue to become hypnotized. A conditioning-like effect may also be instituted. Finally, the request to sit in the hypnosis chair may become tantamount to a request or instruction to enter a hypnotic state.

Usually, the third and subsequent inductions can be abbreviated by the therapist telling the patient that he is going to hypnotize him and that the patient should just listen to him. The therapist then begins to count from 1 toward 20, interspersing appropriate suggestions as needed. From there on, counting is usually all that is needed, and this can be even more abbreviated by counting by twos or threes. Eventually saying to the patient something like, "You know that 2 and 18 add up to . . . 20 . . . ," will be just as effective as an actual count to 20. Incidentally, when initially introducing this suggestion, I prefer to speak to the patient of counting from 1 *toward* rather than *to* 20 because the latter may be understood by the patient that he is to enter hypnosis only when 20 is reached. "Toward" makes it possible for the patient to do so from the very start of the count. From here on, the therapist can introduce other posthypnotic signals for rapid induction, either as substitutes for, or in addition to, counting. In general, whatever signals are used should be such that they are not of a kind that could readily be used by accident. Otherwise, qualifying suggestions should be associated with them to forestall this possibility. For example, when it is suggested that counting from 1 toward 20 will bring about a hypnotic state, one would normally want to include that this will be effective only when the counting is done in the context of a therapy session. Review the pertinent material in Volume 1 as necessary.

One addition I always make, usually in the second or third session, is in regard to the signal for dehypnotization. I keep the backward counting as an option, but add the following instruction: "Whenever I ask you to take a deep breath and to no longer be hypnotized, you will come back to your normal state." When the time comes to dehypnotize the patient, I then say, "Now take a deep breath . . . [*I wait for the patient to inspire*] . . . open your eyes [*if they are closed*] . . . you are no longer hypnotized." If sleep suggestions were given in inducing hypnosis, the last statement could be, ". . . and be wide awake." In this case, as I have explained in Volume 1, it is good to then add, "You are no longer hypnotized." Although this is not required, if the patient's eyes are open when I am ready to dehypnotize him, I usually ask him first to close them.

Problems of Low Suggestibility and Resistance

A frequent question asked is, "What do you do with 'resistant,'" or refractory, patients?" See Chapter 3, Volume 1 for a discussion of this issue. I like to reserve the term resistant to denote cases where psychodynamics (using this term in a broad sense) are responsible for the lack of responsiveness. I include in this individuals who deliberately set themselves out to be unresponsive because, presumably, there are underlying dynamics. I reserve the term refractory for individuals of very limited innate suggestibility. There is a small percentage of individuals who, for reasons unknown, are essentially and innately unresponsive to suggestions. For these, my answer to the question asked earlier is, "One does nothing," because there seems to be little that can be done to change the situation. One problem, however, is that one rarely knows ahead of time who is and who is not refractory. One has to try to hypnotize first or give suggestions, and then, when no response or only a very weak one is obtained, there is the question of whether it is a matter of dynamics and that with a little more time and effort expended, something better would ensue. It is important not to allow oneself to view this as a challenge, especially to one's reputation as a hypnotist. There are some professionals who cannot rest until they have succeeded in hypnotizing every resistant and refractory patient that comes their way. This is an unfortunate and unreasonable attitude. Any practitioner who feels this way should seriously examine his motives for using hypnotism. With few exceptions, I rarely attempt more than four inductions. If I obtain some minimal signs of a positive effect in at least the second trial, or if I obtain some clear indication that the problem was one of resistance and have some understanding of its nature, then I will try again. When one is doing psychotherapy and encounters resistance to hypnosis, it is best to put off hypnotizing the patient until some of the resistance has been dealt with through accepted therapeutic non-hypnotic procedures. Resistance originates and manifests itself in a number of ways. Hartland (1971) sums up the main sources of difficulty that one may encounter as follows:

1. Overanxiety and fear of failure
2. Fear of hypnosis itself
3. Defiance of authority
4. Need to prove superiority
5. Fluctuating attention
6. Physical discomfort

7. Dislike of the method of induction employed
8. Inadequate preparation for induction

The problems discussed previously will not be discussed here. The fear of failure often expresses itself in the patient trying hard to bring about the suggested effects through an act of volition, thus interfering with its occurrence as a non-voluntary action. Others are distracted by their overconcern with whether what they are doing is right or wrong and whether or not they are experiencing the right response. This could be because of inadequate preparation, but regardless, this can best be handled by going back to that step and reassuring the patient.

Resistance can take subtle forms, and one needs to learn to recognize the signs. Some of these signs include fidgeting, becoming increasingly tense, complaints about the lighting of the room, about the chair being uncomfortable, or about noises. The experienced hypnotist knows that a responsive subject can go into a profound hypnotic state under the most adverse of circumstances. Some patients will seemingly begin to enter the hypnotic state, only to open their eyes suddenly and state, "I am not hypnotized." A warning here: Sometimes they are, nevertheless, in a hypnotic state, and one should take care that they are fully dehypnotized before they leave the office. When a patient reacts in this manner, I routinely say, "That's all right . . . Please close your eyes again for a few moments. . . ." Then I ask him to take a deep breath and be back in his normal state. In such cases, it is important to accept the patient's need to escape the hypnotic state and not to proceed further without at least looking closer into what is going on.

The best way to handle patients who challenge the therapist to hypnotize them is to refuse to accept the challenge. A very good reply to such a patient is, "I quite agree with you that I probably cannot hypnotize you, so rather than waste your time and my time trying to do so, I suggest we work awhile on your problem without hypnosis." To a patient who states, "No one has ever been able to hypnotize me," my reply is, "And I am sure neither can I. Now what else can I do for you?"

Resistance when doing hypnotherapy often shows up not at the level of inducing hypnosis, which may present no problems, but at the time specific therapeutic suggestions are given. One needs to be cautious at such times because this is often a sign that the patient's defenses are being breached and that he is not ready for the intervention in question. In such cases, a suggestion may be rejected outright. In other cases, it may have an effect, but only a weak or a transitory one, as when a symptom that has been removed reappears at a later date. Or it may have a totally unexpected effect, having little resemblance to what was suggested, as when a substitute symptom shows up in symptom removal. This matter will be discussed in greater detail in the section dealing with hypnopsychotherapy.

Best Methods of Induction and Deepening

We have already touched upon this question in Volume 1, but it is one that comes up so often in relation to clinical practice that we return to it in this context. At a scientific meeting some years ago, I was scheduled to lead a conversation hour on hypnotic techniques. When the hour began, there were perhaps 50 to 70 people in an overcrowded room. Before I even had a chance to approach my topic, a woman asked me, "What *special* methods do you use to hypnotize?" My answer was that I did not use any special or unusual methods. There was an immediate exodus of about half of those present! The woman was one of those that stayed and, undaunted, she persisted with her query stating now with an air of disbelief, "But, surely, you have a special way of working with people who cannot be hypnotized." To this my reply was, "Yes, I do not try to hypnotize them." Whether or not she felt I was being flippant, which I was not, my questioner angrily walked out of the room with an air of disbelief, accompanied by at least half of the remaining audience. I truly believe that she, for one, continued to believe I had a secret with which I would not part. It is surprising how, in this day and age, many otherwise well-informed, intelligent individuals continue to seek magic potions and their equivalents. Hope springs eternal!

I certainly do not have any secret, magical technique for hypnotizing people, especially those who, for one reason or another, respond poorly to inductions. I doubt that anyone has. I say this even though many other experts in the field swear by this or that method to which they often give rather fanciful, catchy names. The literature abounds with descriptions of these methods. Of course, success is relative and is a function of the criteria one uses to speak of it. Too often, these criteria are not given. If one considers obtaining eye-closure as a sufficient criterion for the presence of hypnosis, then one will, indeed, be able to claim far greater success than when one uses the presence of posthypnotic amnesia. In many instances, the sole criterion used is obtaining muscular relaxation, which is a very weak criterion indeed. Whenever anyone claims to have a highly successful method of induction, we must inquire by just what criteria he judges this success. Lacking this information, the assertion is rather meaningless. I suspect that, if there had ever been a powerful, infallible induction method that had universal application, we would know with certainty of its existence by now, and a well-trodden path would have been beaten to the door of whoever used it.

To date, no universally applicable, fail-proof method exists. Personal preferences, more than anything else, seem to be the basis for consistent use of a given technique by most hypnotists. The only value there is in becoming familiar with the large variety of induction or deepening methods that exist is that a person may find one that is particularly appealing, or may occasionally discover a new idea or step that is useful. Again, the most effective approach is to let each situation dictate how one will deal with it, and allow the hypnotist to modify the procedures as needed.

FURTHER GENERAL PROCEDURES

Once the initial procedures are over, one is ready to undertake the therapy proper. Psychotherapy may be one exception to this statement, because most of the time, the psychotherapeutic process seems to begin with the initial session, even if it is limited to the gathering of personal data. This is even more true when hypnotism is introduced. In any event, we have reached the point where we are nearly ready to look at specific applications. I say nearly because it remains to look at certain procedures of general applicability which are specific to the use of hypnotism.

Posthypnotic Suggestions in Therapy

Posthypnotic suggestions are widely used in a variety of ways in the context of therapy. The nature of the problem is usually the guide to the form these suggestions will take. One routine use is for the rapid reinduction of hypnosis. The signal for this may be given by the hypnotist or someone else designated by him, or it may be the occurrence of a certain event or combination of events. It can even be a signal the patient gives to himself. The termination of this hypnotic state can similarly be controlled. Another wide use is for the production of an anesthesia or analgesia that is to persist either after the patient is dehypnotized, or to occur under certain conditions and at a later date.

In general, any time a therapist has a need to bring about a change or initiate an action that must either take place after a hypnotic session or, having been initiated in hypnosis, is to continue into the normal state, a posthypnotic suggestion will be called for. This could be for a reduction of muscle spasms, increased appetite, increased lactation, a change in attitude, having a dream, understanding a dream, controlling hyperhidrosis, controlling gagging, maintaining a certain posture for a length of time, and many other effects.

Contrary to a common belief, amnesia for a posthypnotic suggestion is not an absolute requirement for it to be effective. As we have seen in Volume 1, there are reasons for it. This is not to say that there may not be situations in which it is imperative to have amnesia. It seems reasonable to think that if a patient is aware of the content of a posthypnotic suggestion, he is in a position to interfere deliberately with it and, in any case, he is likely to develop, without intending to, interfering sets and behaviors. However, this is not what one encounters in practice, at least not in the laboratory and in informal demonstrations. Some posthypnotic suggestions seem to be so compelling that forewarned subjects cannot prevent them from becoming effective sooner or later. At best, they can delay the occurrence of the effects. Assuming that amnesia can be a factor which must be considered, its utility in a therapy setting would be expected to vary and to partly be a function of the nature of the suggested posthypnotic action. In some applications, amnesia seems clearly irrelevant, such as those in which one will tell the patient, after he has been dehypnotized, that a posthypnotic suggestion has been given and what its nature is. This is frequently done when a patient is given, as needed, training in the production of analgesia. Another example is when a patient is given suggestions that will enable him to be hypnotized by other practitioners. In both instances, the patient needs to know, in the non-hypnotic state, what he now is able to do, when he should do it, and how he will go about it. For these situations, it certainly seems immaterial whether or not amnesia can be produced by suggestion. Nevertheless, it is conceivable, although not demonstrated, that even in such applications, the presence of amnesia may increase the potency of the suggestions. For this reason, and unless it is contra-indicated, the practical thing to do is to suggest amnesia any time it is obtainable.

When giving posthypnotic suggestions, it is a common practice to have the patient repeat them back after they have been given. Not only does this insure that the patient has heard the suggestions correctly, but it is generally believed that this makes them more compelling. It is also part of the common practice to follow up immediately such feedback with the statement, "That's right. And you will do it, won't you?" If the patient does not respond to this question, it is reiterated in one form or another until a clear response is obtained. When the posthypnotic suggestion is a compound one, that is, is made up of a number of more elementary suggestions, some hypnotists then take up each element individually and ask for an affirmation for each. Thus, having suggested that the patient will (1) change chairs after being dehypnotized, (2) comment on the weather, and then five minutes later (3) again go into a hypnotic state, and the patient having repeated this, the therapist might then say, "That's right. And you will change chairs. Right? . . . And then you will say something about the weather. Right? . . . And five minutes later you will again become hypnotized. Right? . . ." Although never formally confirmed, it is generally believed that affirmative answers insure that the suggested action will occur. The feeling seems to be that this elicits a particularly strong commitment from the patient.

I have found it a good practice, when possible, to check out the effectiveness of posthypnotic suggestions in the session in which they are given. For example, if the patient is supposed to be able to produce in himself an analgesia on demand, I test his ability to do so right then and there. It may be discovered that one needs to correct certain misunderstandings the patient has regarding what he is to do or what is to happen or that there is a need for reinforcement of the suggestion.

As explained in Volume 1, posthypnotic suggestions can be long-lasting in their effects without having to be reinforced. Some have been known to last 10 to 15 years. But with many patients, usually those of medium or lesser suggestibility, periodic reinforcement is required. One can often do this by means of specially prepared tape recordings that one gives the patient.

As for the production of posthypnotic amnesias, with some subjects, a simple direct instruction of "You will not remember anything . . . ," or, "You will not remember that I told you this . . . ," will suffice. When one knows that this will not work, or one is doubtful that it will, a frequently effective suggestion is in the form of, ". . . but it is not necessary that you remember my telling you this. It will take place just as well . . . ," or, ". . . you will have no interest in recalling this . . . ," or, ". . . you will not have any desire to think about it. . . ." One can be even more indirect, as was Milton H. Erickson (see Chapter 7), by matter-of-factly talking to the patient, before or after other posthypnotic suggestions have been given, about how easy it is to forget something for awhile, about how dreams that are so vivid will be forgotten on waking, how one may forget something because of intense interest in something else, and so on. No references at all are made to the material for which amnesia is sought. There are still more indirect ways in the form of story telling. But this belongs to Ericksonian hypnotism and will not be discussed further at this time.

Telling a patient, "You will be unable to remember (or recall)," and, "You will have no memories of . . . ," may have quite different effects. The first of these may affect only the act of active recall. As a result, the patient may have the on-the-tip-of-the-tongue type of experience. He may feel there are memories right there to be called forth, but which he cannot reach. The experience may be one of not being able to initiate recall or to make the necessary effort. On occasion, a patient will make mouthing movements, and will later state that he could not vocalize the memories. These effects do not occur when the second type of suggestion is given because it is accessibility and not retrieval that is focused upon. The outcome, as with suggestions in general, depends partly upon the patient's understanding of what is communicated and the degree to which he is literal.

One should also keep in mind that "remembering" and being "aware of" can be two different things. Sometime a hypnotized individual who has amnesia may retain an awareness that there is something he should be able to remember but cannot. He may also be fully aware of the suggested effect when it takes place, and may deduce from this occurrence that a posthypnotic suggestion must have been given to him. Unawareness of the effect taking place is most often automatically associated with an amnesia, but not always. In some cases, there is awareness at the time of occurrence, but a spontaneous-like amnesia for what has just occurred immediately follows. The only way to insure that there will be unawareness is to suggest it in addition to amnesia. One way to induce amnesia *and* unawareness of the effect is to suggest something like, ". . . after you wake up [*come back to your normal state*], you will be unaware I have told you this, and you will be unaware of (name effect or action) . . . and of my telling you this now." The reason for the last provision is that what precedes does not necessarily include the total posthypnotic suggestion.

Self-Hypnotism in Therapy

Occasionally, one encounters patients who, on their own, at some point in the treatment, will place themselves in a hypnotic state by reintegrating a previous induction or therapy session. This usually happens when the patient feels the need for it prior to the next scheduled session. For example, one patient who was having a bad time trying to go to sleep imagined that he was back in my office listening to me inducing hypnosis with sleep suggestions. Another patient having a recurrence of pain imagined herself receiving pain-relieving suggestions from me. This may be indicative of the patient's desire or need to have more of a feeling of control. In any case, it is generally an indicator that the patient is a good candidate for training in limited self-hypnotism. Why anything more should be done when the patient is obviously already capable of doing self-hypnosis? There are several reasons. Most patients need some education regarding the proper uses of self-hypnotism. Their ability to do so can often be more effectively channelled by the therapist. There is often a need to incorporate protective limits and safeguards against unintentional misuse of self-hypnotism. For example, an individual with a painful injury might induce an anesthesia and ignore the need to receive treatment. There are such cases on record. Finally, the therapist may be able to formulate the suggestions better.

Most of the time, it is the therapist who initiates the idea of teaching self-hypnosis to the patient. Actually, it can be argued that, if it is true that the actualization of a posthypnotic suggestion is always accompanied by a hypnotic state, it should follow that self-hypnosis is inherent in any posthypnotic suggestion that the patient has been given. Most therapists consider that a patient is doing self-hypnosis when he induces an analgesia in himself as a result of having been told he can do so by thinking, for example, "1, 2, 3, the pain is going away." Unless hypnosis is specifically self-induced apart from any other effects, this may be somewhat of an abuse of the expression "self-hypnosis." As pointed out in Volume 1, self-induced hypnosis in which the induction consists in knowingly employing an implanted signal would probably be more correctly denoted by the expression "pseudo self-hypnosis."

A particularly effective way of using guided, limited self-hypnotism is with the help of audiotapes. This is especially useful with patients who are of medium suggestibility or less and whose treatment calls for much repetition of certain suggestions session after session. This is the case, for example, in the non-analytic treatment of eating and of habit problems in general, of habitually tense and anxious individuals, those with chronic pains, and patients needing ongoing supporting and motivating suggestions. Tapes are also indicated when patients are forced to have infrequent sessions, patients who may be moving to a distant locality, or who may have to interrupt therapy for an appreciable period of time. Another indication for tapes is when a long induction or a complex set of suggestions have to be used. Finally, some patients feel more secure when they have a tape to fall back on between sessions.

The audiotapes I give my patients always combine an induction with therapeutic suggestions. The best way to make such a tape is simply to record a typical session with the patient as one goes through it, adding whatever other suggestions may be called for in order for it to be used for self-hypnotism. This should include suggestions to cover the following: the taped session being interrupted by an equipment breakdown, interruptions (telephone or doorbell), and emergencies. I usually give the patient the option to come out of the hypnotic state in an emergency or to handle the emergency while remaining hypnotized. Equipment breakdown is handled by telling the patient that should he cease to hear the tape for longer than five minutes, he will come out of the hypnotic state. The five-minute provision may have to be changed if, for example, the tape purposefully contains a ten-minute or longer period of silence. I usually discuss with the patient how interruptions might be handled, and then make suggestions in keeping with his preference.

When a patient is instructed in doing self-hypnosis, it is a good idea to follow the instruction with a rehearsal by having the patient go through the procedures while in the office. This allows the therapist to note any difficulties the patient may have with them. In case there are problems, additional suggestions and instructions can be given to counteract them. Not all patients are able to go readily into a self-induced hypnotic state the first few times they try it. The therapist can give aiding suggestions while the patient goes through the steps of the induction. For example, with a patient who has been told to count to himself to 10, I might ask him to demonstrate the procedure, counting out loud, so that I may follow his progress. I also tell him, if it seems a good idea, that I will help him along. If it appears that the counting is not as effective as it could be, I will pick it up at some point and will continue the count out loud with the patient while interspersing various helping suggestions. Before having the patient come out of hypnosis, I suggest that greater success will occur in the future, and may add such other suggestions as may seem needed. I then have the patient try again, and proceed accordingly.

One problem some patients have when they use self-hypnosis is setting for themselves a certain amount of time during which they will remain hypnotized. They may decide, for example, on 20 minutes, and will either run under or over the time set by an appreciable amount. To remedy this, one tells the hypnotized patient that time appreciation is often initially affected by the hypnotic state, and that this can be easily corrected. The patient is then instructed that until it is no longer needed, when he uses self-hypnosis, he will check the time just before inducing hypnosis and will also do so immediately on coming out of the state, noting any discrepancy that may exist between the final reading and the duration he had chosen. He is told that knowledge of any existing discrepancy will help him to correct automatically his time sense in hypnosis. In most cases, I have the patient do this exercise in my office a number of times until the discrepancy vanishes. I tell others to set a time aside at home to do the same.

Distance Hypnotherapy

Over the years, I have had the opportunity to do brief hypnotherapy over the telephone. This is normally a crisis intervention procedure, and certainly not one to be used for routine therapy. The first time I did this was when I received a call from a patient who was highly suggestible and whom I was treating for a weight problem. She had slipped in her bathtub and torn some ligaments in a shoulder. She was in great pain. It occurred to me that I should be able to treat her pain over the telephone. I told her of my idea, to which she was agreeable. I asked her to make herself as comfortable as she could, and no matter what happened, to keep the telephone to her ear. Since I had trained her to go into a hypnotic state at a signal, I told her that when I next gave her the signal to become hypnotized, she would do so, continuing to hold the telephone so that we could keep on talking. I then gave the signal, immediately following it with the instruction to keep holding the phone. The remainder of the work was straightforward. I ended this session by giving the patient appropriate suggestions for possible future inductions by telephone that, incidentally, in this case was not again required.

One could routinely incorporate suggestions in the initial preparation of the patient to allow for the above. I have not done so regularly, but only in cases where I could anticipate a need for it. Patients who are so incapaci-tated that a visit to my office is difficult, who do not have ready access to it, or who have to travel frequently are among those for whom I will make such a provision. I have done this mainly in the case of patients with severe pain problems, although not exclusively so.

If one plans to take the above step, one should do so only after having discussed this option with the patient and obtained his consent. One then suggests that hereafter, if the need should arise, the patient will readily be able to be hypnotized over the telephone. It is imperative to include sugges-tions to the effect that, no matter what happens, the patient, while hypno-tized, will continue to hold the phone in such a way as to maintain adequate communication. As with the use of tapes, instructions are also given to cover equipment breakdown, emergencies, and other interruptions.

For greater details regarding this technique and other examples, the reader is referred to an article I published some years ago (Weitzenhoffer, 1972b).

Ego-Strengthening Suggestions

In preparing patients for hypnotic work, some practitioners make routine use of "ego strengthening" suggestions. That the suggestions are supportive is clear, but it is much less clear that they actually increase ego strength. This has never been satisfactorily documented. To the extent that one can mean-ingfully speak of ego strength, one needs to question whether or not many of the suggested effects would do so.

Patients are typically told in various ways that, as the days pass, they will feel physically and mentally stronger and fitter, that they will feel more alert, more energetic, and more effective in whatever they undertake. They are told that they will become mentally calmer, that their power of concentration will increase, and that they will be able to think more clearly. They will become more positive, more optimistic in their outlook on life, will worry less, and will become less easily upset. They will believe in themselves and their ability to take control of their lives. They will stop dwelling on their problems, diffi-culties, health, and symptoms. They will increasingly turn their attention to the external world and those things they can accomplish in it. Some practi-tioners, like Hartland (1971), spend considerable time doing this. They use a rather broad approach that covers all possibilities. Others, such as myself, prefer to limit themselves to those aspects that are particularly pertinent to the patient, and do not use this routinely, but only as needed.

Although the concept of ego strength is fairly well-defined in the psychoan-alytic literature where it had its origins, many therapists tend to use the expres-sion somewhat loosely. One consequence is that the hypnotherapy literature describes a variety of ego-strengthening methods that, if they increase ego strength, must do so indirectly, or that may owe their effectiveness to other reasons. Some of these methods are described in great detail, often given verbatim. One such method, called "The Serenity Place," described by Hammond (1985), involves telling the patient the following:

1. The patient will find himself in front of a door. The door will presently open, and he will be able to enter a very special, wonderful place.
2. This place will be one where he has previously been, or a totally new one.
3. As the patient enters this very special place, he can experience refreshing feelings of calmness, happiness, contentment, and security.
4. The patient is now given the choice of exploring or of just sitting there enjoying the good feelings that he absorbs and that become part of him.
5. After allowing the patient time to do the above, the therapist tells him that "things can come into perspective," that he can become "aware of actual feelings, with a correct sense of perspective," undistorted by moods or circumstantial sets.
6. The patient is next told that his unconscious mind knows what he needs most and will see to it that the above [5] will be accomplished in some manner or other.
7. The patient is allowed to have more time in the special place for as long as he needs, continuing to revitalize himself by absorbing all the good feelings.
8. The suggestion is now given that in the future, the patient can return to the special place any time he feels the need to do so.
9. Finally, the patient is told he will become dehypnotized when he is ready.

Hammond has a strong Ericksonian orientation (Chapter 7), and consequently his verbatim account goes through the above steps using a permissive and open-ended approach. His reference to the "unconscious" (in step 6) is very typically Ericksonian. If one takes the position that anything that helps the patient to cope better with life situations is ego strengthening, it is probably legitimate to speak of the above as doing this. Whether these procedures truly increase ego strength or help the patient in some other way, the above steps seem reasonable ones to take. For years, I used a somewhat analogous sequence in teaching alcoholics tension-reduction techniques.

Another procedure bearing some similarity in form to the above, and sometimes considered an ego-strengthening technique for patients with negative feelings, consists in having the hypnotized patient begin by searching his memory for a time when he had opposite, positive feelings. He is then instructed to go back to that time and re-experience it, letting the hypnotist know when this takes place. At this point, the patient is told to close his dominant hand into a tight fist, and that as he does so the good feelings will become even more intense. Again, he is asked to signal when this takes place. The patient is allowed to have a few moments to continue having the experience, then he is told that in the future, whenever he wants or needs to re-experience the good feelings, he only needs to close again his dominant hand into a fist.

Repeat at least two more times, with the patient identifying two other occasions in which he experienced the same positive feelings. Then a new step is introduced. The patient is asked to recall a situation in which he experienced the negative feelings in a mild form. He is told he can now transfer these feelings into his non-dominant hand as he makes it into a fist. When he reports that he has made the transfer, he is then asked to make a fist of his dominant hand while he relaxes his non-dominant hand, and he is also told that as he does so, all the unpleasant feelings flow out into the surrounding space and the good feelings replace them. The patient is finally told that he will be able to do the same thing on his own whenever he needs to do it.

Calvert Stein (1963) was probably the first to describe this procedure, and he did so in great detail. His account shows a great deal of the probable influence on him of the thinking of earlier clinicians such as LeCron, Cheek, and, especially, Erickson regarding working with the patient's unconscious. Thus, in Stein's account of the above procedures, it is actually the patient's unconscious that he instructs to locate the past experiences and to regress the patient to them. Likewise, he uses ideomotor signaling as a means of communication with the patient's unconscious.

Reader's familiar with the "anchoring" techniques of NLP (Chapter 8) will probably think that they see a similarity between them and the above. Anchoring per se is not really involved in this because the association between feelings and the closed fist is created by means of suggestions, and true anchoring is posited to take place only through contiguity. On the other hand, there is such a strong similarity between the above procedures and certain uses of anchoring described in the later literature that one cannot help but feel that Stein's description must have served as an unacknowledged model for them.

There is one last procedure that might also be considered a novel approach to ego strengthening. I first came across a mention of it around 1970 in courses developed by Jose Silva that teach and use self-hypnosis. Silva was the founder of an organization devoted to the development of psychic abilities. A special place, called "the laboratory," is created, and in this place the hypnotized person contacts a "consultant" or "guide" of his choosing to whom he can turn for help in resolving the problems in life that he encounters. Many readers will undoubtedly see further similarities with the use of spirit guides and with "channeling." That therapeutic gains may come out of such procedures cannot be denied. However, how consistently this happens and how permanent the results are remain largely unanswered questions. Additionally, it is not at all clear what is actually responsible for the therapeutic results when they occur.

This is the end of the discussion on general procedures. We shall now examine more specific applications of hypnotism. It is not practical to discuss examples of applications under each heading and subheading listed earlier, nor is it necessary. Instead, a sampling of applications will be provided, with enough details that the reader should be able to extrapolate from these to other situations. Keep in mind that every case must be considered as having its unique characteristics calling for appropriate modifications. It is for this reason that no single recipe or formula can be provided for the treatment of any given class, even less so for all classes, or problems.

4

Specific Procedures in Traditional and Semi-Traditional Clinical Hypnotism: Somatic and Related Problems

INTRODUCTION

Having been identified as a psychologist for more than 30 years, it may be natural to wonder about my qualifications to write about how to use hypnotism in medical and dental practice. I have had about 30 years of close association professionally with medical practitioners and dentists, sometimes as a consultant, sometimes as a teacher, sometimes as a collaborator in the treatment of patients, and sometimes as a student. Three years of teaching physiology and pharmacology in a dental school gave me an opportunity to learn a great deal about dentistry and oral surgery. More than 20 years on the staff of a general hospital, and being associated with other hospitals and a medical center, provided me with many experiences of medical problems and their treatments. Some of my most valued first-hand experiences have come from nearly five years of working on an inpatient alcohol treatment unit, where one is exposed to much more than the behavioral effects of alcohol. I also had a medical chief who was very willing to educate me. I may not be able to do surgery, but I have prepared patients and attended their surgeries. I may not have performed physical examinations and made medical diagnoses, but I have conferred with those making them and taken part in planning patients' overall therapies. I did, however, learn to do neurological examinations and have received instruction in neurology. I have never worked with a new medical problem without first consulting the medical literature pertaining to it. I can, therefore, write knowledgeably about a variety of medical problems.

My choice of topics has been selective. This partly reflects my limited experience, but also reflects the selective applications of hypnotism in medical and dental practice. This is understandable when one considers that a great deal of medicine and dentistry deals with problems of the body that are not directly connected with mental functioning, whereas hypnotism is, first of all, mental in nature. Psychosomatic medicine and psychosomatic dentistry are the only areas in which one can expect hypnotism to be a potentially equal partner with somatic therapy, and then, as such, it becomes one with psychotherapy and no longer fully comes under the heading of medical practice.

ANALGESIA AND ANESTHESIA

General Considerations

The use of hypnotism for the production of analgesia and anesthesia is relevant not only to surgery, but also to a number of other specialties, particularly obstetrics and dentistry. Also, as we shall see, it goes appreciably beyond merely suggesting the absence of pain or a lack of sensation.

Pain has many facets and is a very complex phenomenon. Even today, it is not at all clearly understood. It involves more than the pain receptors, the nature of which is also unclear. First, it appears that some pains may be of thalamic origin. There is also referred pain, in which the locus of sensation is not the locus of trauma. Pain has qualities, some of which are known to be associated with the kinds of nerve fibers that conduct the pain. For this and other reasons, one needs to think not of pain, but of pains. According to a current theory, the chemical endorphine, produced in the brain under certain conditions, has properties that can dull the experience of pain. There are also interactions, caused by pain and other stimuli that are believed to occur at nerve junctions, that can exacerbate pain; there are other interactions that can block it. There is considerable evidence that various central nervous activities can have a strong influence upon the perception of pain. There is evidence that muscular tension, often a reflection of psychological tension, exacerbates and can even cause pain. Muscular and mental relaxation work in the opposite direction. There is also evidence to show that the pain experience can be absent in spite of the continued presence of somatic concomitants of pain. It is important to keep this in mind when trying to evaluate the effectiveness of suggested analgesia. Finally, pain appears to cause tissue changes, particularly inflammations, that tend to maintain and exacerbate it and that in themselves are deleterious. Conversely, a side effect of reduced pain may be a reduction in inflammation. All of these factors need to be taken into consideration when thinking of altering the experience of pain by suggestion.

Although there is a basic distinction to be made between analgesia and anesthesia, I will generally speak of anesthesia inclusively of analgesia when the distinction is not critical. Although in practice the primary aim is usually to prevent or decrease pain, thus to produce analgesia, methods used are often of a kind that will produce anesthesia. Be that as it may, frequently it is easier to produce analgesia than anesthesia by suggestion, but I have no hard data to support this impression.

Historically speaking, spontaneous "insensibility" was at one time considered to be a sign of artificial somnambulism and, even earlier, of the mesmeric influence having been obtained. Esdaile is reputed to have performed a multitude of painless amputations on magnetized patients during the nineteenth century. There is also on record a detailed account of a mastectomy performed in the early part of the nineteenth century on a magnetized patient. Whatever the case may have been in the past, it has not been found in modern times that spontaneous anesthesia generally accompanies hypnosis. On the other hand, suggestions can be very effective in altering sensations, and the common practice has been to use suggestions for the production of anesthesias. Pains that may be treated with hypnotism fall into a number of categories. There are the somatic acute pains caused by the trauma of an operative intervention, acute pains due to recent injury, and chronic pains of purely somatic origins resulting from past injuries, surgery, or disease. There are the purely psychogenic (functional) acute and chronic pains. And, finally, there are the acute, but mostly chronic, pains of mixed origin. These are not all treated the same way. In particular, the treatment of psychogenic pain belongs much more to the domain of psychotherapy than of any other medical specialty. On the other hand, even pains of somatic origin can have strong emotional ramifications, and their treatment cannot always be completely divorced from psychotherapeutic considerations. This does not mean that a psychotherapist must necessarily become involved, but it does mean the specialist doing the treatment must be ready to work at this level, too.

I will say a few words about acupuncture and the use of white noise in the reduction of pain. The production of anesthesia or analgesia by the stimulation of acupuncture points was not a part of traditional acupuncture and not even intimated by the underlying ancient theory. It was discovered by accident in recent times. Western neuroscience has offered an explanation of the effect in terms of the gate theory, a modern theory regarding nervous interactions. This theory is only one step better than the Chinese meridian explanation, whose weakness lies in the absence of solid anatomical and physiological evidence for the existence of meridians. The widely accepted hypothesis that it is all a matter of suggestion, while reasonable and appealing, is itself not well-founded.

There is also a lack of solid evidence to support the effects of white noise on the perception of pain. This effect, in any case, appears to be somewhat erratic, and there are only weak hypotheses available to explain its mechanism. Suggestion has been proposed as a possible explanation. While this might account for later reported results, it does not seem to account for the initial discovery.

Hypnoanesthesia for Surgical and Like Procedures

The most direct and, certainly simplest, approach is to say to the patient that he is no longer able to feel anything in the part of the body that one wishes to be anesthetized. Many therapists like to use a signal so that they may say, "In a moment, when I next say 'now,' you will no longer have any pain in . . . ," or, "I am going to count to three and at three you will no longer have any sensations in . . ." Or, if the aim is to relieve the patient from an ongoing pain, one might say, for example, "At the count of five your headache will be gone." There is technically and linguistically a clear distinction between anesthesia and analgesia, and in the practice of hypnotism it can make quite a difference whether one tells the subject he will feel no pain or he will feel no sensations. The first of these suggestions, if effective and taken literally, will cause an analgesia, but other sensations may remain. In this case, the suggestion may appear to have failed. For example, in some of my early research, I had decided to use the neurological technique in which the patient's ability to feel pain is tested with a blunt and a pointed stimulus. My hypnotized subject had been instructed to say "dull" and "sharp," according to what they felt. Much to my initial surprise, subjects whom I expected would develop a good analgesia would report accurately the nature of the stimulus. However, when I began to question them about their experience, it became clear that, indeed, they had felt no pain with the sharp stimulus but had still had the other tactile sensations that accompany this kind of stimulus. Later, when I shifted to the use of an electric shock, subjects who were analgesic were often found to be able to report accurately feeling an electric shock because of their awareness of muscular twitches that accompanied the shock. Had I gone only by their identification of sharpness and of shock, I might have assumed that the analgesia of these subjects had been incomplete, if at all present. Patients who are being prepared for hypnotic analgesia are often initially tested with relatively mild pain stimuli. The therapist must be sure not to misinterpret the patient's response and *infer a failure when there is none.* It is particularly important to remember that a patient who fears pain and is anxious or tense may, by reflex, overtly react to the non-algesic elements of the evoked response, just as he would to the algesia had it been present. One of the best ways to ascertain the true nature of the patient's response is subsequently to use a control test in the absence of suggested analgesia, not differences in reaction, and ask the patient to describe any difference he may have noted between the two situations.

In the light of the above remarks, it might be asked why one should suggest only analgesia. Why not, to be safe, suggest an anesthesia from the beginning? There are a number of practical reasons for this. Although it seems increasingly to be less of a problem, some patients fear the unconsciousness associated with general chemical anesthesia. Although most of the time suggesting, "You will feel nothing," is not interpreted as being unconscious, there are exceptions. More to the point, one may need the patient to be able to have some or all of other tactile sensations intact. A good example of this was the case I mentioned in Chapter 2 of the woman who went into labor without any awareness of doing so because of the broad suggestions she had received. I have known of prospective mothers who wanted only analgesia so that they could retain other sensations during delivery. Such individuals may reject a broad suggestion of anesthesia when it is given. Most women, however, are willing to accept the equivalent of a saddle block. Unusual needs of the patient can sometimes lead to unexpected results. I know of a woman who was capable of developing a very strong glove anesthesia, but who was initially and unexpectedly found to be incapable of developing a suggested saddle block. When the obstetrician eventually explored with the patient what might be interfering, he discovered that she was a religious person who firmly believed that women were meant to experience pain during childbirth. Not to do so would be a sin. It turned out, however, that the patient could concede that it would be acceptable to feel only a small amount of pain. The obstetrician wisely told her in hypnosis that she "would experience only as much pain as she needed to have." Labor and delivery turned out to be essentially painless. On the other hand, I have known of some women who wanted to have no awareness at all of labor and/or delivery. For these, a complete anesthesia is in order.

The manner of producing a glove anesthesia has been described in Volume 1, Chapter 5. For reasons that are far from being clear, glove anesthesias seem to be among the more easily suggested anesthesias. They will often occur when the suggestion fails that an anesthesia will develop in some other part of the body. For this reason, many practitioners will start out by suggesting a glove anesthesia, then will transfer it to whatever part of the body is to be eventually anesthetized. The preferred method of transferring is to have the patient place the anesthetized hand against the part to be anesthetized, and then to suggest that the anesthesia is becoming transferred. Since a glove anesthesia is usually characterized by a feeling of dullness or numbness, a leathery feeling, etc., it is usual to speak of the transfer in terms of a transfer of these sensations, and then of these spreading out, if necessary. Thus, in the case of preparing a patient for dental work, the hand is applied against the face in the vicinity of or over the area where the anesthesia is desired. A gynecology patient who has difficulties with pelvic examinations might be told to place her hand on her stomach below the umbilicus, or even lower, and to think of the numbness flowing and spreading into the perineal region, using, of course, non-technical language.

Another method for inducing the equivalent of a local anesthesia when a patient has experienced actual local anesthesias, as most persons will have, is to remind the hypnotized patient of such past experiences. Have him recall the experiences associated with the absence of feeling, then localize them in that part of their body where anesthesia is desired. One may even suggest that an injection is being made. This is fine, provided the patient does not have a distaste for or fear of injections. Related to this method is the use of past experiences of having a hand, leg, arm, or foot "go to sleep," or of going numb and "dead" from exposure to cold. A popular technique used is to suggest to the patient, or ask him to imagine, that a piece of ice has been applied to the part to be anesthetized, and then suggest the numbing and other effects. One can supplement this by initially applying a cold object to the part in question. A coin, the head of a stethoscope, a dental mirror, and so on will all do. With patients who have previously had saddle blocks or caudal anesthesia, one can use their past experiences to produce the equivalent by suggestion. One word of warning: caudal anesthesia can be followed by violent headaches. A patient who once had this happen to him may end up with as bad of an indirectly suggested headache as the one he previously experienced, unless appropriate suggestions have been given to prevent this. In general, one should acquire sufficient knowledge about the past experiences of the patient to offset by suggestion any renewal of previous unpleasant experiences. Since in the above procedures the sensations involved are universal, the therapist has no problem in pacing and leading the patient.

Rather than speak of the absence of sensations or suggesting certain altered sensory experiences, one can also suggest the absence of awareness for the part involved and what is done to it. For example, to produce a glove anesthesia, one can suggest to the patient that he will become unaware of his hand. A very different process is involved, one that some writers have proposed is a dissociation. The patient can be told quite directly, "When I next say 'now,' you will no longer be aware of the lower half of your body. It will be as if it had no existence, but this interesting experience will not bother you. You will be very comfortable with it." Note the additional suggestions that have been incorporated. They are aimed at preventing adverse reactions that sometimes will otherwise take place. For some subjects, losing the awareness of part of their body can be quite threatening. Milton H. Erickson produced anesthesia by having the patient hallucinate being in a different geographic location than where his body actually is.

One method that may be related to Erickson's consists in having the hypnotized patient experience himself involved in some activity, and in some other locality, than the one he is presently in. Taking an extended trip, being at a concert, enjoying fishing, and so on, are examples. I am inclined to believe that while a dissociation may take place in some cases, as Erickson proposed, other processes may be equally responsible. It has long been known that in everyday situations, if a person's attention can be strongly diverted from certain events, these events will not be experienced at the time. It is the common experience, that everyone has had, of not being aware of certain occurring events because of attending to others. This kind of experience has been used by some researchers in support of their claim that everyone experiences spontaneous occurrences of "everyday" hypnosis. Not only is this argument fallacious, but this hypnotic procedure also makes use of natural non-hypnotic processes to attain a certain goal. An analogy may be helpful. On the one hand, thinking of eating a tasty morsel of food can cause salivation and, on the other hand, this can be used under hypnosis to promote a more intense salivation for a specific purpose. This does not make the naturally occurring process a hypnotic one. Why, then, should this be less the case for the effects of focusing attention? The answer is that it shouldn't and isn't. In any event, when using the above approach, I start out by asking the patient what his favorite activities are. Having been told, for example, that it is traveling, I will then go on to say, "Good. Where would you like to go now if you could take a trip?" Most of the time the patient will name a place or places. "Have you ever been there before?" might be the next question. It is not essential that the patient has been there, but it does make things easier. For this reason, one may start out by saying, "Where have you gone to that you would like to visit again?" Once a place or places have been decided upon, one might go on to tell the patient, "Fine. When I next say 'now,' you will be on the point of taking a trip to _____. You are going to experience taking this trip in its smallest details, starting with your arrival at the airport. You will live your trip minute by minute, hour by hour, day by day. You will live it fully and you will travel until I tell you it is over." The wording of this last suggestion may have to be changed according to the patient's habitual way of traveling, since some prefer to drive, go by boat, or take a bus. In European countries, as well as in Japan and China, going by train is a popular form of traveling. Although this may not be necessary, one may want to add, "You will have no other awareness than of your trip, which you will enjoy very much. Now you are off on your trip." In spite of these instructions, pain stimuli can sometimes become incorporated in odd ways, usually in a masked form, in the subject's suggested experience. This will cause him to have a less than totally pleasant experience. The situation is like that in which real stimuli become incorporated in dreams; it is not usually serious. For surgical or other procedures in which the patient does not have to participate actively, the above will do fine. When it is desired that the patient be able to respond to the practitioner, as in dental work, additional instructions may be given to the effect that the patient will respond appropriately to the dentist without this in any way affecting his travel experience. To do so is particularly important when the hypnotist is preparing the patient for therapeutic work with another person. I will come back to this in more detail shortly.

Hypnoanesthesia for major surgery is effective in probably no more than 10% of cases, and these patients have been very carefully selected and trained. As Kroger (1963) has pointed out, as long as the above limitation exists, it will never replace chemoanesthesia. It is more useful for minor surgical procedures, and one of its main applicabilities is in pre- and postoperative management. Hypnoanesthesia has been found very useful in surgery of the face and head where the maintenance of proper airway can otherwise be a problem. As mentioned earlier, the apposition of parts of the body for tissue grafts can also be facilitated. The standard use of plaster casts to immobilize the parts of the body involved causes skin irritation, sores, and stiffness. It also causes pain and discomfort and eventually requires physiotherapy. It is possible to induce, in some patients, posthypnotic limb catalepsies that can enforce the required immobility without any of the undesirable side effects of casts. Such a catalepsy can be so strong that applied external force cannot displace the cataleptic limb. The reduction of fractures and the setting of bones is readily done with hypnoanesthesia. It has also been found to be particularly applicable for the pain of labor and delivery. Episiotomies are a simple matter. One advantage of hypnoanesthesia in obstetrics is that it allows the physician to have more than normal control over the birth movements. It also eliminates all ill effects of chemical anesthesia on the unborn child. After labor and delivery, shock is also greatly diminished.

Most surgeons and anesthesiologists using hypnoanesthesia are always prepared to back it up with chemical anesthesia, if necessary, because of the former's unpredictability. The knowledge that this will be available is also reassuring to the patient and does not seem to have adverse effects on the success of the hypnoanesthesia. A fair number of patients are unable to develop the kind of anesthesia that is required for certain types of surgery where more than insensitivity to pain is needed and chemical supplementation is a must. However, it is widely agreed that a combination of hypnoanesthesia with chemical anesthesia helps to reduce appreciably the amount of chemicals required. This is an asset. It is also claimed that bleeding and surgical shock are decreased; however, these effects have been poorly documented, especially the reduction in bleeding. Most anesthesiologists who use hypnotism have also found it to be beneficial for the preoperative preparation of the patient as well as for the postoperative recovery. It is widely claimed that postoperative recovery is improved by the use of hypnoanesthesia, even when no suggestions are made regarding the recovery. Hypnotism is particularly useful in allaying preoperative fears and anxiety, and it can be an alternative to preoperative sedation. With regard to the postoperative period, it is an obvious solution to relieving postoperative pain and discomfort. Urinary retention occurring in abdominal surgery can be countered. Postoperative constipation and hiccups can also be aided. Coughing can be facilitated. The latter is largely done by eliminating the pain that patients experience when coughing right after surgery. Retching can be decreased by direct suggestion. The dumping syndrome following gastrectomies can be reduced and even eliminated. Changing surgical dressings in painful situations, as in burn cases, can be greatly aided. Hypnotism can be a great help where debridement must be done. It has been found particularly helpful following hemorrhoidectomies for eliminating the postoperative rectal pain and for facilitating bowel movements. It is an aid to be used in making patients in traction and in body casts more comfortable. It can be useful in facilitating immobility following open-heart surgery.

One should exert care in wording the suggestions. One does not want the patient to feel so good as to overexert himself before proper healing has taken place. This applies to the convalescence period at home as well as immediately after surgery. It is best to allow for some pain, or at least discomfort, being retained. While it is desirable to make the patient as comfortable as possible following surgery, one does not want to prevent new pains or an exacerbation of pain to pass unnoticed, since these can be warning signs of complications. Retention of some degree of pain is therefore to be preferred over a complete postoperative anesthesia. The modern practice with many operations is to require patients to walk and exert themselves in other ways soon after the operation. Since this is at times quite painful, it seems legitimate to give specific suggestions associating fairly complete analgesia with these activities. For example, with surgery for varicose veins, the patient has to get up and walk about frequently as soon after surgery as possible.

For the first 18 hours or so, this is extremely painful. With a responsive patient, one might say, as part of the postoperative instructions given to him in hypnosis, ". . . As will be explained to you later, after surgery you will have to get up at intervals and walk. When the time comes for you to have to do this, you will be completely free of pain. You will, however, get out of bed *gently* and *slowly,* and you will walk *carefully.* If in doing this you begin to move too fast or too vigorously, as you would normally, you will again feel the pain that is there as a warning for you to slow down." Suggestions aimed at relieving postoperative pain in the abdominal region and below should be so worded as to allow the patient to be able to experience the need to void or to have a bowel movement. For example, the suggestion, "You will not feel anything below your navel," would be contraindicated. Even, "You will be comfortable at all times," could have unexpected, undesirable effects. One way around this problem is to specify that such a need as voiding will be felt. In rectal surgery, one should limit postoperative suggestions of anesthesia to the rectum. A suggestion of an absence below the waist would be too general in more than one way. First, it would eliminate the perception of a need to urinate. It might also affect the patient's ability to have sensations in his lower members.

Generally, the use of hypnoanesthesia for major surgery calls for a preparatory period, a maintenance phase, and a postoperative phase. Kroger (1963) and others also recommend the use of a rehearsal phase.

The preparatory phase presupposes that the patient has been previously hypnotized, found to be capable of producing a glove anesthesia, and possibly given a posthypnotic signal for reinduction. Preparatory to surgery, preferably the day before, the patient is hypnotized and spoken to as follows:

> You have been in hypnosis a number of times now, and you know how easy it is to do so. You know that you can do this so well and so completely that you become oblivious to your surroundings. You can also bring about a total insensitivity in your right (left) hand. When the time comes for you to be taken to the operating room, that is, when the attendant wheels you down to it, this will be your signal to enter a deep hypnosis in which you will go deeper and deeper with each breath that you take. At that time, your right (left) hand will develop an anesthesia just as it has before, and you will place it against [name approximate site of surgery], and the anesthesia will transfer from your hand to that part of your body and spread within your body some distance from the point of contact, as I have explained to you earlier. Your insensibility will be complete, and you will no longer feel anything in that part of your body until you are back in your room (or I tell you otherwise). In fact, you will remain hypnotized until that time. As I have explained to you, should you have the least bit of discomfort, you will be able to request the use of regular anesthesia while still remaining hypnotized. Either way, you will have a very pleasant, painless experience. You need not have any more discomfort than you are willing to have. You will have no worries about your surgery or its outcome.

When only an analgesia is suggested, or one is not certain that anesthesia will result, mention should be made that although the patient will feel no pain, he may feel pressure, pull, warmth, cold, and other sensation.

If the hypnotist is to be present during surgery, the following can be added: "I will be present during the entire procedure, and I will do what is necessary to make you comfortable and free of tension." In any case, the preparatory suggestions continue with, "After the surgery is over and you have come out of hypnosis, you will continue to feel good and free of major pain and any other discomfort. You will make a rapid and uneventful recovery." When specific postoperative effects are expected, these should each be dealt with using appropriate posthypnotic suggestions. With abdominal surgery, for instance, it is desirable to make routine suggestions with regard to the ability to void and have bowel movements. Additional suggestions that can be routinely given include those of having a good appetite, being in good spirit, and sleeping soundly. Also, in particular, suggest that if he should have pain, he will be able to get relief by thinking of his hand developing a glove anesthesia and transferring the anesthesia to the locus of pain by applying his hand to or near this locus. Training the patient to do this can be done earlier in the preparation. When doing this part of the training, one should always test the patient's ability to produce the glove anesthesia and transfer it, and not assume that he can do so just because it was suggested.

Also, it is good to place limitations on the patient's ability to do this. Patients have been known to misuse it unintentionally.

The above assumption has been that the hypnotist will be present prior to surgery and even during it. This is not always feasible. As a psychologist, I have been consulted to prepare patients for a surgery at which I could not be present. I have prepared pregnant women (and some who anticipated bearing a child in the future) for a delivery that would take place in a locality much too far for me to be present, or at a time when I might not be available. Likewise, I have worked with patients, with whom I would not be when the work was done, in anticipation of dental work or oral surgery. Obviously, the above instructions will have to be changed accordingly. The biggest trouble I have encountered has been situations in which a totally unknown physician or dentist would be involved who might or might not be open to the use of hypnoanesthesia. The patient needs, of course, to be made aware of this possibility. I always recommend to such patients that they seek out a physician or dentist who is willing and, preferably, one who himself makes use of hypnotism. If the practitioner in question will contact me, I can then provide him with appropriate information. In any event, patients can be given suggestions that will enable them to be relaxed and free of anxiety, and they can even develop an appropriate analgesia whenever they are to undergo dental work, a pelvic examination, or some other potentially painful or very uncomfortable procedure. They can do this regardless of their current therapist's attitude toward hypnotism or his knowledge of it. There is no reason for the patient to experience the discomfort of the injection of a local anesthetic, even if one is unneccessarily used. When I teach a patient limited self-hypnosis for such a purpose, I always include suggestions aimed at enabling him to interact during hypnosis with his new physician or dentist with regard to procedures. I do the same when I train a patient to undergo some specific procedure under hypnosis with a specialist's participation. However, I usually place limits upon the degree of responsiveness that he will have to the specialist in question. The reason is very simple. Unless I am well acquainted with the specialist and know that he is knowledgeable regarding suggestion phenomena, I do not want to leave my patients open to suggestions that could otherwise have potentially harmful influences. I do tell them, however, that if ever they decide to be hypnotized by another therapist who they know is competent, it will be entirely possible to do so.

Any time a patient is to be prepared for treatment in another specialty than the one in which the therapist is trained, it is important that one first become acquainted with what will be involved. For example, when abdominal surgery is to be done, the hypnotist needs to be aware that there is a likelihood of urinary retention and constipation and that gastrectomies can be accompanied by the dumping syndrome. For patients undergoing profound general chemoanesthesia, it is important that they should be able to cough freely after the surgery. If a rehearsal is to be used, the hypnotist should become familiar with the details of the surgical procedures. Again, for the preparation of the patient, it is useful to be familiar with the procedures followed by the hospital where the patient will be hospitalized. Sometimes, acquaintance with the physical layout of the hospital, of the operating room, and of the recovery room can be useful. The same is true regarding labor and delivery rooms. For these reasons, even when the surgeon or obstetrician is not the primary hypnotist, they should, if possible, be involved directly at some point in some of the patient's preparation. The hypnotized patient is placed in rapport with them for this purpose. Physicians will naturally have less to do than, for example, a psychologist, since they will already be acquainted with many of the above mentioned details. Still, there are enough variations among, for example, surgeons regarding a particular intervention, as to make it advisable for even a general medical practitioner or an internist preparing a patient for surgery to follow some of the above recommendations.

Active maintenance of hypnoanesthesia during a surgical procedure is optional with patients who are highly responsive to suggestions. With these, it is more a question of watching for signs indicating that they might be experiencing some discomfort. At such a time, give reinforcing suggestions of greater depth, of continued anesthesia, and of comfort. With those of lesser suggestibility, there may be a need to reiterate such suggestions throughout the procedure. It may be desirable to give suggestions in a continuous and repetitious manner that there is no pain or discomfort, that the patient feels no pain (or nothing), that he is relaxed (deeply asleep), unaware of anything else but the hypnotist's voice (or whatever he is fantasizing), and so on. Actually, in surgical procedures there are only specific times when pain will primarily be produced. In abdominal surgery, for example, this occurs when the skin is incised, pierced, or pinched; when the peritoneum is incised; and when organs are stretched, tugged on, twisted, or pinched. Supplemental suggestions are needed mainly at such times. The only other indication is if there has been a rehearsal and the surgeon deviates from the "script." At such a time, it may be advisable for the hypnotist to make appropriate suggestions.

The postoperative phase includes the dehypnotization of the patient. If the hypnotist is present, he can choose the time for this and give the signal or instructions. In this case, it is generally a good idea, before doing so, to restate any suggestions that were previously given having to do with the recovery. New ones can be added. If a general chemical anesthesia was also used, one should wait until its effects have worn off. One should never assume that hypnosis ceases with the end of the effects of an anesthetic agent. Unless a suggestion was given to tie both effects together, the likelihood is that the patient will continue to be hypnotized beyond the cessation of the general anesthesia. It has not been common for the nursing staff to take any part in the above procedures. It would be a simple and reasonable matter to instruct the patient in such a manner as to make it possible for a nurse to give him the signal for coming out of the hypnotic state when the hypnotist cannot be present. Otherwise, one can always associate the dehypnotization with activities that will occur following recovery from the chemical anesthesia.

It is generally a good idea for the surgical and nursing teams to be alerted to the fact that the patient will be hypnotized. Some members of this staff may need special instructions. The staff should also be impressed with the understanding that a hypnotized patient is fully conscious and will hear and understand anything that is said in his presence and be affected by it in proportion to his suggestibility.

The rehearsal phase is somewhat optional. It is more so if the surgery is minor, and not really necessary if the patient demonstrates high suggestibility. It is more indicated for major surgery and for patients who have difficulty developing a good, sustained anesthesia. it is particularly indicated when the patient can develop only an analgesia. The procedure consists in going step-by-step through the entire surgical procedure to be used, including the motions. This, obviously, needs to be done by a physician, preferably the surgeon. If the patient has been prehospitalized early enough, it can be done after he has settled in his room. Otherwise, it can be done in an examination room at an earlier date. Kroger (1963, p. 187) has very nicely described this procedure in the case of abdominal surgery. His description is reproduced here:

REHEARSAL TECHNIC

During a typical rehearsal session for abdominal surgery the patient is told, "Now your skin is being sterilized." (At this time the abdomen is swabbed with an alcohol sponge.) "I am now stretching the skin and making the incision in the skin." (The line of incision is lightly stroked with a pencil.) "Now the tissues are being cut. Just relax. You feel nothing, absolutely nothing. Your breathing is getting slower, deeper and more regular. Each side of the incision is being separated by an instrument." (The skin and the muscles are pulled laterally from the midline.) "Now a blood vessel is being clamped." (A hemostat is clicked shut.) "You feel absolutely no discomfort. You are calm, quiet and relaxed. Your breathing is getting slower, deeper and more regular. Just relax! Now I am going deeper and entering the abdominal cavity." (For the peritoneum, suggestions of relaxation and assurances of complete pain relief are repeated several times.) "Just relax. You are getting deeper and deeper relaxed; your heartbeat is getting slower and more regular. Just relax. You feel nothing, absolutely nothing." The viscera are relatively insensitive to cutting—one does not have to worry about pain. However, the patient has to be prepared for the discomfort produced by pulling and torsion of the abdominal organs.

The steps for closure of the peritoneum, muscles, fascia and skin are also described in a similar manner. There are really only 3 times when pain can be expected: When the skin is incised, when the peritoneum is incised, and when one is tugging on the viscera.

One deterrent to the use of hypnoanesthesia for many practitioners is the amount of time that can be required to prepare the patient. The process can certainly be quite time consuming in some cases. However, at least for the 10% of patients who can develop deep anesthesia, the initial induction is usually easy and quick, and the necessary skill is developed readily. Many patients can develop a helpful degree of analgesia that is satisfactory for minor surgical procedures, with a minimum of time expended on this. Far more individuals can benefit from these procedures in minimal time than would at first seem. In any event, a short preliminary hypnotic session can usually quickly determine the patient's potentials. If these seem too poor to the physician or dentist, they always have the option of not pursuing the matter. In the case of obstetric and dental patients, much of the initial preparation can be done in group sessions, thus saving much time for the practitioner. A half-dozen patients can easily be treated. At a later date, those that require it can then be given individual attention. In the case of obstetric patients, the introduction of hypnotism should be done early. Although this has not been a standard practice, it could be made a routine procedure in prenatal clinics. Another time-saving approach that has not been utilized would be to involve the nursing staff or dental assistants in the early preparation of the patient. This is much better than the practice of some dentists of using taped inductions that they request the patient to listen to in a waiting room. I am a strong believer in the need for personal contact and attention in the use of any hypnotic technique. On the other hand, I am opposed to the use of so-called "hypno-technicians." They usually have no adequate knowledge of the domain of application. Furthermore, their training in hypnotism is quite inadequate for professional work, falling rather short, in particular, in the area of standards of professional conduct and ethics.

The use of suggested analgesia or anesthesia is not limited to the above kinds of situations. There are medical and dental applications that, while minor compared to the above, nevertheless represent useful and legitimate applications. Sprains, luxations, minor but painful wounds, skin irritations, lacerations requiring a suturing, and so forth, are all candidates. Again, judicious suggestions limiting the patient's actions are usually additionally called for. For these situations, as well as those of the next section, the approach to producing hypnoanesthesia or hypnoanalgesia will, in essence, be the same, but with certain obvious differences. Lesser suggestibility is required, and the process is generally less elaborate. By their nature, many of the applications that have just been mentioned, such as a fracture, will not allow for any preparatory periods. Usually, hypnosis, and then anesthesia, will have to be induced for the first time in the same session as the intervention is performed. Because intervention is a situation that can arise in anyone's life, I routinely, unless contraindicated, include suggestions in my training of the patient that will enable them to produce a temporary and limited anesthesia, should the need for it arise.

Some diagnostic procedures, although of a different order, are sufficiently painful and uncomfortable to be given consideration. Typically, cystoscopies, pelvic examinations for some, bronchoscopies, spinal taps, and so on fall into this class. For the most part, the ability to develop a mild analgesia will suffice to ease the process. It will be helpful if the hypnotist, preferably the physician doing the testing, will give maintaining suggestions while carrying out the procedures.

Finally, patients sometimes have to go repeatedly through a course of treatment that may be very unpleasant, if not painful, and that may have unpleasant and possibly painful side effects and sequelae. Chemotherapy is one example. Again, the ability to develop even a mild analgesia can be of help. In most cases, one can do much more than that to make the treatment more tolerable. Furthermore, with appropriate posthypnotic suggestions or the teaching of a limited self-hypnosis, it is possible to eliminate the need for the hypnotist to be present each time the treatment is given. How often and to what degree the hypnotist will need to keep in touch with the patient will depend upon the nature and course of the problem being treated, the nature and duration of the treatment, the patient's needs, and other factors, such as accessibility.

Finally, although this has nothing directly to do with the production of surgical anesthesia, the preparation of some patients may include relief of anxiety, reassurance, and sometimes more. Actually, there are few patients facing surgery that do not have some anxiety, even when they do not show it. The preparation of the patient for hypnoanesthesia and its production are ideal situations for the above type of intervention. With individuals who are particularly fearful of the outcome of the surgery, an excellent technique is to have the hypnotized patient see himself functioning actively and happily after discharge from the hospital. An example, real but admittedly somewhat extreme, is that of a pregnant woman who feared dying in childbirth. Under hypnosis, she was given the opportunity to see herself giving birth painlessly, holding and breastfeeding her child in subsequent days, going home, and celebrating with the family and her child its first birthday. This was done several times. The delivery not only was successfully done with the sole use of hypnoanesthesia, but her behavior during the remainder of the pregnancy showed positive changes. While earlier there had been little pleasure shown, and an attitude of sad resignation was evident, there now appeared expressions of happy anticipation. I should probably warn the reader that other like cases might have required a more complex approach, including a psychotherapeutic intervention.

Hypnoanesthesia for Chronic and Intractable Pains

The kinds of intractable pains that a practitioner will encounter, and their frequency of occurrence, will necessarily be a function of his specialty and the milieu in which he carries out his professional work. An oncologist will naturally have much exposure to the pain of terminal cancer. Orthopedists will most likely have considerable exposure to back pain problems. General practitioners and internists will be exposed to a wider variety of chronic pains. As a psychologist working in a hospital, I probably had more exposure to terminal cancer cases, as well as to quadriplegics and paraplegics with pain problems, than I would have otherwise had. Because a good portion of my time was spent in a hospital for war veterans, I also had greater exposure to phantom limb problems.

Going by my own experience in private practice, I think that the most frequent chronic pains that come to the attention of professionals in private practice using hypnotism are back pains, neck pains, and headaches. Some of these may be associated with muscular spasms and contractures. Neuralgias and sciatica-type pains are perhaps next on the list. Finally, there are a variety of pains, sometimes bizarre and of unclear origins, including some so-called thalamic pains. Some of these may be referred pains, and, obviously, in such cases medical attention must be given to the true site of origin. *As a psychologist, I will not undertake the treatment of chronic pain until I have been able to reassure myself that the pain has first been given proper medical attention.* Only then can I have a basis for deciding whether the pain is real or functional. The same applies to cases of acute pain of obscure origin. Relief of pain is not relief of the condition causing it. To treat a pain while the disease behind it goes undiagnosed and unchecked is not therapy. Even with the above provision satisfied, there is no absolute guarantee that the pain is not associated with a disease condition as yet undetectable. I know of a number of cancer cases for which this was true. This can also be true with other unusual, odd or aberrant troublesome sensations. The musician and composer George Gershwin complained for years of smelling gas. This was eventually related, unfortunately too late, to a developing tumor involving the olfactory portion of his brain. For this reason, it is necessary for the therapist to be constantly on his guard against making or accepting quick diagnoses.

Many chronic pains are functional. Others do have their origin in actual physical trauma, but subsequently acquire a functional component and may even become completely converted after the physical basis for pain has ceased to be.

Most commonly, the somatic back pains one encounters are the consequence of a damaged spine caused by an accident, over- and improper exertion, and, not infrequently, by scar tissue resulting from back surgery. I have also encountered some cases brought on by spasms and contractures of back muscles. In the latter case, the pain can be a combination of muscular pain and pain from pinched or stretched nerve bundles. One of the unfortunate aspects of back pain is that, in the past, surgery aimed at correcting a spinal condition has often led to further painful conditions, leading to more corrective surgery, the whole thing eventually ending up with equally painful scarring. Surgery for chronic, intractable pain often has unpleasant, if not deleterious, incapacitating side effects, and hypnotism should first be considered. Surgery should be a last-resort treatment. Changes brought about through hypnosis can usually be canceled; not so in the case of surgery. Surgery may be inevitable if the overall physical well-being of the patient depends on it.

The treatment of backaches, as is true for other chronic pain, may run from a few sessions to a series of sessions, at first weekly, then increasingly spaced out. One of my first cases was a man who had undergone much back surgery and who was now probably having more pain due to the side effects of the surgery than due to any residue of the original pain. The first session, lasting an hour, combined an induction and suggestions of analgesia. This resulted in complete relief. On the second appointment, a week later, the patient reported experiencing some pain again, but relatively mild. The previous suggestions were reinforced and the patient told that in the future, if he should experience any recurrence of mild pain in his back, all he would have to do is think, "There is no pain in my back," and the pain would go. He was not given any further appointment, but told to contact me should he need to do so. I was able to ascertain indirectly, several months later, that the patient was functioning quite well. About a year and a half later, the patient contacted me because his back was hurting. I expected a recurrence of the old pain; much to my surprise and satisfaction I learned, when I saw him, that the pain was a new one resulting from having fallen off his bicycle. His old pain had given him no further problems. He had been checked out by a physician who had found only bruises. I gave him new suggestions of analgesia for the new pain, which were fully effective. After the hypnosis session was over, I discussed with him the kinds of activities he should engage in for awhile and then let him go home. The man was obviously a good subject as far as suggestibility is concerned. My estimate is that he could attain at least a medium hypnosis. He may have been much more suggestible, and, had this been important, I could have found this out. I did not do any pretesting, but after a short explanation to the patient of what hypnotism was about, I proceeded with an induction by eye fixation. As usual, I employed the Fractionation Technique with counting for deepening. The analgesia suggestions were given after the patient had gone back into a hypnotic state as I counted to 20.

I once had a woman patient whom I treated for back pain that had a somatic basis. I saw her on a weekly basis three more times after the initial session, then every two to three weeks as needed. This lasted for about a year. This patient was a dentist, which in those days was a profession that often led to back problems and was also bound to exacerbate any other back problem. That she needed continued treatment is not surprising. This woman had a large family, of which she was the matriarch; she was indirectly involved in local politics through her husband, who was an optometrist; she lived a lifestyle that produced much tension. This was probably a factor that prevented her pain from being permanently eradicated. Her use of the sessions partly for catharsis added another dimension to the pain treatment. This situation of a painful injury combined with emotional factors is one encountered fairly often with chronic pain.

The next case is that of a woman in her middle 30s who had sustained a back injury some years earlier while horseback riding. She had never been fully free of pain, but the pain had lately become more severe and frequent. The physicians she had consulted could not find any good reasons for this. They had recommended physiotherapy, which she had not found helpful. She was readily hypnotized, and the pain was relieved just as readily. She left my office feeling "marvelous," with an appointment for the following week. When she came in that day, it was clear that everything was far from well with her. She told me how she had felt "so good" following her visit with me that she had gone horseback riding again, thus stressing her weakened back unduly with resulting pain. Fortunately, no further damage had resulted. Removing the pain was no problem. The rest of the session was spent on discussing with the patient the issue of stressing her body, especially her back. Her next visit was prompted by a recurrence of severe pain. Her account was that she had been free of pain for better than half of the week, and then the pain had suddenly resumed and progressively increased. This is not an unusual occurrence, although a sudden onset of the pain is not usual if it is somatic. Perhaps this was the reason that I questioned her more closely regarding her activities around the time the pain had returned. What had happened was that she had felt so good that the day the pain returned she had decided to do a thorough cleaning of her two-story house, including scrubbing and waxing floors. The return of the pain that evening was now quite understandable. I had assumed that with her years of experience living with a weak back, she would routinely take precautions not to overstrain it. Fortunately, no damage had been done. A hypnotic induction again gave her relief. This time I added protective suggestions to the effect that should she engage in any activity that would strain her back, she would be warned by a momentary pain that would increase if she persisted. I made provisions for emergency situations in the manner that I have already described. Finally, realizing that she had been a very active woman prior to her accident, I included suggestions to aid her in adapting to the new required-activity regimen. After she was dehypnotized, I explained to her the provisions I had made to prevent overexertion and assured myself that this was acceptable to her. I ended the session by reviewing with her the kinds of activities she could engage in and which ones to shun or engage in carefully. I asked her to report to me by telephone in two weeks, unless she needed to talk to me or see me before that. Two weeks later, she reported that she was still free of pain. I had no further contact with her.

A rather different kind of case is that of a 15-year-old female quadriplegic. She had been involved in an automobile accident that had resulted in her having a complete flacid paralysis below the arms. There was some involvement of her upper extremities; she could only make gross movements of her arms, had only minimal control of her hands, and had no control of her fingers. There had also been an appreciable sensory deficit in her extremities. At the time I was asked to work with her, she had developed a great deal of pain in her hands associated with an apparent hypersensitivity to touch, so that any contact was extremely painful. She no longer made the little use of her hands that she had previously done, and she now held them protectively near her midrift. The skin of her hands had become dry and was beginning to deteriorate.

Massaging and the application of ointment to her hands had become totally impossible because of the accompanying pain that the neurologists had decided was probably of thalamic origin. Hypnotism seemed to be the only solution to the problem. She came from a small Oklahoma community located several hundred miles from Oklahoma City, where she was currently hospitalized and where I was located. I was called for a consultation on a Friday and understood that the patient was to be discharged by the end of the following week. There was therefore limited time in which to work. This is clearly the kind of case where it is not possible to use the Hands Together Suggestion nor a Hand Levitation Induction. Because a relaxation induction technique depends greatly on obtaining a felt muscular relaxation, this kind is also not useful here. Suggestions of relaxation, if used, should qualify the relaxation to be "mental" or "of the mind." About the only kind of test that could have been done would have been of eye closure and/or eye catalepsy. If one is going to use an eye fixation induction, which is a logical approach, such tests are essentially included in the induction and do not need to be done separately. I elected to use a visualization technique. My main reason for this at the time was that I did not feel that an eye fixation technique without suggested muscular relaxation would be satisfactory. With the patient's help, it was decided that she would visualize herself on a sailboat on a lake. The outcome was probably to be expected, and would probably have been the same no matter what other topic had been chosen. The patient readily visualized, and while doing so, tears began to stream down her face. The patient was able to grieve over the loss of her mobility and, essentially, of much of her body, for the first time since it had happened. She began to talk about her feelings of having sinned at the time of the accident and having been punished for it. The details are unimportant here. The incident, however, points out the type of complications that may arise when using hypnotism for what is expected to be a straightforward application. It also shows that hypnosis is frequently found to free suppressed feelings and emotions. Any therapist, whether a psychotherapist or not, must be ready to deal with this. Much of that first session, which was on Saturday, was devoted to allowing the patient to ventilate. I did induce hypnosis by means of a modified eye fixation technique with suggestions of sleep, and I gave some preliminary suggestions of decreased pain and sensitivity. The next day, I did a second induction by visual fixation with the Modified Fractionation Method. I suggested she would be able to bring her hands together comfortably and painlessly until they touched without pain. She was able to accomplish this, and I then proposed she could rub one hand against the other without discomfort. This was again accomplished. The next step was to suggest that lotion could be applied to her hands, that she could rub the lotion in, and that all of these would be quite painless. This, too, was accomplished, and she was left with the posthypnotic suggestion that she would continue to be able to use her hands and to have them manipulated without pain. Suggestions for general comfort were added. The next day, I found the patient in the process of doing some typing. She had a small portable typewriter and her father had made her an ingenious device that allowed her to peck the keyboard. I saw the patient a few more times before she was discharged. By then, the skin of her hands had become healthy looking. In addition to reinforcing the suggestions previously given, I used the sessions for giving her ego strengthening suggestions and also for training her in the use of self-hypnosis for pain control. I lost track of the patient for many years. Then one day I received a typed letter from her. She had by now attained womanhood, had gone to college, and was a teacher. Her reason for writing me these many years later was because she had some recurrence of pain and wanted my advice.

The next case involves a phantom pain. The patient, a male veteran from the Korean War, had been amputated above the left knee. He had developed a phantom leg and foot in which he experienced constant pain. On the first session, I did an induction by visual fixation with sleep suggestions. I was able to obtain a satisfactory glove anesthesia and suggested its transfer to the stump. I made no effort at this time to eliminate the phantom leg and foot, but only the pain. Partial relief was obtained, but by the second session, a week later, it had returned full strength. The patient had described the pain as burning. After hypnotizing him, I suggested that now he was receiving a special injection in his blood stream of a cooling anesthetic agent that would course into his entire right leg, starting above the knee, and that this would extinguish the burning. This was quite successful in eradicating the pain, and the relief was sustained posthypnotically. The patient was hypnotized a second time. The suggestion was reinforced. He was then given the posthypnotic suggestion that, should he have a recurrence of the pain before the next session, he would be able to remove it by thinking about receiving another injection of the cooling anesthetic. This action would briefly place him back into a hypnotic state of a few minutes duration, out of which he would awaken free of pain. This step was, of course, reviewed with him after dehypnotization. At the next session, the patient reported having been free of pain most of the time and having successfully used the self-hypnotic procedure a number of times. He added that he had modified the color of the injected fluid to blue and visualized it as flowing throughout his phantom leg. The session was devoted primarily and unsuccessfully to removing the now painless phantom limb. Because the presence of the phantom did not seem to be a major issue, it was decided that nothing more would be done in regard to it. No further appointment was scheduled. I only saw the patient once more many years later, by accident, on one of his visits to the hospital where I worked. He indicated that he still had some pain at times, but was able to deal with the situation to his satisfaction and that he did not feel the need to see me again.

Psychological and social considerations can enter in odd ways in the treatment of chronic somatically-based pain problems. One of the first cases brought to my attention, after I moved to California, was that of a woman suffering from a trigeminal nerve neuralgia, otherwise known as a *tic douloureux*. The patient had been referred by her personal physician to a psychiatrist of my acquaintance, who in turn consulted me regarding the possibility of using hypnotism. We agreed to work jointly with her. I was to concentrate on the hypnotic work, while my colleague would proceed with individual therapy, for which there appeared to be a need. The woman was a good hypnotic subject, and temporary relief of the pain was found to be possible, but refractory to full control. It was soon established that recurrences and exacerbations of the pain were closely associated with events in her marital life. As my colleague probed into the matter, it became clear that a sado-masochistic relationship existed between her and her husband,

and that the *tic douloureux* played an important part in it. My colleague came to the conclusion that there was a likelihood the husband would become psychotic if his wife was completely cured. This presented us with some serious questions, some ethical, others having to do with the long range welfare of the patient. This ended in a compromise in which the patient was allowed to retain a milder neuralgia with less frequent attacks, and these of much shorter durations. A total of about four sessions of hypnotherapy were involved. It was left to the patient to request further sessions if necessary. As far as I know, the individual therapy sessions were also discontinued.

Not all of the cases of chronic pain I have treated have been successful. Far from it. I probably have had as many total failures as I have had successes. In many cases, complete relief was never attained; only some amelioration. One area in which I have done poorly is in the treatment of terminal cancer cases, because, as in most cases I have attempted to treat, the patients were unable to develop a satisfactory degree of suggestibility. It is not possible to conclude from these cases that the pain of terminal cancer is itself not readily countered by suggestion. I would expect that at least the same 10% of individuals capable of developing good surgical anesthesia would do well in the case of cancer. It would appear from my experience that this percentage is much less for terminal cancer cases. I have wondered, at times, whether or not metastasis and/or toxins produced by the cancer cells and affecting the brain might not have a contrary effect on suggestibility. In any case, although there are many reports in the relevant literature of the successful use of hypnotism with cancer cases, they also seem to indicate that the pain from cancer is not particularly easy to deal with, and its treatment can be taxing on the therapist.

Although a good many of the cases of intractable pain were associated with emotional issues and problems of everyday life that I also had to take into consideration, I have encountered very few cases of purely functional pain. Establishing that a problem is purely functional can be quite difficult. The case of the quadriplegic I mentioned earlier may have been such a case, rather than one of a thalamic pain, as neurologists had proposed. Usually, unless the underlining dynamics are dealt with, a functional pain will resist treatment completely, will repeatedly subside only to recur shortly thereafter, or will vanish, and the patient will develop a new, usually incapacitating, and, at best, unacceptable symptom. My conclusion, arising out of my work with intractable pains, is that there is a small number of individuals who are probably borderline psychotics, and who develop pains that are of a purely hallucinatory nature, but nonetheless quite real. These individuals can sometimes be hypnotized, and their pain can even be briefly ameliorated while they are in the office, but the relief does not persist beyond it. They tend to be paranoid and tend to incorporate the pain in their paranoia.

They are obsessed with it and often show a compulsive personality. They also tend to exhibit an undercurrent of generalized anger. I respect any symptom that is refractory, and, in these cases, I feel the best one can do is not to push the issue. Usually the patient drops out of therapy on his own.

To conclude this section, I will describe three special ways of handling pain with hypnotism that have proven to be quite effective, especially with chronic, intractable pains. The first of these may have grown out of the observation that when anesthesia or analgesia are suggested to an individual, sometimes he reports having felt pain, but that it did not bother him. The experience, as described, resembles that of lobotomized persons. It has been referred to as a psychic lobotomy in which the affective component of pain has been removed or dissociated. The application of this observation consists in suggesting to the patient that he may feel pain, but that it will not bother him anymore. Sometimes, suggested anesthesia and analgesia cause a person to experience the pain as externalized. That is, they will state, "the pain did not bother me . . . It was outside of me . . . out there . . . As if it was in someone else." The obvious use of this observation is again to suggest this very thing. The third method consists in using suggested time distortions. As will be recalled from Volume 1, it is possible to alter a hypnotized person's perception of the passage of time. Various ways of doing this were then discussed. When a patient has intermittent pain, sometimes the best way of dealing with it is to suggest that the duration of each attack of pain will be experienced as shorter and shorter, and the intervals of time between attacks will be experienced as being of increasing length. It is usually not necessary to train the patient first to do time distortions; however, the technique is a little more involved than might appear from the above. Having hypnotized the patient, I might say to him something like this:

> I am going to remind you of a fact you know. This is that for each of us there is a clock time, marked by clocks and watches, and there is a personal time, which is not dependent on time pieces. Personal time, your personal time, can be slower or faster than clock time. You have experienced this fact many times in your life. Think of the many times when you have had a good time for hours, and it seemed to you hardly any time had passed, possibly just minutes. And then there have been times when you were anxiously waiting for something to happen, and each minute you waited seemed like hours. We will use this ability that you have of experiencing events in a personal time. The next time you have a pain, no matter what its duration actually is by clock time, you will experience it as shorter, and thereafter you will experience in your personal time the duration of each pain as being less and less. And again using our personal time, the time between pains will progressively increase in your personal time. There will come a time when, in your personal time, each pain

will be like a flash, and there will be an eternity of time between their occurrences. Only the pain will be thus affected. For other events, your personal time will match clock time except, naturally, when you would normally experience a different time, such as when enjoying or waiting for something.

This suggestion can be modified in various ways. It can be expanded, and key elements in it can be repeated any number of times.

HYPNOTIC TREATMENT OF SOMATIC, PSYCHOSOMATIC, AND SOMATOPSYCHIC DISORDERS

There is a great deal of material available in the hypnotism literature on the symptomatic treatment of purely somatic diseases. There is little available on treatment aimed at the underlying somatic causal factors. This probably reflects that hypnotic suggestions appear to have a very limited power with regard to directly bringing about physiological and tissue changes. Even if this were not the case, the complexity of the known bodily changes that constitute a disease would be a barrier to this type of action. Furthermore, even when we know, as in the case of diabetes, that it is the breakdown of certain glandular cells that is the causal element, we still do not know what causes the breakdown, what steps are involved at the histological and cellular level, and what needs to be done to stop the degradation process. Tissue and physiological changes resulting from bacterial, protozoan, virus, and fungus infections do not appear to be particularly treatable by hypnotism, if at all. The same is true for sustained physical injuries due to physical or chemical action and endogenic malfunctions of organ systems. Pneumonia, dysentery, appendicitis, gunshot wounds, poisoning, drug overdose, renal failure, and many others fall into these categories. In such instances, hypnotism is, at best, useful for making the patient more comfortable and helping to create in him a positive frame of mind. I recognize that there are practitioners who hold the belief that general suggestions of healing and suggestions focused more specifically on the ailing process or part of the body involved have the power to bring about beneficial changes in, even reversal of, the disease process. The techniques used often include visualizing the changes taking place or the end result, such as a healed organ, body part, or the total body. A fairly widely-accepted hypothesis is that there is a "wisdom of the body" that is somehow tapped. One further hypothesis is that the suggestions activate the patient's unconscious, which in turn accesses the source of this wisdom. Another hypothesis makes the unconscious the container of this wisdom. In either case, the unconscious proceeds to do what, so far, no human brain aided by the best of computers has been able to accomplish. There are, however, no hard data to support any of this, anymore than there are to support the miracles of Lourdes as being true miracles. This is not to say that authenticated cases of such seemingly miraculous cures are not available, but what is missing in each case are details that would allow one to distinguish those that were cures of pure somatic disorders from those that were cures of psychosomatic and functional disorders, not to mention spontaneous remissions. The most reasonable scientific guess one can make in regard to such cases is that many were not purely somatic in origin. Likewise, while it seems reasonable that a positive attitude toward recovery would promote it, and a negative attitude interfere with it, here, too, hard data are difficult to obtain. Such evidence as is available is largely anecdotal, but is massive enough to force one to take notice and not altogether discount as possibilities some of the above. It is not unscientific to keep an open mind. Since we cannot say with certainty that there cannot be any positive effects in connection with the above practices, the best tactic seems to be to go ahead and make suggestions of favorable tissue changes, of healing taking place, and of promoting a positive attitude toward recovery while also proceeding with accepted medical somatic interventions. To treat a streptococcal throat infection by suggestion alone, as I have once seen it done, is malpractice. To use an antibiotic and aspirin, while at the same time using hypnotism to make the patient more comfortable and adding suggestions for quick reduction of the fever and quick recovery, is reasonable and acceptable practice. The suggestions may or may not affect the fever or the recovery, but it costs little time and effort to do this, especially with a patient who has been previously trained for the use of hypnotism, and it should be done on the premise that we cannot be sure that it has no effects. We shall come back to this in Chapter 8 when we discuss mind-body healing, which is the latest development in the domain of Ericksonian-style hypnotherapy.

In any event, when the literature on the uses of hypnotism in the treatment of medical and dental problems is examined, it becomes clear that reported successful hypnotic treatments have either been directed at the control of somatic symptoms rather than a cure of the underlying causes, and/or, as is more often the case, have been directed toward bringing about changes in the patient's lifestyle and his affective life. If a cure has thus been effected, it was because the problem was psychosomatic or behavioral. In the latter cases, the situation becomes reversed, with somatic treatment being aimed at symptom relief and hypnotism being aimed at the underlying psychic causes.

In the light of these remarks, it appears that a great many medical problems call for psychotherapy, and that their discussion, perhaps, more appropriately belongs under the heading of psychotherapy. If I discuss these now, it is because they usually first come to the attention of a physician, even when, eventually, the patients may seek the help of a psychologist or psychiatrist.

Secondly, they are basically medical problems, even if their treatment turns out to be primarily or entirely psychological. Finally, in my experience, most medical practitioners who use hypnotism proceed with the psychotherapy in their own way rather than make a referral. The following pages present a sampling of typical treatments of somatic problems.

Weight Problems

The treatment of *obesity* and *overweight* is a good place to begin discussing specific forms of treatment with hypnotism. Some individuals with this problem seek help for psychosocial reasons or for health reasons. Others seek help for both reasons. In some cases, the problem may be purely metabolic, but more often than not it is behavioral and emotional in origin. Furthermore, when it is purely metabolic, there are often somatopsychic ramifications because of the way the problem affects the patient's life and because of social and other pressures emphasizing the desirability of being thin. The practitioner confronted with a case of overweight is rarely going to know initially how the patient should be classified. Sometimes, the issue may seem clear from the beginning, as when the patient declares, "I just love sweets of all kinds. I know I should not eat them, but I can't help myself." There is a good likelihood that the problem is psychological in nature; still, it could reflect something organic that first needs to be checked out. It is often said that one way to distinguish a physical from a psychological craving is that, when direct suggestions countering the symptoms are given, the first can be easily and "permanently" countered; the second will tend to be resistant to suggestion, or other symptoms will develop. This is only partially true. A somatic craving can be strong enough to overcome a suggestion and, if not, because the organic need is still there, physical tension may develop that will manifest itself in such ways as irritability, headaches, and hyperactivity.

The abundance of individuals with weight problems has led some practitioners to use a group approach. Ideally, for this to work well, the group should consist of members who are uniformly capable of attaining the same degree of suggestibility and whose weight problems are closely similar in nature. This situation is not likely to occur. Disparity will usually be the rule, and the more disparity is present between patients, the more individualized therapy will become a requisite. A reasonable compromise is to do an initial group induction with a small group of, at most, eight patients. Each patient is then seen on an individual basis for awhile and provided with an appropriate individualized audio tape to be used daily between sessions. If indicated, group work with them can be continued at intervals. Weekly sessions are advocated by many therapists. Others advocate weekly sessions for the first four to six weeks, subsequently spreading the time between successive visits. The needs of the patient should certainly be a guide, but in my experience, I have found that the physician's personal preferences seem to be as much of a determinant.

Some practitioners combine individual hypnotherapy with other, non-hypnotic, group activities that have been considered effective by some specialists in weight problems. This includes weekly group weighing with posting of the results, getting up before the group and confessing one's relapses or reporting one's successes, and so on.

This is probably a good place to comment upon certain weight-control clinics and courses that have flourished in the United States in recent years and that advertise having a success rate of 90% and better using hypnotism. These are usually conducted by hypnotists with no professional accreditations, who either do this on their own or as members of a business chain. Their success rates are probably highly inflated figures. These courses, or clinics, are usually conducted in a small auditorium or a conference room, with an attendance of a hundred or more participants. That there is a natural distribution of suggestibility is a guarantee that, to any onlooker, it will seem that there has been a high percentage of successes, because the inductions usually amount to no more than inducing relaxation. Since hypnosis is usually presented to the participants as being nothing more than attaining a relaxed state, a majority of the participants also feel that the sessions have been successful. The hypnotist uses broad suggestions that attempt to cover all grounds. Frequently, the patients are given (or more often sold) an audio tape of the induction and "therapeutic" suggestions, with the recommendation that they listen to it daily or as needed. It is, of course, pure chance whether or not a participant will receive suggestions that pertain to his specific problem. The odds are somewhat improved because most of the patients tend to fall into a relatively small number of categories with respect to causation of weight problems, and because a wide variety of effects are suggested. Because these treatment sessions are a one-time affair with no follow-up, there is, of course, no opportunity for the operator to gather any significant data in regard to the effectiveness of the treatment. Again, one can expect that a percentage of those attending will experience some more-or-less lasting results. I have had the opportunity of subsequently treating individuals who had taken part in such group sessions. With a few, there had been positive effects lasting up to a year; with others, no effects at all.

Many patients seeking to lose weight through the use of hypnotism have the expectation that all that needs to be done is to tell them, when hypnotized, that they will lose weight, and this will take place. This is not so, at least for the majority. Unfortunately, there are also some practitioners who believe this. Some do so in the belief that through hypnosis, one contacts the patient's unconscious, and that once it is apprised of what is desired, it will do the rest. Both therapist and patient need to accept that, in most cases, if weight is going to be reduced, an appropriate diet will have to be followed, and that the food and calorie intake will have to be controlled. Burning up calories with exercise is undoubtedly helpful, but controlled food intake remains the primary key. When extensive hypnopsychotherapy is not involved too, the main function of hypnotic suggestions is of facilitating appropriate food intake. Although the latter is also the ultimate goal when hypnopsychotherapy is carried out, many of the suggestions will then be directed at other issues.

The first step that should be taken in the treatment of weight problems is to obtain not only an adequate personal history, but also one that covers, in fair detail, the patient's eating behavior and weight problem. If there are periodic binges or cravings, it is important to explore the circumstances under which they occur. Information regarding weight problems among family members can be important. A single statement made by a patient during this exploration can be of crucial importance in diagnosing the nature of the weight problem more precisely, as well as in deciding the course of therapy. For example, I once worked with a young woman who wanted help in controlling her weight. There was no question that she was somewhat overweight, but not to the extent of her having a problem in this area. However, talking of her eating behavior, she described how, "I stuff myself until it hurts!" And beyond question, it did severely hurt. From this simple statement, it became clear that weight was not the primary problem. When such a situation arises, it is important to steer the patient carefully in the proper therapeutic direction.

In general, in the absence of information leading to the contrary, the most direct and simplest approach is to tell the hypnotized patient something like, "From now on, you will stay with your diet. You are firmly resolved to lose the weight you need to lose and to do whatever you have to do for this. Nothing will make you break this resolve. At no time will you diverge from your diet until you have attained your goal. When it is reached, then you will be able to change to and stay on a maintenance diet. You will eat only [state number of calories] calories a day (or per meal). At no time will you eat between meals. Even though you will eat less, you will end each meal with a satisfactory feeling of fullness, and you will have no desire to eat at other times than mealtimes. You will have no thoughts about food except at mealtimes. The sight of tempting food and of people eating it will have no effect upon you because you will not pay attention to them. You will be able to ignore them. Should you go to a party, you will refrain from eating more than you should. You will have no difficulty in doing this. Should you go to a restaurant, you will eat only as much as you know you should eat, even if it means leaving food on your plate and passing up some items of food. Each time that you become aware that you have lost some weight, you will feel very good about yourself, very much encouraged, and even more determined to carry out your weight reduction program."

If the prescribed diet specifically calls for eating certain things and not others, the therapist may want to add to the above specific suggestions regarding them. Hypnotherapeutic steps can be combined with other kinds of steps that the patient can take. For example, substituting carrot and celery sticks for candies, potato chips, nuts, or popcorn can be recommended. In this case, suggestions can also be given to reinforce the use of these substitutes and make them more appealing and satisfying. Many diet foods are not particularly appealing, and there are others for which the patient may have never developed a taste. Suggestions can often be used to increase the appeal of these foods.

Many overweight individuals can relate their weight problem to special cravings, such as cravings for sweets (or specific sweets), for bread and butter, for so-called junk foods, and so on. Unless these can be related to a metabolic-induced need, cravings should be considered to be of the order of compulsions and to indicate the probable need for a psychotherapeutic intervention, which can often be quite minor and brief. However, sometimes the mere suggestion that the desire for these foods will decrease and cease to be can be effective and should be tried first.

Unless there are reasons for doing otherwise, one should start treatment with a direct approach, such as the one described earlier. If this is failing after a few sessions, one should then consider a different approach. One that is very popular among therapists is modeled on a conditioning paradigm. Eating properly is associated, through suggestions, with good, pleasant feelings and experiences, while the opposite is associated with eating improperly. In doing this, one should refrain from stimulating guilt and self-deprecating feelings. When specific foods are abused by the patient, the suggestion may be given that from now on the patient will no longer get satisfaction from them, or even that these foods will have a persistent bad taste and odor. Some therapists will go so far as to use worlds like "vile" and "disgusting." It is usual to counter this with suggestions that the foods the patient should eat will become increasingly palatable and satisfying, and that he will acquire a taste and desire for them. One should be careful, because with individuals with compulsive personalities, a suggested desire can turn into a craving of its own. The same can be true with the use of strong descriptive words like "vile" and "disgusting." The response of a patient may be one of nausea and worse. I once saw this happen at a demonstration. A smoker had been told that her cigarettes would have a "vile taste." The subject became quite ill upon taking the first puff from a cigarette shortly thereafter.

The above method can be elaborated on in many ways. A hypnotherapist of my acquaintance would first ask the hypnotized patient to imagine (see) an empty theatre stage. An actor of the patient's gender was then to appear on this stage and do and say things that would cause the patient to develop very unpleasant feelings. The patient was next told that whenever he strayed from his diet or ate the wrong foods, he would immediately develop these same feelings. The next step consisted in having the patient see another actor come on the stage who said and did things that caused the patient to develop very pleasant feelings. These were then associated, by further suggestions to the patient, with his resisting any tendency or urge to discard his diet or to eat the wrong foods, and with eating the right ones. I have used this method quite effectively with some patients.

One needs to realize that there are few rules one can give regarding when to use this or that approach. Some therapists, because of training or because of personal preferences, will consistently use one approach above the other. I usually start with a fairly direct approach customized to the patient. If it works poorly or not at all, I then shift to some other approach. I find that in the early sessions, it is important to start each one with the patient reporting in some detail upon his eating activities since his last session. Any failure to follow the diet should be explored. Frequently, information comes out of these conversations that throws a useful light upon the patient's eating problem and that can be used as a basis for making effective modifications in the treatment procedures.

Some therapists, such as Hartland (1971), consistently begin the treatment with the use of ego-strengthening suggestions. Most patients that seek hypnotherapy for weight control are individuals who have consistently failed to accomplish this goal. They are, therefore, often discouraged, have low self-esteem, may be depressed, and may be pessimistic of the outcome. While not an absolute necessity in all cases, doing this routinely is probably a good idea. In my practice, I tend to give such suggestions in the course of the treatment rather than at the start. This is more of a personal preference on my part than a theoretically or empirically based choice.

I do not believe in crash diets. They severely tax the patient's body, and, if they are to be done, should definitely be undertaken under close medical supervision. I also believe, on theoretical grounds, that a much more enduring eating-habit change is brought about when weight is gradually lost over a reasonable length of time. This also often permits the uncovering of elements in the patient's life that have an adverse effect on their weight control program and allows the therapist to deal with them. For this reason, I aim, with the patient's consent, for an average loss of two pounds a week.

Weight problems which are of a behavioral nature come into being for many different psychological reasons, some, admittedly, of a speculative nature. Anyone planning to work with weight problems should thoroughly acquaint himself with the relevant psychological and psychiatric literature. In many instances, nothing less than a psychotherapeutic approach will resolve the weight problem. One of the best ways I have found of getting at psychological factors is by having the patient dream about their weight or eating problems. I will simply tell the hypnotized patient that he will have a dream about eating or about his inability to control his eating. Sometimes I have the patient do this in the office, sometimes at home. Sometimes I tell the patient that a thought will come to his mind that will help him, and me, to understand his problem better. These techniques, which are useful in most areas of psychotherapy, will be detailed in the section that discusses psychotherapy.

A case in point is that of a middle-aged woman who was definitely overweight; she needed to lose sixty pounds. She ascribed her weight problem to her love for bread spread thickly with butter. She was an excellent hypnotic subject, and for this reason, I decided to go directly to the source of the problem. I suggested that she would cease to eat bread and butter, that she would no longer have any desire for either bread or butter, and that she would develop a dislike for them and their combination. I added that she would no longer experience pleasure in eating bread and butter and that she would discover new pleasures in eating non-fattening foods. The following session, she reported that she, at first, had no desire or urge to eat the bread and butter, but that during the week there had gradually been a return of the old habit. However, it was not nearly to the degree that it had been when I had first seen her. This was encouraging, and I devoted the session to reinforcing the previous suggestions. Following this session, she, again, initially did quite well, but eventually went back to eating appreciable quantities of bread and butter. The third session was essentially a repetition of the others, and was no more successful. On the fourth session, I shifted to a different approach. I told the hypnotized patient that I would count to three, and at three, a thought would come to her mind that would help us understand this craving for bread and butter. I counted and a few moments later heard the patient say, "If you don't eat you'll starve!" Then she added, "My mother said that. She was always telling me that." On inquiry, she remembered that when she was a child, her mother constantly worried about her not eating enough, and repeated the above statement at nearly every meal. In an age-regressed state, when asked what she understood this to mean, she stated, "I will die if I do not eat!" I ascertained that she was willing to retain this forgotten material on being dehypnotized. This was done, and a discussion ensued regarding how a small child might misunderstand her mother's statement and grow up with a message to eat or die. This was the end of her difficulty in dieting, and the patient went on to lose the sixty pounds and to maintain her ideal weight. At least two years later, she was still in control of it. Interestingly enough, the significance of eating bread and butter was never clarified. There was no need for this and, curious as I was about the matter, I could not see any purpose in pursuing it.

I am a strong believer in letting well enough alone. Although I feel that the above incident was the turning point in gaining control of the patient's weight problem, it should be said that she stayed in therapy with me for other problems for a period of about a year to 18 months. One cannot discount the strong possibility that the ongoing therapy had additional positive effects with regard to the initial problem, although it was never touched upon again.

I have often encountered, in working with weight problems, individuals who requested help in quickly losing weight just before the holidays or before a special occasion such as a wedding. One might think that these are highly motivated individuals who will respond well to treatment. They rarely do! Furthermore, they are not serious about weight control. The best way to handle them is to tell them that it is rather unlikely that their weight can be reduced by the desired amount in the allotted time. They should go ahead and enjoy eating all they want, and then come back after the feasting is over to begin serious work on their weight problem. Most do not return for treatment!

Smoking Problems

I have generally found smoking to be much more resistant to therapy than weight control, and have had much less success with it. The traditional hypnotic treatment of excessive smoking bears many similarities to that of obesity, and the reader should have no difficulty in adapting the techniques that have been described.

One rather brief and apparently successful treatment I once undertook was that of a woman smoker in her early 50s who had been advised by her physician to stop smoking because of an asthmatic condition. Fairly early in the therapy, I asked her what smoking did for her. She divulged that the cigarette smoke "opened up" her nasal passageways and allowed her to breath more freely. Although dubious about the reality of this effect, I suggested to her, under hypnosis, that, hereafter, whenever she felt the need to breathe more freely, she could imagine that she was smoking a cigarette, and that this would have the same effect as a real cigarette, except that it would be a much more lasting one. I had her next do this while hypnotized, then after being dehypnotized. She reported, in both instances, a satisfactory result. I heard no further from the patient after this session, and can only assume that this continued to work.

A technique which can be very effective with some patients is to have them visualize their lungs at present, and then a year later if they continue to smoke, and, if necessary, later in the future. Some patients have hallucinatory experiences that have sufficient impact on them as to inhibit all further smoking.

There is another approach that works fairly well when a patient is willing to accept less than a 100% cure. Begin by asking the patient, under hypnosis, how many less cigarettes he could consider smoking during the following week. Most patients will come up with a figure. If they cannot, the therapist arbitrarily chooses one cigarette less. Using his usual consumption minus the agreed on figure, it is suggested that during the coming week, he will smoke only that particular number of cigarettes. The suggestion is also given that he will smoke more slowly and that the effects of each cigarette will be more lasting, so that he will not feel the need for another one as soon as he usually would. If the procedure has worked, at the next session the process is repeated, again letting the patient choose the number of cigarettes he can give up. If the patient is successful in doing this, he is allowed to stay on this schedule another week. If he fails, he is taken back to the previous schedule and allowed to stay on it another week. Then the next step is tried again. If the patient is able to proceed to smoking half or less of what he had been smoking, this is pointed out to him, and it is now suggested that in the next two weeks he will be able to cut his smoking down by another half, and that when he is ready, he can altogether stop smoking. Otherwise, he can continue to cut his smoking by half during the following weeks. The patient is then told to report on his progress, by telephone, in a month's time. The figures I have used are somewhat arbitrary, and the therapist will want to change them according to how many cigarettes the patient initially smokes and how many he is willing to give up. Frequently, the patient goes on to give up smoking altogether. Others do not, but are able to greatly reduce their smoking.

As with weight control, there is no single method that one can say is the best one. Knowing the smoking pattern of the patient is very helpful, since some individuals tend to smoke excessively only in certain situations, and the hypnotic work should concentrate on these. Some patients are found to overestimate greatly the amount of smoking they do by counting how many cigarettes or packs they use, without realizing that they actually smoke only a fraction of these. They may light up a cigarette, take a puff or two, and put it down. Sometimes they take occasional puffs, but mostly let it burn itself out. They light up a cigarette when waiting for a bus, and when it arrives, they throw their cigarette away. These are individuals for whom suggestions of smoking less in fractional amounts can be very effective. One can also use this smoking pattern by suggesting that the first puff, or the second, at the most, will satiate their smoking need for a long time, and that they will then discard the cigarette. Adding time distortion has been reported as helpful in some instances.

Many smokers light up a cigarette without much awareness of doing so. With some, it seems to be an automatic act. Forcing them, with appropriate suggestions, to become conscious of this act can sometimes be of considerable help by giving them the opportunity to exert voluntary control over their smoking behavior.

The smoking behavior of some individuals is intimately connected to their emotional life, and treatment will not succeed unless this is taken into account. Unfortunately, it seems to be a characterological feature of many of these individuals that they are not open to psychotherapy.

Chronic Headaches

Complaints of chronic headaches are fairly common. There are many kinds of headaches, which is often confusing. The two most frequent types are migraines and tension headaches. Of the two, tension headaches are easier to treat with hypnotism. As their designation implies, they are usually associated with physical tension that, in this instance, manifests itself most often in a tenseness of the muscles of the neck and scalp. This tenseness is usually palpable and is often accompanied by tenderness. Suggested analgesia, even when self-hypnotically produced, is rarely a satisfactory solution because the effects tend to be transitory. Controlling the underlying physical tension through relaxation training is the more productive approach. When a tension headache is found to develop in specific situations, as is very often the case, stress desensitization combined with relaxation training can be highly effective. Desensitization will be discussed later in the section devoted to the treatment of stress in general. Since physical tension is believed to be most often a reflection of a psychic counterpart, it is always a good idea, when suggesting relaxation for relief of physical tension, to suggest that mental relaxation will take place, too. Thus one might say to the patient, ". . . As your muscles relax, so does your mind, and as your mind relaxes, so do your muscles . . . ," and variations of this.

Migraine headaches are much less susceptible to hypnotic treatment. Teaching the patient self-hypnosis for producing analgesia may help. Also, training the patient to develop a feeling of warmth in their hands can be helpful. In my experience, the use of biofeedback monitors is quite unnecessary when doing this. Some migraine headaches are clearly related to events in the patient's life, and in such cases, this aspect needs to be considered when planning the treatment. Stress seems to aggravate migraine headaches, and stress-relieving hypnotic suggestions should also be used. In some instances, the best treatment is a combination of hypnotism and medication.

Insomnia

Most insomnias encountered in practice are largely functional. There are some somatically based insomnias, but these are unlikely to be amenable to hypnotic interventions. In any case, there does not appear to be any reports of attempts to treat them thus. Again, because insomnias in general are likely to come to the attention of physicians rather than psychotherapists, it seems best to discuss them in this section. This problem takes a number of forms. There are individuals who have difficulty falling asleep. Others fall asleep readily, but sleep poorly; they wake up frequently and sleep lightly. Still others wake up after a few hours and are unable to go back to sleep. In some instances, this early waking is connected with a need to void. The patient gets up, and in the process, awakens himself more completely and cannot go back to sleep. Insomniacs often retire anticipating a bad night. They become upset, if not ahead of time, at least when they find themselves unable to sleep. This anticipation and upset become contributors to the insomnia, and frequently, not only does a vicious circle develop, but often there is a spiraling effect. When the problem is of fairly recent occurrence, or is sporadic with no clear causation, breaking the circle, or spiral, is often all that is needed. Doing this with hypnotism is certainly one way of dealing with the problem. Taking a mild sedative or hypnotic at bedtime for a week or two will also often suffice. I have found that 10 mg. of Valium taken by the patient for a week or two, ten minutes before retiring, is quite effective for those having difficulty falling asleep. For those waking up in the early morning, a 5 mg. Valium tablet taken upon waking will often be effective. When the waking is not related to a need for voiding, the patient should keep the Valium and a glass of water by his bedside so that he will only have to engage in a minimum of activity. I give preference to Valium because it is the least likely to have effects that carry over into the waking hours. Because of this problem with even mild hypnotics, it is the only kind of medication that is advisable to take with early-morning waking. Of course, as a psychologist, I cannot prescribe medication, and when I encounter such cases, I necessarily must obtain the cooperation of a physician. It may seem strange to some readers that in a book such as this, I would advocate a pharmacological approach over the use of hypnotism. To clarify the matter, let me say that for most physicians, as well as for the patient, this will be the more expeditious way of handling the matter. If the insomnia is a long-standing one with a chronic repetitive occurrence, particularly one that has been resistant to a pharmacological approach, or one where there are reasons to believe there are psychic elements, then hypnotism, with or without psychotherapy, is indicated.

For insomnia, the use of a passive type induction, particularly one in which sleep suggestions are given, is the method of choice. With a responsive patient whose problem is falling asleep, I usually suggest that when he is ready to go to sleep, he will take his favorite position for sleeping, and that this will be the signal for him to enter a hypnotic sleep like the one in which he now is. This hypnotic sleep, I go on to suggest, will then quickly turn into a restful, undisturbed night sleep from which he will awaken at the appropriate time. I usually treat patients who sleep fitfully in the same manner, but place more emphasis upon sleeping profoundly and undisturbed. With those who wake up with a need to void, I first find out what their pattern of fluid intake is. If I find that they take an appreciable amount of fluid during the evening, especially near bedtime, I recommend they limit themselves unless there is a medical reason for doing otherwise. In any event, I suggest that they do not have to be wide awake in order to relieve themselves, but can do this remaining partly asleep, and that when they return to their bed, they will return to a deeper sleep. For those who become wide awake in spite of these suggestions, I proceed the same as I do with patients having problems falling asleep.

Unless there is some underlying pathology, the worst insomniac will sooner or later fall asleep. Also, many insomniacs misjudge the amount of time they are awake. Many sleep a good portion of the night, but do not realize it. With individuals who fail to respond to the above approach, or do so poorly, I begin by reassuring them that their physical health will not suffer from their sleeplessness. I point out that many individuals do well with relatively few hours of sleep, and that under certain conditions, normal persons have been known to stay awake and active through several nights without any harm. I usually tell them about our current understanding of the sleep cycle and its phases, emphasizing that periods of very light sleep are quite normal, and that dreaming is, physiologically, very close to being awake. I emphasize that they should not worry about not getting enough sleep, and that getting upset over being awake is almost guaranteed to keep one awake. I then propose that the next time they find themselves unable to sleep, they will get up and go to some other part of their home where they can read a book, write a long overdue letter, watch an unexciting late TV show, or listen to gentle music that they like. I add that since they most likely will become sleepy at some point, they should be prepared to remain where they are and let themselves go to sleep. For this reason, they should sit where they can be comfortable, and they should have a cover they can pull over themselves before they fall asleep completely. They are also instructed not to be concerned about turning off lights or the TV, since this would probably awaken them. Better to waste a little electricity and have a good rest! These instructions can be used effectively even with patients not undergoing hypnotic treatment. With those in hypnotherapy, they should be given in hypnosis first, then following dehypnotization.

Warts

There are a number of reports concerning the successful eradication of warts. There is, however, some question regarding the reality of this success because the percentage of cures is the same as that of spontaneous remissions of warts. I have encountered relatively few cases over a period of about 30 years. Many warts seem to come and go on their own. Plantar warts have come more to my attention than others, but possibly because, of all warts, these are the most painful, the most difficult to eradicate, and their eradication is the most painful. My approach is to suggest anesthesia for any pain associated with them. I also train the patient in the use of self-hypnosis, on a daily basis, in which he visualizes the wart growing smaller and smaller, and then vanishing, while healthy, normal skin tissue fills in the space. I also have the patient think of the blood supply going to the wart as being reduced and pinched off. There is no question that hypnosis can effectively give the patient relief for the pain of plantar warts. Their eradication is another matter. I have had only two instances of it, and these could easily have been spontaneous remissions. The suggestions I used have no other basis than that they seem reasonable ones to use in this situation.

A Case of Reynaud's Disease

While the etiology of this disease remains obscure, it is clearly established that it is a painful progressive vascular disorder that affects the extremities. It involves a constriction of the peripheral blood vessels leading to eschemia and eventual degeneration of the tissues serviced by the blood vessels. Cooling of the hands and feet are particularly likely to trigger painful attacks. I had the opportunity to work with a male patient, about 30 years of age, who was a veteran. He had begun to show signs of Reynaud's disease while stationed in Alaska. When I saw him, he was an inpatient at the Oklahoma City VA hospital where I was employed. He was being treated mainly with physical therapy and physiotherapy. He was referred to me only for treatment of the pain he experienced in his hands. One of the striking features of this man when I first met him was the protective way he held his hands close to his midrift. He moved about slowly because he was afraid that his hands would make painful contacts with his surroundings. The man had become a successful hairdresser after leaving the armed forces, but in recent times, he had to give up his profession because the constant immersion of his hands in cold water had become impossibly painful, and he had been advised against continuing this line of work. Unable to do so anyway, he had liquidated his business. With this condition, he did not see any future for himself, and he showed signs of a natural enough depression. He turned out to be a very good hypnotic subject, and I was able to relieve him of the pain without any difficulty. I explained to him that he did not have to be as protective of his hands as he was, and that because his problem was one of decreased circulation in them, allowing them more movement would be helpful. When I saw him the next day, I explored his ability to experience a feeling of heat in his hands. Having found he could do this, I suggested that he would be able to do it when not hypnotized by visualizing his hands as being immersed in a container of hot water of a bearable temperature. I also suggested that he would allow his hands even more freedom of movement. After assuring myself that he could carry out the posthypnotic suggestion regarding the hot water, I prescribed that during the remainder of the day he would do this every hour for ten minutes. The next day, I canceled the suggested analgesia and instructed him to use the hot water exercise any time he began to reexperience pain in his hands. Additionally, he was to keep up the exercise I had previously given him. Finally, having noticed that he still had a tendency to inhibit hand and arm movements, I suggested this was no longer necessary, and that he would now allow his hands to hang by his sides and to swing freely when he walked. I allowed two days to pass before seeing him again. He reported having had a small number of attacks, but that he had easily controlled them. He was now using his hands quite freely. His hospital chart contained several notes regarding observed improvements. By now, all signs of depression were gone. The session was devoted to reinforcing previous suggestions with two modifications. The patient was to use the hot water exercise only as needed, and it was added that each time he did so, the effects would be more lasting. I saw the patient on a weekly basis thereafter. He quickly progressed in physical therapy to doing woodwork and intricate leather work, and he was discharged a month later. During that time, he had a small number of attacks that he readily controlled, and by the time he was discharged, he was using his hands as if there had never been any problem. Just prior to his discharge, he told me of his plan to move to Maine to live with a relative. Knowing something about winters in Maine, I was somewhat concerned about this move. I certainly would have picked a different climate for him. However, I did not share my concern with him. I lost track of the patient until about 15 years later when, through a relative, I found out that my former patient had moved back to Oklahoma City. He was now a successful businessman engaged in repairing and refinishing antique furniture and making custom frames for pictures. There were no entries in his hospital records that he had had any further problems with his hands.

This particular case calls for further comments. Research data dispute the possibility that one could control blood circulation in a person's hands by directly suggesting this effect. On the other hand, there are research data that support the possibility of affecting blood circulation indirectly through its association with other effects. Warmth will cause the dilation of blood vessels. Although by no means demonstrated, one can reasonably hypothesize that over a lifetime, a conditioned response will develop that associates the dilation of blood vessels with the idea of a localized warmth. This can be viewed as a second level or derived ideodynamic action, or more specifically, an ideo-vasomotor action. The idea of warmth gives rise, through ideosensory action, to an experience of warmth that in turn produces a motoric response, in this case a vasomotor response. Be that as it may, research data not only support, but also suggest, the above approach. In the early stages of Reynaud's disease, the pain is associated with episodic constriction of blood vessels. Merely suggesting analgesia would leave the effects of the disease process unchecked. Something more needs to be done. On the other hand, part of the time the blood vessels are as they should be, and there is no need for any action on the part of the patient. This action is needed only when overconstriction takes place. How can one make the patient aware of this? Possibly, suggesting he will sense the constriction *per se* would work, but there is little to support the feasibility and reliability of doing so. On the other hand, pain always accompanies the constriction and is an unambiguous signal. The logical thing to do is to use this pain as a signal that the constriction is occurring and that counteraction is needed.

Was a cure affected in the above case, or were the symptoms merely kept from manifesting themselves without the underlining causative process being itself affected? Because the etiology of the disease remains unknown, this question cannot be answered. The question is of some importance in understanding the course of the disease. If the cause of the constriction is itself not affected, the above results might indicate that the progressive deterioration that is usually seen in unchecked instances of the disease is itself a by-product of the resulting ischemia and/or the changes it induces. Since the treatment was entirely aimed at counteracting the constriction when it occurred, one would not expect the basic cause to be affected. It is interesting and possibly significant that the patient did not continue, at least consciously, to practice the original suggested task for the simple reason that the attacks of pain ceased. This can mean that either the disease condition did indeed cease to be, or that at some point a conditioned-like response became established whereby subliminally perceived ischemic pain became a trigger for a vasodilation. This hypothesis has, in turn, implications for the question of what the eventual fate is of posthypnotically induced effects that are supposed to go on indefinitely over a long period of time. I once discussed the matter with Milton H. Erickson in a somewhat different context. He had demonstrated that the actualization of a posthypnotic act is accompanied by the reinstatement of a hypnotic state. The question I put to him was as follows: Suppose that I were to give a patient suffering from tachycardia an effective posthypnotic suggestion slowing up his heart, in which each heartbeat was a signal for the heart to continue to beat at a slow rate. Would this effectiveness mean that the patient would have to be in a perpetual hypnotic state? Erickson answered that he thought the suggested slowing process would quickly transform into a non-hypnotic process and become incorporated as a normal automatism, just like all other acquired behaviors. I am inclined to believe that something of this type does take place in situations such as that of the case just discussed.

A Case of Diaphragmatic Myoclonus

I reported this case in detail in a journal some years ago and have reproduced the article in its entirety in an appendix to this chapter because I believe it has particular pedagogical value. It is a good example of a situation in which a traditional, direct approach to symptom control was particularly indicated and most effective. But it also shows that a direct approach does not necessarily mean that an immediate resolution of the symptom by the use of direct suggestions will take place. The right suggestion to be given may first have to be found by a process of trial and error mixed with some judicious considerations. The case is also a good example of the importance of flexibility in treatment. It also demonstrates that flexibility can be quite compatible with a traditional approach. It further shows that utilization procedures are not unique to Ericksonian hypnotism, but are a natural step in traditional hypnotherapy. Finally, the reader will find that the case demonstrates rather well the relevance of the seven questions I recommended in Chapter 2, and that one should consider in undertaking any treatment.

I would add two other comments to the above for the benefit of readers already familiar with non-traditional hypnotherapeutic methods. First, one might think that the use of such a technique as reframing (this will be discussed in a later chapter) would have been simpler and more direct, and thus more effective. That is true, if it would have worked. It may or it may not have, and it could have required just as many treatment sessions. Also, the use of metaphors plays a big part in non-traditional hypnotherapy. It could be argued that part of the treatment involved the use of metaphors and that this was what affected the amelioration. I cannot say that this was not the case. I certainly did not use metaphors intentionally, and it is only in retrospect that I recognize this possibility. However, the muscular contractions and the analgesia that were produced by direct suggestions as part of the treatment were very real, and there was nothing metaphorical about the reasons for producing them.

STRESS AND ITS TREATMENT

We have referred to stress a number of times. Stress is loosely said in the literature to be of two kinds: mental and physical, with the understanding that these two forms interact and are even capable of engendering each other. But what, exactly, are we talking about?

As defined in *Taber's Cyclopedic Medical Dictionary* (1981), stress, in medicine, is "the result produced when a structure, system, or organism is acted upon by forces that disrupt equilibrium or produce strain." Just what "strain" specifically refers to is not covered. The "forces" which are involved also lack specificity. The term "system" gets extensive coverage. The parts of the definition most useful for us is that it is an organized grouping of related structures, parts, or organs functioning together in the performance of certain functions. The term "structure" remains undefined. Equilibrium is said to be a state of balance, that is, one in which contending forces are equal. The definition unfortunately goes on to say that in health care, stress denotes the physical and psychological forces that disturb the equilibrium. Thus we end up with the term "stress" denoting both a force and its effects!

According to English and English (1958), who are authorities on the terminology of psychology, stress is a force applied to a system and is sufficient to cause "strain," or a distortion, in the system, and even to alter its form. One of the many definitions of "system" that they give essentially matches the one above. The reader may want, at this point, to review the discussion of systems given in Volume 1 and that essentially agrees with these definitions.

To get a more precise understanding of what is involved, we must go to the physical sciences, particularly since other usages of such terms as "stress," "strain," and "tension" seem to have their origins there. The physical sciences state that stress is the resultant internal force that resists change in the size and shape of a body acted on by external forces. Deformation will result until the stress checks the effects of the external forces. However, the maximum stress that can be developed may fail to do this, and in this case, the body in question will break down and rupture. Strain is often used as a synonym of stress, but more correctly refers to the resulting deformation, if one occurs. Tension is the name given to a stress that resists forces tending to increase, or stretch, the "length" of a body. The physical definition expresses an important feature of the stress-strain phenomenon that the first two definitions have missed: that there is, indeed, no stress *unless there is resistance or opposition to a force or a change.* Without going into detail, it is also appropriate to say, in a more general way, that when stress is present, there is, effectively, a disturbance of the equilibrium of the system involved that culminates either in a new equilibrium becoming established or in the disruption of the system. In the more general treatment of systems, one can speak of static and of dynamic systems, and that in the case of the latter, the term equilibrium can refer to the existence of a balance between other elements beside forces. The balance, for example, may be one between the polarization on the two sides of a membrane or the oxygen saturation between tissues in contact.

Properly speaking, a system should be said to be "strained" only when deformation is associated with stress, but recognize that the former can be infinitesimal. It is conceivable, however, that a stress situation could exist in which there is a balance of forces without deformation taking place. There would, therefore, be no strain even though stress was present. Although this is not part of the language of physics or engineering, it would seem reasonable to say that the object in question had been "stressed." It also seems to be a reasonable word to use in those cases in which there are shifts in equilibrium but no corresponding material deformation, such as would be the case in a physiological system. It is also convenient to adopt the term "stressor," that was proposed by Selye, to denote any agent causing stress.

The concept of strain as a deformation was originally in reference to a change in the relative position of the particles making up a physical object. Strain has not adequately been defined for the case of a disturbance in equilibrium, but its counterpart might be the nature and extent of the shift in equilibrium that results. However, things get somewhat more complicated when we look at non-material systems, such as a mental system. Can the concept of deformation apply to it in a meaningful manner? One can conceive of ways in which it could, but only by doing a great deal of speculation about the nature of the mind and its physical counterpart. Likewise, the application of the word "tension," as when we speak of "emotional tension," "nervous tension," or of "tension" resulting from "stress," is rather questionable. The one way in which "feeling tense" may make some sense in the above context is when the experience can be clearly related to actual muscular tension. This can frequently be done. Pressure from within an enclosed space is often referred to as tension. The tension must be understood to be associated, by extension of the concept, with the enclosure that is being stretched in all directions. It is not too hard to see how one can speak metaphorically of people being under pressure and being tense in a more general sense. I do not think it is necessary to expand on this.

But can one stressed system engender stress in another? Only if they are interconnected in some manner, and then it may be more appropriate to speak of a single system of which they are parts, or subsystems. Psychosomatic medicine is founded on the hypothesis that an interconnection exists between mental and physiological processes. This is certainly a reasonable hypothesis, and one for which there is considerable support. The interconnection would presumably be inherent in the further hypothesis that all mental processes have a physiological substrate and thus are associated with physiological changes. This is a hypotheses that also has considerable support.

I have discussed these details because, when we speak of using hypnotism to treat stress problems, it is obvious that we are dealing with a rather complex situation in which the picture is somewhat hazy with regard to what it is that hypnotic procedures should focus upon. We must distinguish between somatic and mental (psychic) stress. If we assume that any abnormal stress is undesirable, then there are somatic situations in which hypnotism can be useful and others in which it is unlikely to be effective. We can prevent an individual from creating undue stress on a weak or defective body part. On the other hand, the somatic stress or stresses created by a virus infection seem to be less likely candidates for hypnotic treatment. Mental stresses, by their very nature, seem to be generally more widely amenable to hypnotic interventions. However, because of the interactive nature of mental and somatic stresses, it is also clear that there will be many situations in which hypnotic stress-reducing interventions in one domain will be indicated for the relief of stress in another domain. In some cases, a double intervention will be indicated because of the vicious circle that is involved whereby a somatic (or a mental) stress causes a mental (somatic) stress, and similar to a circular positive feedback, both maintain and even exacerbate each other. The case of tension headaches is typical. Emotional responses to a psychological stress-producing situation are associated with muscular tension that produces pain referred in the head. There are reasons to believe that pain itself has deleterious physiological effects that create additional somatic stress. Equally important, pain is also a source of further mental stress. In this situation, a multi-pronged approach is indicated, but because the primary cause is the mental stress, treatment is primarily aimed in that direction. In the Reynaud disease case, mental stress brought about by anticipated pain in the hands had led the patient to keep his hands in a position that hindered the already defective circulation in them. It also seriously limited his ability to participate in everyday activities. Part of the treatment was therefore aimed at eliminating this factor, even though it in itself was not expected to alleviate the problem. As was also seen, a consequence of his incapacitation was a state of depression. It is impossible to say what its course would have been had the treatment not been instituted and been successful. My prediction is that there would have been progressive deterioration. Direct treatment of the depression would have been difficult.

Since there can be no stress if there is no opposition by a system to the forces acting upon it, one way of preventing or removing stress is by working on the opposition. Changing the individual's perceptions and attitudes through hypnotic intervention is one way of doing this with some individuals.

Stress and its control is an important issue in "mind-body" healing, and in Chapter 8 we will come back to it, as well as to a number of the issues that have come up in this section.

APPENDIX

Limited Hypnotherapy of a Case of Diaphragmatic Clonus*

The case that follows is offered as an instructive and interesting example of a methodical application of hypno-suggestive methods to an unusual and challenging clinical problem. It is given in some detail in the belief that what went on from moment to moment in each session, as well as from session to session, contributed significantly to the success of the hypnotherapy. This case clearly shows that there is much more to hypnotherapy than hypnotizing the patient and giving the "appropriate" suggestion. Determining what the appropriate suggestions are can turn out to be a key problem all of its own. Other issues also have to be dealt with that are not necessarily pertinent to the use of hypnotism.

Case History

The patient, J. C., was a 30-year-old, married, white woman, with two children, from a small Texas community, and hospitalized in Oklahoma City for an intractable condition described as a severe, uncontrollable "stomach flutter" of about 18 months duration. Bilateral crushing of the phrenic nerve was being seriously considered as a last resort. Because of the attending risks, however, her physician consulted me about the possible use of hypno-suggestive methods first. On January 9, 1973, I saw her for the first time.

   J. C.'s medical history included long-standing constipation, complicated more recently by nausea, vomiting, and stomach cramps. These last three symptoms had appeared in late summer, 1971. The following February, the patient began to suffer postprandial abdominal pain and bloating. On March 7, 1972 she underwent a vagotomy and pyloroplasty. At that time, the surgeon discovered a superficial duodenal ulcer. Three weeks after operation, the postprandial bloating of the abdomen recurred, but in much more severe form. On May 24, spasms of the anterior abdominal wall appeared, associated with increased abdominal pain. Severely depressed over her worsening condition by July, the patient was hospitalized for 2½ months in a psychiatric clinic where she received psychotherapy and nine electroshock treatments for both the depression and her physical complaints. The depression was greatly ameliorated. Physically, however, she worsened, having developed dry heaves, dizziness, and increasingly severe headaches

---

* Reprinted with permission from *The American Journal of Clinical Hypnosis*, Volume 16, Number 3, January 1974, pp. 147–154.

accompanied by diploplia, palpitations, and skipped heartbeats. She also complained of poor memory and poor reading comprehension.

After further unsuccessful treatment in her hometown and nearby communities, J. C. finally traveled 450 miles to Oklahoma City where she was hospitalized on December 18, 1972. By January 9, when I first saw her, whenever she ate she invariably suffered severe abdominal clonus and pain within 5 to 10 minutes. This could be controlled only by an intramuscular injection of 10 mg of diazepam (Valium) (for the spasms) and 5 mg of morphine sulfate (for the pain). Even then, the spasms took 10 to 15 minutes to subside. The spasms could also be readily elicited by having the patient drink a glass of water and giving her a sharp slap on the epigastrium. In addition, some spontaneous episodes of abdominal clonus occurred. The clonic movements were so pronounced that the hospital bed shook. They seemed to involve the entire abdomen in a massive, convulsive, churning, wavelike series of movements. Fluoroscopy and bilateral block of the phrenic nerve had clearly established that abdominal movements were caused by a diaphragmatic clonus involving an excursion of the diaphragm of two intercostal spaces.

Neurological examination of the patient had yielded essentially negative findings. The consensus of the physicians who had seen her was that this diaphragmatic clonus probably had an obscure physical basis, and was possibly aggravated by long-standing emotional problems centered around her home life. The only psychological test that the patient took was the Minnesota Multiphasic Personality Inventory. Her profile was of type 13'; hence showed the neurotic triad most frequently associated with conversion and psychosomatic problems.

Treatment

The patient was seen in her hospital room daily before lunch for 10 days, except for one day when she was seen three times (a total of 12 sessions). The sessions lasted from 1 to 1 ½ hours, with the patient usually reclining or half-sitting on her bed.

Session 1. The first session was devoted to getting acquainted with the patient who knew that I was a psychologist and a specialist in hypnotism. I had been warned that J. C. had strong negative feelings toward psychiatrists and psychotherapy, rejecting any intimation that her illness might be partly or wholly psychogenic. Indeed, no sooner had I introduced myself than she pointedly and suspiciously, asked me what a psychologist does. I explained that a psychologist is a specialist in human behavior, including such manifestations as her abdominal spasms. I stated that, as far as I was concerned, all behavior, including emotions, had a physical basis in the functioning of the body, particularly the brain as an organ. Presently she asked how hypnotism could help her. I explained that suggestions, especially those given in the hypnotic state, often enable the hypnotist to help the patient gain special control over muscular responses. What I proposed to do, with her help, was to use a technique to control her painful abdominal spasms. Pointedly, I then reverted to inquiries about the physical aspects of her problem.

Apparently satisfied that I would not encroach upon her emotional life, the patient opened up considerably. The rest of the session was spent with J. C. talking at some length about herself, her home life, and her feelings. She brought out the fact that, until the onset of her illness, which she felt had really begun four years ago, her domestic life had been unhappy. She chose not to elaborate on this, and I did not pursue the matter.

The interview ended with my telling J. C. that, during the next session, I would hypnotize her and start treatment.

Session 2. After a preparatory discussion, in which I explained the hypnotic process, I attempted Spiegel's eye-roll technique. She responded poorly to this and I shifted to a standard technique, combining visual fixation with suggestions of relaxation, eye-closure, and sleep. The patient closed her eyes and relaxed quite readily. In a sleepy voice, she reported that she felt very relaxed and drowsy. Hand and arm levitation was, thereupon, induced as part of a deepening procedure. J. C. was then given the posthypnotic suggestion that she would, henceforth, enter a deep hypnotic state whenever I counted from one toward ten.

The patient was dehypnotized and, after a brief exchange, rehypnotized by counting. The hypnosis was deepened, during which I made direct suggestions of well-being and freedom from tension. Suggestions were also given that, after each meal, the patient's abdominal muscles would become extremely relaxed, to the extent that they would be incapable of contracting. This would last at least 20 minutes. J. C. was again dehypnotized, without any suggestion of posthypnotic amnesia. After opening her eyes she commented on how relaxed she had felt and still felt. She then volunteered the important information that in the past she had tried to relax before and during the attacks, but this only made the spasms more severe.

Session 3. The patient's condition was unchanged. The session was devoted largely to training J. C. to attain as deep a hypnotic state as possible at a signal. Some time was also spent allowing the patient to talk about herself and ventilate her feelings, as she seemed to desire to do so.

Session 4. To explore the nature of the stimuli triggering the clonus, I hypnotized J. C. and gave her the suggestion that she was eating a meal. She reported experiencing this quite vividly (but without overt corresponding movements) and within five minutes, announced that she could feel the precursors of the spasms. A few moments later, a light flutter of the epigastrium appeared, increased rapidly, and developed into the usual clonic movements, accompanied by much pain and involving the entire abdomen. Direct suggestions aimed at decreasing the spasms and controlling the pain were ineffective, and the usual injection of diazepam and morphine sulfate had to be administered.

It now seemed quite clear that actual physical stimulation, particularly that associated with the ingestion of food, was not essential to trigger the spasms. When I mentioned this to J. C., she retorted angrily, "You mean it's all in my mind and I'm crazy!" I responded that this was not my meaning at all. Obviously, I pointed out, the spasms were real and unquestionably painful. However, they could be due to any of a number of causes, and in order to help her we needed to explore them. I then briefly, and in highly simplified fashion, explained the conditioned reflex theory. Emphasizing the physical nature of the mechanism, I particularly pointed out how even thoughts, images, feelings, and emotions could act as stimuli, with the power of evoking physical responses from the body. This seemed to reassure the patient. At the end of this session, I told her I would return at lunch to do something that might help her.

Session 5. While working with J. C. earlier that morning, an idea occurred to me for indirectly controlling the spasms and giving her some relief. Accordingly, just before her lunch, I hypnotized her, successfully suggesting left arm rigidity. I then told her that similar muscular rigidity could be elicited just as easily in other parts of her body. I went on to suggest that the onset of any spasms after her lunch would signal all her abdominal muscles to tense up. They would, I said, become tight, stiff, and rigid, thus forming a tight belt of muscle, like a girdle, around her abdomen.

The patient was dehypnotized, ate her lunch, and was rehypnotized as soon as she finished eating. The suggestions regarding her abdominal muscles were reiterated. As usual, within 10 minutes of the end of the meal, the spasms began—at which time I proceeded to repeat and reinforce these suggestions. As a result, definite tensing of the abdomen became apparent, to the extent that it was quite hard to the touch. More important, the spasms were much less severe than usual. Indeed, within another 10 minutes, they ceased without the aid of the diazepam injection. Suggestions were then made to extend this effect to future meals. The patient was left with the understanding I would return at supper.

Session 6. Essentially the same procedure was repeated right after the evening meal, with equal success.

Session 7. At my visit the next morning, J. C. reported having successfully controlled the spasms after breakfast by using autosuggestions modeled after the suggestions I had given her earlier. I expressed my delight at this news. Then I hypnotized her again, spending some time helping her attain a deeper hypnotic state than she had previously reached. She was given suggestions for enhancing her ability to use autosuggestions, as well as instructions for training her in the technique of self-hypnosis. In this session, suggestions were also given that the counterabdominal tension would, henceforth, automatically be initiated by the first signs of impending spasms, rather than by actual spasms. I was prompted to attempt this because of J. C.'s report that she could feel the onset of the spasms about a minute before muscle movements became observable.

As I was ending this session, J. C. asked whether she would have to continue using this maneuver for the rest of her life. I answered that I could give her no definite answer, but that if this proved to be the case, the procedure would become so automatic that it would not intrude significantly in her conscious life. On the other hand, I continued, if the spasms were indeed a long-established conditioned reflex, as she became more proficient in blocking her abdominal spasms, the association between food intake and the spasms would eventually break down. I went on to briefly describe a typical experimental extinction of a conditioned reflex.

Session 8. Because Session Seven was on a Saturday, J. C. was not seen again until two days later, Monday. Although she reported continued success with the technique, she had trouble keeping her muscles tight when lying on her side. Under hypnosis, she was told that she would be able to make her abdomen taut no matter where she was or how she was positioned. This was then tried successfully. J. C. was also told that henceforth her abdominal muscles would begin tensing as soon as she had finished her meals, well before any signs of impending spasms. The automaticity of this effect in response to the end of a meal as a cue was re-emphasized. Then, dehypnotized, she had her lunch sitting up in a chair. A hardly noticeable, fine abdominal flutter, lasting less than 10 minutes, was the only event following the meal.

Sessions 9, 10, 11, and 12. The training of this patient in the production of abdominal countertension really ended with Session Eight. On my ninth visit, J. C. reported experiencing a tight band of sharp, gnawing pain around her entire midriff earlier in the morning—"like hands squeezing me." It had interfered with her efforts to tense her abdomen after breakfast because the procedure aggravated the pain. Noteworthy, however, was the fact that her abdominal muscles were relaxed when the pain appeared. She added that the pain closely resembled that she had experienced for a period of time before the first episode of clonus. The session was devoted to further exploring with the patient the variety of symptoms from which she had suffered (and was still suffering from). No hypnosis was used. Because past and current headaches stood out prominently, we agreed to focus future sessions on these, their control, and on relief of the band of pain.

The last three sessions were used essentially for this purpose. After trying several methods for producing analgesia, we found that the band of pain could be most effectively controlled by having J. C. reexperience, in her mind, saddleblocks she had had in the past. On the other hand, no satisfactory method could be found for controlling the headaches by direct suggestions. Giving up the latter for the time being, I decided to use the autogenic (temperature) feedback technique recently described by Sargent et al. (1971) devoting part of the last two sessions to this. The twelfth and last session was also used to review and consolidate, under hypnosis, the patient's gains.

Follow-up

Because the patient's home was so far away and I thought she might need to see me a few more times, we agreed that after discharge from the hospital she would stay with her sister, 70 miles away. I felt this might also offer a useful transition from hospital life to home life. She was discharged on Saturday, January 20. She was to call me for follow-up the next Tuesday, which she did—but from her own home in Texas, where she had returned on Monday. She claimed she simply felt too ill at ease in her sister's home.

Since then, J. C. has been seen twice (in February and May) on the occasion of follow-up visits with her Oklahoma City physician. There have been two major developments. Since March, the clonic movements have become infrequent and completely disassociated from eating. Although they do occur occasionally they are related to nothing in particular. The patient still controls them by tensing the abdominal wall. On the other hand, she has been subject to more frequent attacks of the "band" of pain, about which she had complained earlier. When it is present during clonus, she finds it more difficult to control the clonus because tension of the abdominal muscles aggravates the pain.

Inquiry revealed that J. C. could still induce hypnosis in herself as well as the saddleblock experience, but that she had not done so when in pain. When asked why, she replied, "It just doesn't enter my mind." She was unwilling or unable to elucidate this somewhat peculiar remark further. Her headaches were also as severe as ever. She admitted that the autogenic training method she learned in our hospital sessions had helped, but that she had not been using it, nor had she been practicing several self-hypnosis exercises I had prescribed. Her explanation was that constant intrusions from her neighbors and the members of her household deprived her of the necessary privacy.

The follow-up sessions quite clearly indicated that J. C. plays a variety of transactional games, including "Yes, But," "Victim," and "If It Weren't For (Him) Them."

Despite her complaints, however, the patient seemed to be in fairly good physical and emotional condition. A course of psychotherapy, along transactional analytic or Adlerian lines, would probably be helpful. This would be difficult to institute, of course—partly because of the patient's attitude toward psychotherapy, but largely because of geographical factors. Nevertheless, my feeling that even a single or infrequent exposure to such therapy might be beneficial led me to devote a fair portion of the last follow-up session to examining with J. C. the kinds of transactions she made, and more constructive alternatives.

Discussion

Myoclonus (DeJong, 1950) is a relatively poorly defined neurological disorder of obscure etiology. Almost any part (or parts) of the central nervous system can apparently be involved in its production. Myoclonic movements can be activated by emotional, mental, tactile, visual, or auditory stimuli. The literature makes no mention of diaphragmatic clonus, except for hiccups, and certainly none of the type and severity seen in J. C. Symptomatically, myoclonus seems the best term to describe the spasms she exhibited and one must consider the strong possibility that she had a rare case of myoclonus. A possibility exists, of course, that her spasms were hysterical in origin. It is said (DeJong, 1950) that movements hard to distinguish from true myoclonus can be seen in hysteria. The patient's very real distress, however, in combination with her active participation in her treatment, inclines me to view the disorder as possibly having psychosomatic elements, but not as being hysterical in nature.

When a patient is this severely distressed by a symptom, I often begin by working directly with the symptom. Not only does this often help me understand the nature of the symptom better, but if relief can be promptly provided, dealing with the psychodynamics of the case can advantageously wait a short while. In J. C.'s case, this seemed to be the only sensible course of action because of her negative attitude toward psychotherapy and toward the idea that psychological factors might underlie her problem. Anyway, with the available information on J. C. the probability of her problem being organic was about the same as it being functional. If the disorder was organic, it could easily have been aggravated by emotional factors. But clearly little chance existed for dealing with the latter without some initial groundwork. With that in mind, I felt the only approach to her problem, one acceptable to the patient, would be organically oriented. By presenting emotions to her in the list of behaviors having a physical basis, I hoped to prepare her to deal with her emotional life eventually.

At the start of the treatment, I was unsure how best to deal with the clonus. There were no precedents. The spasms seemed much like a self-sustaining reflex act. Neurological considerations, as well as established facts (Weitzenhoffer, 1953), made it unlikely that direct suggestions could lessen or prevent the diaphragmatic movements. The suggestion of muscular relaxation was partly intuitive, but also partly guided by the involvement of the abdominal muscles. These muscles seemed to go into clonic movements on their own, presumably triggered and driven by the diaphragmatic clonus itself. I thought that possibly, if sustained relaxation or lessened reactivity were present in the abdominal muscles at the onset of clonus in the diaphragm, the diaphragmatic clonus might not be communicated to the abdominal muscles, or at least might lead to a weaker response. Even though this would not eliminate the diaphragmatic movements themselves, such partial control might be very valuable for at least two reasons. First, much of the pain experienced by the patient apparently originated in the abdominal movements, which were violent and undoubtedly stressful for the viscera. Second, J. C. had clearly voiced her distress over the high visibility of the abdominal movements and their incapacitating effects, which interfered with her social life and, to some extent, that of her family. Other considerations included my feeling that effects could be more easily produced in the abdominal musculature by direct suggestions, these being voluntary, skeletal muscles. Also, any positive effects obtained early in therapy would help later therapeutic efforts.

As already reported this approach failed. It did, however, produce the important remark from J. C. that relaxing usually made things worse. This, coupled with my observation of her abdominal movements during the clonus, led me to conceive of using, instead, a general tension of the abdomen to counter the movements. Her abdominal muscles behaved much like a rope tied to a post at one end, held slack, and flailed at the other— producing wavelike movements. Briefly, the large displacement traveling up and down such a rope lessens in amplitude as the rope is made more taut. Eventually the waves cease when it is sufficiently taut. With a rope sufficiently taut at the start, the movements do not take place. Might not the same phenomenon occur with J. C.'s abdomen? As seen, this intervention did turn out to be most effective.

Of course, the above partial solution to J. C.'s problem was not quite that methodically arrived at. Indeed, had I been truly methodical, I would probably have eliminated the first solution without a trial and gone straight to the second.

My suggestion that the clonus might be a conditioned response was initially part of an effort to overcome the patient's negative attitude toward any intimations her psyche might be involved in the problem. Getting her to accept the idea of a relationship between emotions and somatic changes via the mechanism of a reflex arc seemed a good way to prepare her to deal with her emotions and feelings, if this became necessary. Probably at the time I had no clear notion that her ailment might be a conditioned response. Soon, however, I began to consider this possibility. Although the eventual disassociation of the diaphragmatic clonus from eating could be an indirectly suggested effect, it does support the notion that an extinction of the association took place. One might speculate that the patient's phrenic nerve and/or diaphragm initially became hyperreactive to stimuli arising in the alimentary tract or stomach from purely organic causes. This then led to an association between diaphragmatic responses and one or more stimuli originating in the ingestion of food, the abdominal musculature being activated secondarily by the diaphragmatic response. A reflex association may also have emerged directly between abdominal muscular responses and alimentary stimuli. If so, the eventual extinction of the primary association may have occurred through an inhibitory effect of the immobilization or tensing of the abdominal muscles upon the diaphragm. At the same time, immobilization of the abdominal muscles may also have led to the extinction of any independent established association between their spasmodic contractions and alimentary stimuli. While this all remains speculative, it did serve as a useful model for developing a procedure that worked.

I rarely, if ever, administer any of the accepted test-scales of hypnotizability or hypnotic susceptibility to patients. I find it not only unnecessary, but a digression from the therapeutic process. Nearly always, I can estimate a patient's hypnotizability satisfactorily from his responses to procedures used to induce and deepen hypnosis and to prepare him for its utilization. Thus, while I used suggestions of arm levitation, of arm rigidity, and later of glove anesthesia on J. C., and these proved to be useful indicators of hypnotizability, they were initiated for completely different reasons. Particularly, the arm rigidity and glove anesthesia were introduced (a) to ascertain how completely the patient could develop a stable muscular contracture and a limited analgesia, and (b) to serve as a foundation for the production of similar effects in other parts of her body. In my estimation, the patient was of medium hypnotizability and was found capable of producing other effects. Had she been able to produce only these two phenomena, however, or even the muscular rigidity alone, this would have sufficed. I make this last point because I am often asked how suggestible an individual should be for hypnotherapy. My answer invariably is that if he can produce only one effect, which can be used to advantage, he is sufficiently suggestible.

In a case like J. C.'s where a specific effect can be suggested to counter a symptom, I not only use posthypnotic suggestions to this end, I also instruct the patient in the use of appropriate, limited self-hypnosis and autosuggestion to supplement the posthypnotic suggestions. As noted, J. C. anticipated me in the use of autosuggestion, a not-infrequent response in individuals of above-average intelligence who have developed no posthypnotic amnesia and are positively motivated. Such persons ordinarily work actively on their problems between therapy sessions, and will often start using auto-suggestions and self-hypnosis on their own to do so. Often these patients are found to have no prior knowledge of the existence of auto-suggestions and self-hypnosis. This certainly was true for J. C. When asked about this, J. C. rather typically replied: "Well, I thought that if I pretended you were talking to me like you did during your last visit, I could get my stomach muscle tense again." Therapy usually progresses well with this type of patient.

Two more comments are in order. Insofar as J. C.'s specific original symptom of "stomach flutter" is concerned, about which I was initially consulted, the therapy appears to have been successful. More specifically, the patient was beset with a highly distressing, incapacitating abdominal clonus immediately after every meal. The patient is now free of this problem and can control, reasonably well, the infrequent unpredictable occurrences of the clonus that still occur. The patient, on the other hand, now complains more of episodes of a severe band of pain around her midriff. Could this be a symptom substitution? Conceivably. Yet, one must bear in mind that this band of pain is described as resembling that which preceded the onset of the myoclonus. This pain may have been present throughout later stages of the disorder, but may have been masked by the myoclonus—and especially the severe pain specific to it. Control of the myoclonus may simply have allowed this other co-symptom to come back into prominence. The extent to which the nervous system can apparently be involved in myoclonus seems compatible with the view that the pain also had, and still has, an organic central origin. This, as well as other considerations about J. C. and the course of her illness seem to indicate that the pain is not a case of symptom substitution.

As pointed out earlier, definite reasons existed, initially, for using hypno-suggestive methods in the limited way they were. Granted, the patient has emotional problems that could benefit from psychotherapy with a broader aim. She was not ready for this and may never be. In any event just because hypnosuggestive methods were successful on her, this does not mean that hypnotism should constitute the core of future psychotherapy. As already indicated, a transactional analytic or Adlerian type of therapy would probably be the most likely to succeed, at least initially, perhaps with hypnotism being used occasionally as a supportive agent.

Good hypnotherapy, in my opinion, lies in the judicious use of hypnosuggestive techniques (Weitzenhoffer, 1973). While these can sometimes be the whole of the therapy, as often as not they should be coordinated with other, different techniques. In some cases, like the present one the use of hypnosuggestive methods may be essentially a one-shot affair, other techniques then superseding them if further psychotherapeutic work is necessary.

References

Dejong, R. N. *The neurologic examination.* New York: Hoeber, 1950.

Sargent, J. D., Green, E. E., & Walters, E. D. Unpublished research report titled: "Preliminary report on the use of autogenic feedback techniques in the treatment of migraine and tension headaches," The Menninger Foundation, 1971.

Weitzenhoffer, A. M. *Hypnotism: An objective study in suggestibility.* New York: Wiley, 1953.

Weitzenhoffer, A. M. *Hypnosis and hypnotherapy.* Six lectures on cassettes. Fort Lee, NJ: Behavioral Sciences Tape Library, 1973.

5

Specific Procedures in Traditional and Semi-Traditional Clinical Hypnotism: Psychiatric and Psychological Problems

INTRODUCTION

The major psychological disorders can be roughly classified as neuroses, psychoses, personality (including character) disorders, and habit problems. Theoretically, one can conceive of many ways that hypnotism could be used in their treatment. In practice, however, it is found that the psychoses are among the least amenable to such a use, and the neuroses are among the most responsive. Personality disorders and habit problems fall somewhere in the middle. The utility of hypnotism in psychotherapy is, however, also very much dependent upon the kind of therapy one is using. Therefore, it may be useful to tabulate the kinds of therapies that are available. Following Wolberg (1967), one can classify therapies as being *supportive, re-educational,* and *reconstructive.* Under supportive therapy, one can list guidance, environmental manipulation, externalization of interest (occupational, music, dance, etc.), reassurance, pressure and coercion, persuasion, confession and ventilation, and symptom removal (by somatic or psychological means). The re-educational category includes behavior therapy, therapeutic counseling, client-centered therapy, directive therapy, casework therapy, relational and attitude therapy, psychodrama, family therapy, conjoint (couple) therapy, existential therapy, and some group therapies. Finally, under reconstructive therapy, we might list Freudian psychoanalysis and its immediate derivative, neo- and non-Freudian psychoanalysis, dynamic psychotherapies (psychoanalytically oriented), transactional models, and experiential therapy.

It is possible for some therapeutic approaches to belong to more than one of these categories. This is particularly true for so-called Ericksonian psychotherapy (not to be confused with therapy as done by Milton H. Erickson early in his career which was largely a dynamic therapy). Ericksonian psychotherapy is mostly a combination of re-educative and supportive therapies.

Short of writing an encyclopedic work on this subject alone, there is no way that the majority of the techniques in question, and their particular applications to various classes of psychological problems, can be discussed in the context of the use of hypnotism. A selective sampling is the best that can be done. Furthermore, there is no way that one could be an expert in each and every kind of therapy that is practiced, even if one wanted to do so. My sampling has been guided largely by the limitations of my knowledge of and personal experience in many existing therapies. For this reason, I have left many therapies out of my discussion and have made only general comments about others.

This volume has not been written as a textbook of medicine, psychiatry, or clinical psychology. The present chapter is written with the understanding that the reader interested in doing hypnopsychotherapy will already have received training in conventional psychopathology and psychotherapy.

As in the case of somatic problems, hypnotism is always used *within the framework* of an accepted non-hypnotic psychotherapeutic approach. Whatever the rules, concepts, and methods that belong to this framework, *these are retained and come first* when hypnotism is used. Hypnotism must be fit into them, not the other way around. Hypnotism is strictly adjunctive, and not a therapy per se.

While it is clearly and uniformly defined by state laws who shall practice medicine and dentistry, this is unfortunately not the case when it comes to psychotherapy. State regulations allow psychotherapy to be practiced, on the one hand, by self-styled, untutored charlatans and, on the other hand, by highly trained, accredited therapists. Between these are well-meaning but misguided lay individuals of various professions who are well-trained in their respective specialties, *but not necessarily* in the practice of psychotherapy; they are, nevertheless, incorporating this into their more legitimate work.

A great part of the problem seems to lie, as one might expect, in just how we define psychotherapy. In reviewing existing definitions, Wolberg (1967) was able to list at least 26 definitions, some so broad as to allow just about anyone to call himself a psychotherapist and to allow every positive interaction between people to be called psychotherapy. With such a definition, one can maintain that some married couples do psychotherapy on each other. I would argue that a good marriage can be psychotherapeutic, but I am not willing to go further than that. However, the majority of these definitions have certain common delimitations that are well-summarized in the following definition given by Wolberg (1967):

> Psychotherapy is the treatment, by psychological means, of problems of an emotional nature in which a trained person deliberately establishes a professional relationship with the patient with the object (1) of removing, modifying or retarding existing symptoms, (2) of mediating disturbed patterns of behavior, and (3) of promoting positive personality growth and development. (p. 3)

However, without the further clarifying comments with which Wolberg follows this definition, it has a weakness because it does not clearly state what constitutes a trained person. Again, I turn to Wolberg for further clarification on this issue.

> Assuming that safeguards are maintained in regard to the medical and psychiatric status of the patient, *professionals trained to do psychotherapy and who have had sufficient supervised clinical experience may be able to do psychotherapy under such supervision of the psychotherapeutic process as their level of training demands.* (p. 346)

In brief, the determination of who shall do psychotherapy is not so much a matter of possessing professional diplomas in this or that field, as one *of accredited training in psychotherapy,* a view proposed a good 20 years earlier by Lawrence S. Kubie. Unfortunately, many professionals possessing diplomas qualifying them as health providers consider these diplomas as a sufficient credential, particularly if they have a small amount of knowledge of psychopathology and psychotherapy. Furthermore, many who are qualified to practice in one area of psychotherapy will, after reading a few books regarding some other form of psychotherapy, and especially after attending one or two weekend workshops, consider themselves fully qualified to practice the new psychotherapy. Few, if any, really are.

I cannot change the situation. There seems to be an inordinate need among people to play psychotherapist; to many onlookers, psychotherapy appears to be misleadingly simple. Although I have written this volume for qualified professionals, it is the kind of work that will find its way into the hands of lay individuals as well as professionals who must be considered to be lay persons with respect to the practice of psychotherapy. I can only hope that they will read the present volume only out of curiosity, or to increase their knowledge, with no intent to go further with the material without *first* getting appropriate training.

Because I think that degree of suggestibility is the only objective, empirical meaning that one can attribute to the concept of "depth" of hypnosis, I will refer, in the following pages, to various levels of suggestibility *where others would speak of hypnotic depth.* Readers who wish to do so should have no difficulty in making the translation to depth as they read.

HYPNOTISM AND RECONSTRUCTIVE THERAPIES

Material available in this area centers around Freudian psychoanalysis and Freudian psychoanalytically-oriented therapy. I have found relatively little, if anything, written about the uses of hypnotism in the contexts of the many accepted forms of neo-Freudian and non-Freudian psychoanalyses; Transactional Analysis, however, is the only one of the above that I have additionally studied to any extent. While I can say with some certainty that hypnotism has not been used in any major way in connection with Transactional Analysis, if at all, I cannot say this with any certainty for the other forms. Although my knowledge about these psychotherapies is limited (I have none at a practicing level), I can see no reason why hypnotism could not be advantageously used in many of them. In some, such a use would probably be fairly limited; in others, much less so.

There are a number of psychotherapists who, like myself, take an eclectic approach. In such an approach, concepts and methods taken from various analytic schools may be used, but not uniquely so. As a consequence, there may have been many unreported uses of hypnotism in a partial neo-Freudian and non-Freudian psychoanalytical framework. For example, I have frequently used concepts and methods of Transactional Analysis with patients in combination with hypnotic techniques. I can say from experience that this can be a highly useful form of psychotherapy, but I have never published my work in this area. While all eclectic therapeutic approaches are not fully psychoanalytically oriented, dynamic psychotherapy can be placed in the category of eclectic approaches to the extent that, while it adheres closely to psychoanalytic principles, it is not totally focused on reconstruction; instead, it accepts much more limited goals as legitimate.

These remarks should make it clear why the rest of the discussion will be largely focused on the use of hypnotism with orthodox psychoanalysis. There have also been uses of hypnosis by proponents of ego psychology, but the details of procedures have not been widely disseminated. The procedures that will be discussed are eminently suitable for *any* psychoanalytically oriented therapy (dynamic psychotherapy).

I have never used hypnotism when doing pure Transactional Analysis, but only when using some of its concepts and techniques in doing individual therapy. Sometimes I present some of its concepts during hypnosis, but most of the time I do this work in the non-hypnotic state in the first half to three quarters of the therapy session. The patient is then hypnotized with the suggestions that he will absorb and more completely integrate what he has learned during the session and that he will be able to apply unconsciously his new learnings in his interactions with others during the weeks to come. Of course, this is all done in plain language. According to the case, these suggestions may be stated broadly or may be much more specific. For example, if a patient is consistently caught up on a daily basis in playing a destructive game with a family member or a business associate, suggestions are specifically oriented toward this situation. In this case, the patient may even be given an opportunity to rehearse, in hypnosis, appropriate ways of handling the situation; that is, to practice *not playing* the game. For this particular application, one should devote a session or a good part of one, to it. Frequently, more than one session needs to be used. I have also found that age regressions can be very useful in confronting parental messages. Having detected one in the course of therapy, one can hypnotize the patient and ask him to go back to the time he first received this message. Occasionally, the situation becomes reversed in that one uncovers material by using hypnotism for other reasons that suggest a transactional analytic approach. This, for example, happened in the case I have already described of the overweight woman who spontaneously heard her mother telling her to eat or starve. This example of a parental injunction was partly my reason for later introducing Transactional Analysis in her therapy.

A great deal of confusion seems to exist, even among professionals, regarding what distinguishes Freudian (classical) psychoanalysis from other "analytic" psychotherapies. I will, therefore, review the essential characteristics of this particular therapy. It focuses upon giving the patient insight into his unconscious conflicts and bringing about an extensive alteration of his character. This is done by integrating and incorporating this unconscious material into the conscious level of functioning. Uncovering, interpreting, and, especially, analysis of the transference are the major features distinguishing psychoanalysis from other psychotherapies.

Hypnoanalysis

Hypnoanalysis is perhaps the best known application of hypnotism in the domain of reconstructive psychotherapy.

When originally coined, the term hypnoanalysis was intended to denote the application to or the use of hypnotism in classical psychoanalytic therapy. Actually, hypnotism was never accepted by orthodox (Freudian) psychoanalysts as an appropriate tool. Their explanation for this rejection has usually been that free association, around which Freudian psychoanalytic therapy centers, and hypnotism are incompatible. Another argument that has been offered is that the use of hypnotism introduces a foreign element in the transference, the analysis of which is a crucial aspect again of psychoanalysis. Both of these contentions are arguable points. Finally, a particularly weak argument that has been offered, if a valid one at all, is that a somnambulistic state is a requirement for effective hypnoanalysis and that this seriously limits the use of hypnotism. This opposition is really founded in the allegiance of orthodox psychoanalysts to Freud who, after all, developed psychoanalysis as *his alternative* to hypnopsychotherapy, which he had originally used and then rejected. It is perhaps also founded in the inability of some psychoanalysts to cope with the kinds of countertransferences the hypnotic situation can evoke.

Hypnoanalysis proper is psychoanalysis in which hypnotism is primarily used to facilitate the freeing of unconscious material and to speed up the transference. *In all other respects, the therapeutic process remains unchanged.* It probably would, therefore, be more appropriate to speak of "psychoanalysis with hypnotism" rather than of "hypnoanalysis," which has an implication of being a radically different kind of therapy.

Many therapists believe that uncovering unconscious material, with or without hypnosis, alone constitutes psychoanalysis. Even when interpreted (analyzed) for the patient, this is still not psychoanalysis. Even less is any analysis, using this word in any other sense, of material already present in the patient's conscious mind. This misperception has led many therapists to unintentionally present themselves as doing psychoanalysis and hypnoanalysis when they use hypnotism. Others have done so knowingly in the willful perpetration of a deception.

Hypnoanalysis can be used in a number of ways. It is widely used for desensitization. This consists in eliciting unconscious memories, using techniques that will be described. When hypermnesia cannot be directly produced, automatic writing, induced dreams, and other indirect techniques will often succeed. Repeated evocation of deeply repressed material in hypnosis is believed to allow the patient to become increasingly emotionally inured to the memories. Even when the patient continues to repress the material on being dehypnotized, this recollection in hypnosis seems to facilitate eventual conscious recall. Such a recall should never be forced. Rather, the patient should be told to remember in his normal state only such material as he is ready to remember. Even when the patient is hypnotized, there are times when it is preferable to allow him to recover the memory in fragments, as he can tolerate them, with these eventually becoming integrated as a full memory. For the extensively trained psychoanalyst, hypnoanalysis is very useful in facilitating and analyzing the transference neurosis. Practitioners lacking extensive training in psychoanalysis, and for whom analyzing the transference is therefore inappropriate, can still use hypnoanalysis to desensitize the patient by facilitating the uncovering and interpretive process and to reeducate him through psychoanalytic insight.

Regarding the formation of the transference, no specific techniques are involved because the effects of hypnosis on it accrue directly out of the establishment of the hypnotist/subject relationship. Any attempt to use hypnotism to mold directly the patient's conscious behavior is forbidden. As a consequence of these considerations, any discussion of the use of hypnotic techniques in relation to psychoanalysis focuses mainly on their use in the uncovering of unconscious material. Those techniques that can be used outside of hypnoanalysis proper include the following:

Free Association

Even after a patient has learned to free associate, there are times when both conscious and unconscious blocks will interfere in a noticeable manner. Simply inducing a hypnotic state will often be all that is needed to get around this. When there is severe blocking, a useful additional technique is to tell the hypnotized patient that on a given signal, a pertinent thought or image will come to his mind.

Initially, the patient's normal resistance will reappear once he is no longer hypnotized. It is generally believed, however, that repeatedly breaking through the resistance with hypnosis gradually breaks down the normal resistance.

Dream Production

Insight into the nature of repressed material and of the transference is provided by the patient's dreams. These also contain information regarding the forms resistance takes, and can even be used to gauge therapeutic progress.

The production of dreams has been discussed in Volume 1. As was pointed out, they can be made to occur while the patient is hypnotized, or, at a later date, by means of a posthypnotic suggestion. In the latter case, it is usually suggested that it will be a night dream. With some patients, it is possible to specify, with some exactness, when the dream will take place, such as the night following a session, the night before the next session, and so on. With others, however, the best one can do is to suggest that the dream will occur sometime over a specified period of time, such as during the week before the next session. One is not limited to a single dream, but multiple dreams can be suggested. The subject matter of the dream can be left open or specified. Because the patient is in therapy and the suggestion to dream is given during a session, it is practically insured that the dream will be highly pertinent to the therapy, even if nothing is said regarding its content. Not infrequently, material the patient blocked out during a session will come through in a suggested dream the night following the session. This can usually be aided by suggesting this. This is one way to overcome a stubborn blocking in the midst of a session. If the induction of hypnosis does not free the material, the patient can then be told to have a dream. Suggested dreams can be used to recover forgotten natural dreams or missing portions of such dreams. Dreams can also be used to recover forgotten material. In such cases, they may border on an age regression, for which reason I have called them *regression* dreams. A particularly interesting and useful way of using suggested dreams is to obtain a new dream that elucidates a particularly cryptic dream (natural or induced). To do this, it is usually sufficient to tell the patient he will have a dream that will explain the meaning of the one in question. Insight can frequently be promoted by suggesting to the patient he will gain insight in some specific area through dreaming. Another use of dreams is for elucidating the meaning of symptoms. Finally, suggested dreams are useful for uncovering trends in the transference.

Although not suggested, an important class of dreams are those that often occur spontaneously following the first attempt to induce hypnosis, whether it is successful or not. Like those that can occur following the first therapy session, these dreams may divulge the essence of the problem being treated. It is also generally believed that even when not directed at producing dreams, the use of hypnosis in other ways promotes productive spontaneous dreaming.

It is generally held that dreams obtained under hypnosis should not be interpreted to the patient when he is no longer hypnotized. If an interpretation seems in order, it should be made to the patient while hypnotized. In this case, the patient should be told that he can accept or reject the interpretation according to whether he feels it is correct or incorrect.

Many patients will have amnesia for dreams that are produced while they are hypnotized. This is especially true if they are not ready for a conscious exposure to the unconscious material that has come through in the dream. Some therapists take the position that it is best to insure this amnesia by suggesting it. My feeling is that it is better to tell the patient that he may remember the dream, if he is ready for this, and otherwise that he can forget it.

To make the most effective use of induced dreams, the patient needs to be able to attain a medium suggestibility. However, I have found that a surprising number of individuals require much less than that to have productive suggested dreams. If dreams are to be produced in the same session in which the hypnosis is induced, one should use a passive, sleep induction form. If an active form has been induced, it is good to convert it first to a sleep form.

There is one other use of induced dreams that I refer to as the *dream work.* There are reasons to believe that not only do dreams express conflicts and reveal some of a person's inner thoughts, feelings, and personal history, but that they also provide a path for the release of some of the tension that has accumulated. A person may use dreams to work through a conflict, as well as to develop solutions to problems in general. They also provide a means for a person to become desensitized with regard to anxiety-producing situations. In this case, repeated dreaming may be required because the desensitization is progressive. With this in mind, I have made it a practice, when using dreams, also to suggest to my patients that the dreams will help them to understand and resolve their problems. Sometimes I specify the problem, but often I simply refer to "your problem." I usually add that the patient may or may not be aware of having these dreams, but that, if he is not, they will be just as effective. I also remark that it is not necessary that he consciously understand the dream content. I have no data to show that using dreams in this manner is especially effective, because they are always part of an overall therapy that involves other steps that may be the effective elements. As with many other therapeutic steps one may take, the above seems reasonable. There seems to be nothing to lose in doing so, and there may be much to be gained.

Projection Screen

The patient is told that a movie screen is in front of him and that he is going to see something on it. What he is to see can be left open or can be specified to varying degrees. This procedure is very useful when the subject has been severely blocking and hypnosis alone does not overcome the resistance. Frequently, nothing more has to be said regarding what he will see, because what has just been going on will give the right direction. It is often helpful, if one has been talking about the patient himself, to suggest that he will see a man (or woman) appear on the screen. The specified gender usually should be the same as that of the patient. One might thus say, "There is now a movie screen in front of you. . . . Can you see it? Good. In a moment something [someone] is going to appear on it . . . a man [or woman] . . . The man [woman] is beginning to appear . . . Can you see him [her]? . . . Fine, now tell me what he [she] looks like . . . And what is he [she] doing? . . . What is his [her] name? . . . How old is he [she]?" One can, of course, suggest other subject matter according to the situation.

One frequently used modification consists in suggesting that the patient is in a theatre waiting for the curtain to rise. Instead of a screen and a projected picture, one can suggest that actors will appear on the stage. Some therapists who use this method will often add that the patient is alone in the theatre. A possible reason for doing this is that the patient will more readily see highly personal matters. When I use the theatre routine, I usually ask the patient to describe the theatre to me before going on further. Unless I specified that he will be alone, I will also ask him to look around and tell me whether he sees others in the room. When suggesting that there is a screen, one may want to specify that it is blank. If this is not done, occasionally the patient will see a screen with something on it right from the start. I see no problem in that. Such spontaneous material is often significant, and, in any case, one can readily change the material by a suggestion to that effect.

The screen approach is an excellent way to make it possible for the patient to distance himself from the material that is thus freed. Sometimes one gets spontaneous regressive material this way. For example, a female patient, after I told her that she would see something on the screen, reported seeing a small girl. When asked what the child's name was, she gave a name that she had been called as a small child, but that had later been abandoned.

Mirror and Crystal Gazing

In contrast to the screen method, which can be and usually is done with the patient's eyes closed, the present method requires a patient sufficiently hypnotized to be able to open his eyes and remain hypnotized. A high degree of suggestibility is therefore a requirement. The best way to pretest the patient for this is to see, in a previous session, if he has the ability to open his eyes and remain in the hypnotic state. Crystal balls remain the best tool for this approach, but are not as easy to obtain as they once were. They can still be located in large cities from stores that specialize in occultism, from some novelty stores, and from stores that sell supplies to stage magicians. A mirror can be substituted. It should be placed so that when the patient gazes into it, he will see only the reflection of the blank ceiling. One substitute that has been used for the crystal is a glass or a bowl of water.

The technique consists in asking the patient to gaze into the crystal; it is suggested that he will see a vision that he will report to the therapist. The nature of the vision can be left open, or can be specified to varying degrees.

Some therapists begin the crystal gazing with the patient in his normal state. They use the crystal or mirror as a fixation target to induce hypnosis, and sometimes suggest from the beginning that the patient will become hypnotized without closing his eyes. In any case, the rest of the procedures follow. The visual hallucination that results, especially when left open, will often contain forgotten or repressed material.

In the past, this method has been a fairly popular one among hypnoanalysts who feel that it is an especially potent one for the freeing of unconscious material. Unless a crystal is used from the very beginning for the initial induction of hypnosis, there is not too much danger that its use in the course of the therapy will give it an occult flavor. (This is one objection that one might have against using the crystal.) There are some theories that the optical properties of crystals and mirrors facilitate the visionary process. They may, but the fact that patients with whom they are used have to be of a high degree of suggestibility may be as much the reason for the efficacy of the method.

Automatic Writing

Material that is not available to consciousness can often be obtained through automatic writing. The techniques for producing this effect were described in Volume 1. The required suggestibility to do automatic writing is the patient's ability to produce strong ideomotoric effects; this, in many cases, is sufficient.

Automatic writings tend to be highly cryptic and difficult to read. It is generally recommended that the patient be asked to translate it either while still hypnotized or posthypnotically. For this, appreciably more suggestibility is required than that necessary to obtain the writing, especially if the patient does the translation while in hypnosis, as this entails his opening his eyes. The usual procedure in either case is to ask the patient to write the translation down under the cryptic material.

Like dreams, automatic writing can be used to explain the purpose of symptoms and the meaning of dreams.

Drawing and Related Activities in Hypnosis

The use of drawing, painting, and modeling clay are among methods that are often very productive when used with hypnosis. Because the first two are best done with the patient's eyes open, a fairly high level of suggestibility is needed. Clay modeling can be done with the eyes closed. In general, these media of expression can be used like dreams, and they do not require more than medium suggestibility.

Some hypnopsychotherapists have based their whole approach to therapy on the extensive use of these media, and then speak of doing "hypnography" and "hypnoplasty," according to their choice of medium. To limit oneself as a therapist means not to avail oneself of all that hypnotism has to offer; but perhaps this is the only way some therapists can use hypnotism effectively.

There is a theory that the faith a psychotherapist has in the efficacy of a method is a strong element in its effectiveness. If so, this may counterbalance what they lose in not making fuller use of hypnotism.

Age Regressions and Progressions

Regressions are undoubtedly one of the most potent hypnotic devices that one can use. Techniques and types of age regressions were discussed in Volume 1. There are basically two kinds of age regressions. One is a role playing of a past period of life. It involves a nearly complete hypermnesia for past events, but with the patient responding to the memories with attitudes and judgments that belong to his chronological age. Much of his behavior is a product of an adult conception of childhood. This should probably be spoken of as a *pseudo age-regression*. Some patients, however, go back mentally to an earlier period, and the patterns of behavior, thoughts, and emotions that existed then are *reinstated* with a partial ablation of later influences. The individual now reexperiences the past with appropriate child-like perceptions, attitudes, and judgments. In some cases, actual physiological conditions then existing are also reinstated. These are age regressions proper and have often been appropriately called *revivifications*. As pointed out in Volume 1, a paradoxical situation exists in their regard because hypnotic rapport with the therapist is retained, thus showing there is less than 100% ablation of the future. Revivifications have a strong potential for abreactive reactions.

The approach to age regressions varies. The therapist frequently chooses the age, age period, or incident to which the regression is to take the patient. Or he may allow the patient a choice as to which one of a group of target periods or dates he will return to. Regressions can be used to explore the patient's past, to explore the origins of symptoms, and to open channels for forgotten memories and experiences. They can also be used for the express purpose of producing a therapeutic abreaction.

There have been some rather creative uses of regressions, although I question their appropriateness in a truly Freudian psychoanalytic framework. One of these is the use of play therapy with regressed persons. Even though the purpose may be merely to elicit information regarding childhood conflicts, there is an injection of alien material into the patient's past that, while possibly beneficial, may become the source of a paramnesia. Some therapists have gone so far as to attempt to alter the patient's past traumatic experiences by giving suggestions to the regressed patient aimed at creating an alternative, non-traumatic experience. Although it may be useful, I do not perceive this type of reconstruction of the patient's past to be in the spirit of the psychoanalytic process.

Some presumed regression can be more fantasy than reality. Regressions in which the patient describes his supposed experiences in the third person should be considered highly suspect, especially when the patient is extremely vague and reticent in his report and must be constantly prodded with questions. For any age regression to be useful, the therapist must *refrain* from putting words into the patient's mouth. This rule is often broken when the patient must be constantly questioned to obtain details.

There are two related modern developments: One is age *progressions* and the other is age regressions to birth, the foetal life, conception, and particularly, to *past lives*. Both effects were originally mentioned in the literature during the nineteenth century by de Rochas d'Aiglun, a French engineer and lay hypnotist with a leaning for the sensational. However, he was a good enough scientist to make a limited effort to check the validity of his subjects' experiences and report his findings, even though they were mostly negative. His work had relatively little impact, and it was quickly forgotten. Interest revived in the subject of regressions to past lives with the early 1950s publication, by an American business man and lay hypnotist, of a report that came to be known as *The Case of Bridey Murphy*. It received a great deal of publicity, was eventually proven to be a hypnotically induced fantasy, and was forgotten, too. Then, in the late 1970s, there was a renewed surge of interest in the United States in regressions to past lives. This interest was not revived just because it was a fascinating phenomenon, but because it could be used as a form of therapy. Today, there are a number of professionals who have centered their entire therapeutic practice around the production of such regressions.

In age progressions, the patient is sent into the future to see himself when older. In some cases, patients have spontaneously seen themselves as reincarnated. Although there are a small number of therapists that intimate a prophetic aspect to progressions and give credence to the reported reincarnations, the majority do not, and it must be stated that the initial use of the method was in that spirit. There is little available of a factual nature regarding the implications of progressions for psychoanalysis. One can surmise that they may serve as a medium for the expression of unconscious material, and that they may throw light on the likely outcome of therapy.

Scientifically speaking, regressions to non-verbal age levels, to a prebirth period, and to previous lives can, at best, only be viewed as fantasies that, unfortunately, are too often partly a product of the therapist's own fantasies and needs and of the patient's conscious and unconscious strivings. Professionals practicing this kind of regression will go to extremes, even in the face of blatant evidence of their fictitiousness, to convince themselves, the patient, and any observers that are present, of the reality of these productions. This is unbelievable, and a rather sad reflection upon the profession. I had the opportunity to witness a perfect example of this taking place on a popular talk show at the time of my writing this chapter. I will not claim that cures, or, at least, ameliorations, cannot result if these experiences are properly handled. *They probably can.* Thus far, no efforts seem to have been made to use these kinds of regressions in any kind of analytic framework. My surmise is that any therapeutic effects they have is because they constitute a corrective emotional experience.

Induction of Experimental Conflicts

This is considered to be an insight-producing technique. There are relatively few detailed examples of the use of this method in the literature. One of the best is to be found in Erickson's treatment of a case of *ejaculation praecox* (Erickson, 1944).

Basically, an experimental neurosis consists in creating and implanting, through hypnotism, a fictitious conflictual situation that parallels the patient's own situation. Initially, the existence of this artificial neurotic complex is kept out of the patient's awareness by means of suggested posthypnotic amnesia. The patient is then given the opportunity to come to a conscious understanding of the unconscious mechanism causing the new symptomatology. This is usually done by first explaining to the hypnotized patient the meaning of the experimental conflict, then allowing him to remember this material after he is dehypnotized.

For example, a patient suffering from bruxism may become aware that he has a great deal of suppressed anger, but be unable to relate this to the bruxism. A fictitious situation might then be created that is associated with unexpressed feelings of hostility and that also leads to clenching and grinding of the teeth. It is important to understand that the method goes beyond merely suggesting this behavior. That is, one might consider giving the patient the suggestion that he will feel anger at a certain signal, and when he does so, his anger will express itself as teeth gnashing. This can actually be useful, but only at a rather superficial educational level. In most cases, it is too remote from the actual underlying dynamics to be very effective. A somewhat better approximation would be simply to suggest that the anger will occur at a signal, and that the patient will be unable to express it openly; no reference is made to the bruxism. In this case, the clenching and grinding of teeth that might result would be dynamically determined, rather than the possible result of only a suggestion. The third and best way of inducing a conflict in this situation is demonstrated by the following case: A divorced man in his forties had a long-time employer who was appreciably older and was a petty, rejecting tyrant. There were encounters between the two men almost every day. These left the patient full of contained rage against his superior. The patient had no outlet for his anger and hostility, and he felt unable to change jobs. I first tried to desensitize the patient by suggesting the ability to ignore his employer's actions and remain calm; next, I helped him gain insight into the origins of his problem. This, however, had very limited effects, and I decided to use another approach. In hypnosis, a fictitious incident was suggested. The patient was told that he would remember an incident that had actually happened to him, but that he had forgotten because it was too painful. Several days earlier, he was told, he had received an unfair traffic citation by an unpleasant, overbearing policeman who reminded him of his boss. He had experienced the same kind of impotence and the same kinds of feelings of resentment and anger as he did with his employer, and had felt equally impotent to express them. He was then told that on being dehypnotized, he would suddenly recall the incident and reexperience some of the feelings he had had. He would want to share this memory and his feelings with me, but would realize that I probably had other plans for him, and he would feel resentment in anticipation that I might not allow him to do this. He was also told that no matter what happened, he would go back into a relaxed hypnotic state, as usual, when I gave the signal for this. Appropriate selective posthypnotic amnesia was, of course, also suggested. On coming back to his normal state, the patient stated that there was something he wanted to talk about. Somewhat tersely, I replied that this would have to wait; thereupon, an attack of bruxism took place. Hypnosis was reinduced, the attack stopped, and he was told that he could now fully understand the origin of his current attack and relate this understanding to past attacks. The patient did this quite successfully under hypnosis, and he was able to carry his understanding over to the non-hypnotic state. The attacks did not disappear immediately, but became progressively less frequent and intense. As therapy progressed, it became clear that the situation with his employer was a repetition of one that had existed during the patient's childhood between him and his father. He was able to recognize that his boss strongly reminded him of his father. However, with his chief problem under control, the patient indicated his unwillingness to probe further. Therapy was continued for a while longer, mainly along reeducational and supportive lines. Hypnosis was used to desensitize the patient to his employer by suggesting an increasing ability to ignore his behavior and his resemblances to his father. He was also encouraged to consider making changes in his life situation. He presently decided to seek a more satisfying position, took steps to do so, and eventually found a much better one. I had no further contact with the patient, because he moved some distance away to his new job, but subsequently, at his recommendation, one of his daughters came to me for help and informed me that her father was doing well.

Wolberg (1948) has described in detail the treatment of a case of psychosomatic headaches. It had become clear that these headaches were related to the patient giving in to his wife's wishes instead of satisfying his own desires.

Wolberg suggested to the hypnotized patient that he was in a situation in which his wife insisted that he go shopping with her, instead of going bowling as he wished to do. The additional suggestion was given that on being dehypnotized, he would feel exactly as if he had carried out her command. Following dehypnotization, the patient, who was amnesic for the trance events, was found to have developed a violent headache that he could not account for. The patient was then rehypnotized, and his headache was interpreted for him.

There are a number of disadvantages to this technique. It requires considerable skill and understanding on the part of the hypnotherapist, and should be used only by one with considerable experience. It can be rather time consuming, as it requires much preparation on the part of the therapist. Finally, the patient needs to be a very good hypnotic subject; essentially, a somnambule.

Finally, it might be noted that the method is not strictly a hypnoanalytic one because it can suffice, in itself, to cause a symptom to vanish. In such instances, it really belongs under the heading of symptom removal.

HYPNOTISM AND RE-EDUCATIVE THERAPIES

From the list given earlier, it is clear that therapeutic re-education involves a great many techniques. Theoretically, hypnotism can probably find applications in most, perhaps all, of the re-educative methods that have been used. In actual practice, the reported uses have been much more limited. My experience with specific re-educative therapies has been with behavior modification; I shall therefore discuss the use of hypnotism in greater detail only in its connection.

The primary goal of re-educative therapy is to modify behavior through positive and negative reinforcers and/or interpersonal relationships, thereby bringing about modifications in goals, a better and greater use of inherent potentialities, and readjustments to the environment. It may or may not include obtaining insight into conscious conflicts, and rarely brings about a resolution of unconscious ones. Except for behavior therapy, the effectiveness of hypnotism with re-educative methods is attained mainly through the strong positive influence that evolves out of the hypnotist/subject relationship. Hypnotism is particularly useful whenever confrontation, guidance, and the clarifying of feelings is involved.

Hypnotism with Behavior Therapy

In 1956, I spent a year as a fellow at the Center for Advanced Study in the Behavioral Sciences. Joseph Wolpe was also a fellow that year, and had just finished writing his book on reciprocal inhibition. Early in our acquaintance, he told me that he used hypnotism in his practice. Much to my surprise, I discovered that at that time his *only* use for it was to relax his patients. The reason for my surprise was that it seemed so obvious that it could be very useful in creating by suggestion the hierarchy of stimuli he used for the systematic desensitization of the patients. Relaxation can be produced in just about everyone, but the creation of a hallucinatory stimulus is limited in application to patients of fairly high suggestibility. Understandably, suggested relaxation is of broader application, but why not take advantage of the higher suggestibility of some patients, thus eliminating, in their case, the use of the paraphernalia that is otherwise required? Wolpe never used this idea, and I have noted that, as the years have gone by, the above potential use has remained largely potential in behavioral therapy. By behavioral therapy, I mean the use of classical and instrumental conditioning in changing unhealthy behavior into a healthy one. In Wolpe's (1969) terms, classical conditioning includes counterconditioning, positive reconditioning, and experimental extinction. Instrumental conditioning includes positive reinforcement, extinction, punishment, and negative reinforcement. Wolberg (1948, 1967) has aptly referred to these approaches as "reconditioning." I view behavior therapy as going beyond the use of conditioning, and prefer to define it as the systematic use of learning principles and/or theories to eliminate unadaptive behavior.

On the other hand, as I pointed out some years back in an article on the subject (Weitzenhoffer, 1972a), hypnopsychotherapists were doing behavioral therapy long before it was recognized as such. Just as behavioral therapists have failed to avail themselves of all that hypnotism offers them, so many hypnopsychotherapists have failed to avail themselves systematically of all that learning theories have to offer.

One of the earliest forms of hypnotic behavior therapy was that of associating an undesirable habit with an avoidance response to a noxious stimulus. The patient was simply told that he would have a very unpleasant experience whenever he gave in to his habit. This was commonly done during the nineteenth century with alcoholism and excessive smoking. We have also discussed earlier, in the treatment of obesity and smoking, a milder use of negative reinforcement combined with positive reinforcement by suggested pleasant experiences. An interesting way of doing aversive conditioning is to exaggerate the patient's symptom to the point of oversatiation. For example, a patient who abuses sweets can be not only given permission to eat all the sweets he wants, but encouraged to overindulge. Hypnotism can be used quite effectively to increase the compulsion and even create binges. I once cured a patient of excessive eating of chocolates by having her go on a binge that resulted in her becoming quite ill and losing her taste for chocolates and other sweets for an appreciable amount of time. Sometimes, the process has to be repeated.

We discussed earlier, in connection with the treatment of obesity, the use, under hypnosis, of aversion-evoking imagery. Readers already familiar with behavior therapeutic techniques may have been reminded of Cautela's "covert sensitization." The only difference seems to be that he did not use hypnotism.

"Counterconditioning" was Wolpe's (1969) term for denoting the conditioned inhibition of maladaptive behavior through the use of reciprocal inhibition. This process, or rather, principle, can be stated as follows: If a response, R1, inhibitory of another established one, R2, can be elicited by a stimulus that also elicits R2, repeated elicitations of R1 will weaken the stimulus-response bond. When R1 and R2 are incompatible and R1 is prepotent, the result may be the elimination of R2 and the substitution of R1. Stated more briefly, an undesirable behavior is replaced with a competitive incompatible and desirable behavior. Antedating Wolpe, Wolberg effectively applied this, then an unstated principle, in his treatment of several patients. One, for example, felt great unease and discomfort when in the presence of people. Wolberg hypnotically associated induced feelings of pleasure, happiness, relaxation, and peace with this situation. Milton Erickson has similarly described the cases of two patients whose dental defects had caused them to develop strong feelings of inadequacy and self-deprecatory behavior. Using hypnotism, he suggested that these patients associate positive feelings with their dental defects, and was thus able to counter their previous negative feelings. Franz Baumann, a pediatrician who uses hypnotism extensively, has described how he offers young drug abusers the possibility of inducing more satisfactory hallucination through self-hypnosis than they can obtain through drugs. This posthypnotic training is, of course, accompanied by instructions placing limits on this self-induction of hallucinations. I have already described the treatment of an asthmatic smoker for whom the substitution of briefly smoking a hallucinatory cigarette was quite effective. In making such a use of hallucinations, it is important to protect the patient against overtly exhibiting that they are hallucinating. In the case of my patient, when the hallucination was first tested in my office, she overtly went through all the motions of lighting and puffing on a totally invisible cigarette. One can well imagine the potential consequences of her doing this in public. Solutions for this problem are usually fairly easy to develop. The simplest is, of course, to train the patient to hallucinate without overt accompanying actions.

Many "symptom substitution" and "symptom transformation" techniques could probably be considered to be a form of counterconditioning. For example, Milton Erickson described one of his cases, in which a moderate stiffness of the patient's right wrist was substituted for a highly incapacitating hysterical paralysis of the entire arm. The premise is that the symbolic value of the symptom is what is important, and that a lesser symptom with the same symbolic value will be just as good. Such an approach would probably not have worked had the secondary gains from the paralysis been dominant. In another case, also described by Erickson, anxiety caused by a patient's enuresis was relieved by suggesting anxiety for other matters. Obviously, this did not cure the enuresis, and the patient continued to have anxiety. The anxiety, however, was much less of a problem, and Erickson followed up this substitution with specific treatment of the enuresis.

"Thought stopping," which might be viewed equally well as a use of induced distraction, can be very effectively instigated with hypnotism. Ludwig, for example, has described treating drug addicts by causing hallucinations to occur whenever the addict thinks of using drugs. One treatment for smoking (Spiegel, 1970), claimed to be very effective, consists in teaching the patient, in hypnosis, a meditative exercise, to be done in self-hypnosis, associated with the carrying out of a ritualistic-like use of certain acts that the patient performs whenever he feels the need to smoke or thinks of doing it.

The effectiveness of such techniques is sometimes hard to determine because the therapist, more often than not, combines them with other techniques that may be more important in producing the end result, and, in any case, may contribute appreciably to it. For example, Ludwig also used suggested relaxation in a framework of standard desensitization. In the treatment for smoking just mentioned, the meditation focuses on all of the potential ill-effects of smoking, including death; thus, an aversive action is added.

I have found thought stopping to be quite effective with certain phobias. For example, I had a patient who had a phobia of going on elevators because of the fear that the elevator might become stuck between floors. I suggested that the minute she began to think of this possibility, she would become distracted by other thoughts, or, if in the elevator, by something in the elevator, and as a result, would lose her fearful thoughts. Until she reached her destination, she would find herself unable to think about anything else than what had caught her attention. Another technique I have found effective for thought stopping is to suggest that the minute the undesirable thought occurs, the patient will immediately become amnesic for it.

More often than not, hypnotherapists combine a number of behavior therapeutic approaches. For example, in the case of a dyscopresic child, the therapists used a three-pronged approach. First, they employed a schedule of reinforcement with reward to encourage the child to have bowel movements. To this, they added a suggested good feeling with each act of defecation. Finally, relaxation was produced by suggestion to counteract the child's anxiety regarding bowel movements. Von Dedenroth (1964a, b) has described a three-session approach that he claims is very successful in the treatment of smoking. First, various good feelings are associated with a particular sequence of activities in which smoking is prohibited. Second, the patients are instructed, in both the hypnotic and nonhypnotic state, to engage, instead, in various other activities when they have the urge to smoke. Finally, aversive therapy is introduced. The patient is instructed to use brands of cigarettes progressively lower and lower on his preference scale. He is also made, in hypnosis, to associate smoking with all of its deleterious effects. Later in the treatment, it is suggested that each puff will become less enjoyable and eventually disagreeable. Finally, the patient is instructed, in both hypnosis and the normal state, to abstain from cigarettes at times when he is most likely to smoke, according to a schedule of increasing abstinence. This step may be viewed as a conditioning of abstinence with specific stimuli. Since this can be a self-rewarding action, operant conditioning can also be seen at work.

Extinction of behavior through lack of positive reinforcement is another avenue. When suggested dominant unpleasant experiences are associated with a behavior, that behavior may be diminished because there is an absence of positive reinforcement. It may also be diminished by the possible creation of an avoidance reaction. Suggesting the absence of the positive reinforcer should be expected to lead to extinction. Milton Erickson once used an ingenious approach that might be considered to have produced a one-trial extinction. Erickson himself did not use this interpretation, but instead, viewed the treatment as a "pseudo-orientation in time," in which the patient sees the therapeutic goal as having been accomplished. Why or how this worked was not his concern. In any event, the patient felt compelled to make a daily visit to his mother's grave. This interfered greatly with his daily life. Erickson projected the patient two weeks into the future and had him experience himself as having failed to visit the grave during that time. He was brought back to the present with a suggested amnesia for the hypnotic experience. An appointment was scheduled for two weeks later. At that session, the patient stated that he had not visited the grave or even thought about it. This was brought to his attention, and it was emphatically asserted to him that now he knew that he did not have to visit the grave. A 10-year follow-up showed that the patient was still free of the compulsion. What actually happened is subject to interpretation. What appears to have been a one-trial extinction may really have been one resulting from 14 trials, since the two weeks amounted to that many trials. One could also argue that instead of extinction, a strong posthypnotic command not to visit the grave was hidden in the projection, and that it effectively prevented the patient from visiting the grave, with a consequent deconditioning.

Erickson has given accounts of many therapies in which he made a much clearer use of extinction. Unfortunately, his *modus operandi* were so involved that it is not possible to discuss his procedures in any reasonable space. Interested readers should consult some of the collections of his works that have been listed at the end of Chapter 7. The reading of his treatment of an enuretic couple is highly recommended.

The effectiveness of induced artificial conflicts and some of the more complex forms of symptom removal can be interpreted as an application of transfer of learning (stimulus generalization).

In utilizing learning principles, it should not be overlooked that motivation, attitudes, and emotions appear to be important determinants of learning. These are elements that can be easily manipulated by suggestion. Ericksonian therapy makes considerable use of this kind of manipulation. I have found in my own practice that changing attitudes can be very helpful in promoting the acquisition of desirable responses.

HYPNOTISM AND SUPPORTIVE THERAPIES

The success of supportive therapies depends primarily upon the existence of a strong positive patient/therapist relationship that is not allowed to develop into a neurotic transference. Hypnotism is useful because it promotes the formation of this kind of relationship. It is particularly useful in enforcing the utilization of pressure, coercion, persuasion, and the externalization of interest. It can greatly facilitate ventilation and confession and can be used to promote positive desires, likings, satisfaction, and pleasure. Desensitization and re-education, already discussed under other headings, can also have a supportive function.

Supportive therapy is particularly well-suited for physicians and other therapists who have not received the highly specialized training required for psychoanalytic work. Unless one is a strict adherent of behavioral therapy, it can be very effectively combined with the latter. Although less demanding of the therapist, supportive therapy is not suited to every practitioner, because for many, the development of the transference can become a major stumbling block. The success of this form of therapy will depend upon the ability of the therapist to recognize its development and to handle it without analyzing it. Because the transference often develops more quickly and intensely with the use of hypnotism, there are some therapists who do much better using supportive therapy without hypnotism.

In general, a small-to-medium suggestibility is all that is required to use hypnotism with supportive therapy. The suggestions are given both in and out of hypnosis. Posthypnotic amnesia is not desirable, and, should it occur spontaneously, the patient should usually be given posthypnotic suggestions for recall. While hypnotized, the patient should be instructed to carry the suggestions into his normal state. The patient should also be given an opportunity to react to the suggestions that are given to him and to discuss his problem while hypnotized. Once the patient has learned to go rapidly into a hypnotic state, each session should be started with a brief review of the patient's experiences since the previous session. Some discussion of the patient's problem in relation to these experiences should follow. Hypnosis should then be induced and utilized. The last ten minutes or so of the session should be spent with the patient dehypnotized, usually to summarize the session. By following this procedure, one can make maximum use of the *pre*hypnotic suggestion effect. The therapist also has an opportunity to demonstrate that to tell a patient to "wake up" is often not the same thing as to tell him "he is no longer hypnotized." As was explained in Volume 1, in the first instance a "mild" state of hypnosis may persist, even though the patient may seem to be awake. This state of affairs can be promoted if, in training the patient, the therapist routinely instructs him first to "wake up," then a little later tells him he is no longer hypnotized. This procedure becomes an indirect suggestion to remain hypnotized until specifically told not to be.

Symptom Removal with Hypnotism

The primary goal of supportive therapy is to bring about relief of symptoms that are seriously interfering with the patient's life. Removal of symptoms, or at least amelioration, allows the patient to function at a level approximately his norm, and this can be done in a variety of ways. Hypnotism is only one of these. In a manner of speaking, all psychotherapies can be viewed as having this aim. But most psychotherapies do this indirectly. The symptom is viewed as being an outward, superficial manifestion of a much deeper seated dysfunction, and many therapies are aimed at this. When we speak of "symptom removal" in psychotherapy, we have in mind an effort to deal directly with the symptom itself. One major disadvantage of doing this is that, while it may bring immediate relief to the patient, it does not usually eliminate underlying behavior tendencies that sooner or later may cause the same or other difficulties for the patient. The case of bruxism I discussed earlier was clearly associated with a neurosis that had led the patient to form relationships that duplicated the one that had existed between himself and his father as a child. Arresting the bruxism did not change this tendency, and it left the patient with the potential to initiate and/or maintain this kind of relationship. Bruxism might not reappear, but other deleterious effects were a likelihood.

One of the earliest and often most dramatic ways of removing symptoms was to order, or exhort, the hypnotized patient to give up his symptom. Today this approach is usually referred to as the authoritarian, or prestige, approach. It can be done as a posthypnotic suggestion, or first in the hypnotic state with posthypnotic suggestions following. The case of back pain I described in the previous chapter can be viewed as such an application. Symptom removal is particularly easy with conversion hysteria cases. Once, a favorite method was to remove the symptom under hypnosis and let the patient experience its removal on being dehypnotized, thus confronting him with its functional nature. For example, a patient with a paralyzed leg might be ordered to walk, and then be dehypnotized while in the process of walking. As many readers will realize, such "cures" have a tendency to be evanescent.

Extending symptom removal over a period of time is usually more effective than removing it at a single session. In the latter case, sessions of two and more hours are often required. Periodic reinforcement is frequently required and can often be done by means of audio tapes designed for limited self-hypnosis. Although patients of low suggestibility will sometimes respond satisfactorily, a medium-to-high suggestibility is preferable. All suggestions should be specific and to the point, and generally repeated several times, with the patient repeating them back. It is usually better to suggest a gradual disappearance of the symptom than an immediate one. In some cases, complete disappearance should be left to take place in an indefinite future. Initial supplementation with medication is not only permissible, but sometimes indicated.

Regarding specific procedures other than direct removal by authoritarian suggestion, an effective method consists of inducing a like symptom in another part of the patient's body, then removing the actual symptom, and, finally, removing the suggested symptom. Wolberg (1948) recommends inducing first the artificial symptom, then partially removing the real symptom. If this succeeds, the artificial symptom is increased in intensity, and a strong suggestion is made of complete recovery of the lost function. Wolberg has recommended letting the patient shift the symptom through self-suggestion. Presumably, this teaches the patient that he is not as helpless as he thinks.

When the symptom is recalcitrant because of the patient's need for it, or the therapist judges that complete removal is not indicated, partial removal is often an acceptable solution. For example, in the case of a woman with an ugly, large psoriasis lesion on her chest just below the base of her neck, a satisfactory solution was to suggest its gradual reduction to a lesion the size of a quarter, located where it did not normally show. The *tic douloureux* case mentioned earlier was another example of the above. Displacement of the symptom to some other body part where it is a lesser problem, or substituting a symptom that is less incapacitating, are alternative solutions. A manual laborer, with a total hysterical paralysis of his right arm, was able to accept, instead, a stiffness of his little finger. A semi-professional woman who blushed violently in the region of her neck when giving public lectures was relieved of this problem by developing in its place a twitch of her right big toe. Finally, it can be helpful to explain to the patient, both in and out of hypnosis, the dynamics of symptom formation.

Symptom removal is most likely to be successful when the symptoms are minimally defensive and/or the patient has a strong incentive for getting rid of them. Psychosomatic symptoms and habits such as nail biting, insomnia, and excessive eating, are good candidates. Symptom removal is indicated when the symptom dominates the patient's life and when he is not open to or responsive to any other therapeutic approach. It is particularly indicated when the patient's ego defenses are too weak to tolerate an analytic approach. Frequently, the removal of a symptom can also have positive ramifications that lead to positive alterations of personality structure and open the door to depth therapy.

Always keep in mind that functional symptoms are expressions of inner conflicts. They are means of defense and adaptation; one of their functions is to bind psychic energy that would otherwise express itself as anxiety. When anxiety is very high, symptoms will usually not be given up readily. Forcing the issue (and this can be done) will often result in a symptom substitution, which is no improvement. A catastrophic reaction may also result. This is particularly likely if the therapist also removes the substituted symptom.

HYPNOTISM IN ECLECTIC PSYCHOTHERAPY

The need for an eclectic approach in psychotherapy, especially if full use of hypnotism is to be made, grows out of a number of factors. First, there does not appear to be any single therapy that will work with all patients or with all ailments. Second, in the course of therapy, a patient who is not responsive to a type of therapy at one point may become so at a later point. Third, as one works with a patient, one may become aware of some aspect that now calls for the use of one particular approach in preference to another. Fourth, a patient who is not ready for a certain therapeutic approach early in therapy may become so later on. Typically, patients with weak ego defenses are not suitable for a psychoanalytic therapy, but after their ego has gained strength through the use of supportive and re-educative methods, psychoanalysis may become suitable. Finally, the nature of the disorder being treated will dictate,to some degree, what will be done. The following is a brief discussion of the uses of hypnotism with the disorders a psychotherapist is likely to encounter.

Psychoses

As I have previously stated, hypnotism has little to offer for the treatment of psychoses. Any use is in the context of supportive therapy. It should not be used for uncovering.

Psychosomatic Disorders (Psychophysiological Reactions)

On the other hand, psychosomatic problems are good candidates for hypno-psychotherapy. They have already been discussed to some extent in the previous chapter. Because of their nature, they often require a joint somatic and psychotherapeutic treatment. Anxiety, hostility, and generalized tension are at the root of psychosomatic disorders. Neuroticism is frequently associated with them. Some well-adjusted individuals who are overstressed tend to develop diffuse somatization responses in which the organ that becomes involved does not appear to have any particular meaning. Its breaking down merely reflects a constitutional weakness. On the other hand, when neuroticism is present, the choice of organ is generally believed to be related to the character structure of the patient and his habitual way of resolving conflicts. Personality types appear also to be a determinant. With severely neurotic individuals, psychosomatic ailments will occur in the absence of unusual external stress because the neurotic individual is in a state of high internally generated stress at all times. With many neurotics, the choice of organ frequently has symbolic significance, but does not necessarily involve the same mechanism as is involved in hysterical somatization reactions. Some patients with psychosomatic problems, however, can have a hysterical make-up, too.

Suggestions are particularly effective with psychosomatic symptoms that are symbolic. However, suggestions are relatively ineffective when the disorder is the result of a diffuse autonomic draining of tension, anxiety, and hostility. The same thing is true when the symptom is an important defense against anxiety.

Hypnotism can be useful when employed in conjunction with persuasion and guidance aimed at helping the patient live with his problem and avoid situations that arouse conflicts.

Desensitization, in which the patient is exposed to graded degrees of anxiety-producing situations, can be useful, as can the production of experimental neuroses.

Hypnosis may be used with advantage to facilitate ventilation and confession and to uncover forbidden impulses. Recall under hypnosis, with or without age regression, is another useful approach.

With very neurotic individuals, psychoanalysis, with or without hypno-analytic techniques, may be the only solution.

While there can be one session "cures," the treatment of psychosomatic disorders (and this will be true of other disorders to be discussed) most often requires an appreciable number of sessions, many of which will not involve the use of hypnotism, or only to a very small extent. A typical treatment might start out with two or three sessions free of hypnotism. The next one or two sessions might be devoted to introducing the patient to hypnosis and training him. The last of these sessions, or the following one, might then be used to show the patient how determinants he is not aware of ("his unconscious") can produce somatic effects. For example, a posthypnotic glove anesthesia might be induced. This might be followed up, in another session, by the production of an artificial conflict to relate more definitely the previous demonstration to his problem and to allow him to recognize the basis of the disorder. With the patient now open to the possibility that his problem has emotional roots, free association under hypnosis might be tried over several more sessions. By now, some transference should be manifesting itself, and a superficial analysis of it will be made. On the basis of material obtained from the free association, the therapist may proceed to stimulate recall of past experiences by suggesting hypermnesia or inducing age regressions. Sessions that follow might then be used for ventilation, more recall and insight, and for doing some interpretation and guidance. This work will be done with and without hypnosis being induced. A dozen sessions may be required. With highly neurotic individuals, a more prolonged psychoanalytic treatment may be embarked upon in which the various hypnoanalytic procedures discussed earlier can be used.

Conversion Neuroses

These have traditionally been considered highly responsive to hypnotic interventions. The symptoms are easily removed by authoritarian suggestions, but, unless further psychotherapy of the type used with character disorders follows, the symptoms have a tendency to come back. As with psychosomatic symptoms, the choice of organ involved in hysterical conversions is now believed also to be partly determined by constitutional organ weaknesses, but more so by fixations in childhood and, sometimes, identification with an ailing significant figure. Repression is the characteristic mode of solving conflicts employed by hysterics and, in general, the patient uses conversion symptoms both as a means of expression and as a defense against inner unacceptable strivings that have to be repressed. Treatment, therefore, needs to focus on the adaptive role played by the symptoms. Treatment must also take into account that hysterics tend to act out their personal conflicts and demands. In many instances, secondary gains must be considered in the treatment, too. Long term re-educative and psychoanalytic treatment, supported with hypnotic intervention, are recommended in conjunction with symptom removal.

Anxiety Hysteria

Phobias are the main expression of this disorder. In general, phobias do not respond well to authoritative suggestions. Re-educative or psychoanalytic treatment using hypnoanalytic techniques is necessary.

It is important to keep in mind that some phobias arise out of a conditioning-like situation. For these, the use of a reconditioning and desensitization through repeated and gradual exposure to the object of the phobia is the treatment of choice. Sometimes, recalling the traumatic experience under hypnosis and reevaluating it in terms of current understanding will be a successful approach. A method that can be very effective for discovering the origins of phobias is to age regress the patient to a time before the phobia appeared. The patient is then progressively moved forward in time to later life stages until the phobia develops.

Follow-up therapy aimed at reorganizing the patient's personality may be necessary when the phobia is related to character patterns that originated early in his life.

Compulsion Neuroses (Obsessive-Compulsive Neuroses)

These are among the most difficult disorders to treat. The character structure of obsessive-compulsive individuals is such that they may strongly resist becoming hypnotized. Teaching self-hypnosis as a first step will sometimes get around this initial resistance. Wolberg (1948) recommends using a directive re-educational approach along psychoanalytic lines, with guidance, persuasion, and reassurance used in and out of hypnosis. "Thought switching," in which the patient is made to switch to other subject matters when he begins to obsess, has been found to be useful. Thought stopping may also be effective.

Traumatic Neuroses (Post-traumatic Stress Syndrome)

Although they can grow out of a single highly traumatic event, most cases involve an individual who has gone through a series of stressful events to the point that his adaptive resources are nearly exhausted, and who then is confronted with one more highly stressful situation. This is essentially a case of the proverbial straw that broke the camel's back. Traumatic neuroses may be acute or chronic. Chronic cases are usually more difficult to treat than acute ones because the symptom has had a chance to become entrenched and to become reinforced by secondary gains.

It is generally agreed that individuals with neurotic tendencies superimpose the neurotic reactions that are characteristic of their habitual modes of response to anxiety upon those responses that are specific of the stress syndrome. Thus, phobic, compulsive, and conversion symptoms may be seen in traumatic neuroses as well as the more characteristic symptoms of irritability, nervousness, insomnia, and others.

Post-traumatic stress syndromes have traditionally been found very responsive to hypnotic interventions. Hypnotic symptom removal can be very effective. Intensifying, diminishing, removing, and transferring somatic symptoms to other body locations, and teaching the patient to do this through autosuggestion, is a useful technique, presumably because it reduces the patient's feelings of helplessness.

Uncovering techniques are indicated when anxiety is extreme. Removing amnesias and allowing the patient to relive the traumatic incidents is a particularly effective approach with acute cases. However, reliving under hypnosis does not necessarily mean acceptance of the event. Furthermore, having accepted the event under hypnosis, it may remain for the patient also to accept it in his normal state. Various hypnoanalytic techniques discussed earlier, such as dramatization, regression, and automatic writing are useful here. Usually the above processes must be repeated a number of times.

Further therapy normally needs to follow symptom removal, just as in other situations. Hypnotism associated with a re-educational approach using psychoanalytic insight is useful.

Character (Personality) Disorders

Possibly because they are too deeply ingrained, hypnotism does not appreciably help the therapy of these disorders.

Individuals with character disorders who seek hypnotic treatment are poor prospects. They often use the patient/therapist relation to satisfy their neurotic needs. The first aim of hypnotic intervention, if it is attempted, should be in solidifying the patient/therapist relation. Analytic probing and interpretation should be avoided at the start and should not be done until much later, after a positive transference has been established without analysis of its source.

Transient Situational Disturbances

Hypnotism can be used with advantage in the overall treatment of this kind of disorder. A supportive and re-educational approach is often all that is required.

Depressions

In general I have not found hypnotism to be particularly useful with depressions. The reactive depressions (depressive neuroses) are one exception. Hypnotism with a supportive and re-educational approach can be quite effective in these cases. Where deep rooted conflicts are involved some reconstructive therapy may be indicated. With very depressed persons antidepressants are useful at the beginning of therapy.

Case Examples

Case of J.B.

This is the case of a Vietnam War veteran who was a Caucasian in his late twenties and an inpatient on a psychiatric unit. He had a severe sleep disturbance. After falling asleep, he would frequently get up extremely agitated, ometimes several times during the night, and would move about wildly, running blindly into objects and walls. He had suffered fairly serious injuries in this process. This action was always accompanied by loud unintelligible vocalization. Every night he had to be placed in restraints. He had no memory of his sleep activities and could not report any dreams. His war records showed that he had been an officer and had been in charge of a platoon that had been ambushed in the jungles, and that he had been one of the few survivors. J.B. had no memory of this incident, and it was assumed that his sleep problem was related to it. It was also noted that when J.B. did sleep without attacks, he could not report ever having any dreams. At the time I was consulted about the case, the problem had progressed to the point that, unless kept constantly active, he would fall asleep during the day and immediately have one of his typical attacks. I had the occasion to witness one of his day attacks shortly after I had trained him to go into hypnosis. At the time, I was doing EEG research on hypnotism, and I invited the patient to participate in it. The attack occurred while J.B. was in the subject room and I was in the instrument room. An intercom connected the two rooms. Two video cameras gave me a good view of the subject. I had placed the electrodes on his head and was making preliminary adjustments and tests. He was not hypnotized as yet. The first intimation I had that J.B. had had an attack came from an abrupt change in the EEG; it showed the appearance of sleep. Nearly simultaneously, I heard over the intercom what sounded like loud cursing. I looked at one of the monitors and saw J.B. lurching out of his chair. Fortunately, I had with me in the instrument room a resident who was quite husky, and with his help, it was possible to subdue J.B. and prevent him from harming himself until he "woke" up. Although J.B. could normally go into a hypnotic state at a signal, this was found to be totally ineffective during the attack. Moreover, no communication of any kind was possible at such a time. Apparently, the patient had dozed off during the short time I was making adjustments, and the attack had followed. That the signal to enter hypnosis was ineffective is a good indication that the state J.B. was in was not his normal state. Going by the EEG changes, I observed that it was not distinguishable from natural sleep. I must, however, qualify this statement. The electrodes became immediately disconnected, so there could have been a further EEG change that remained unobserved. This might have shown that he was no longer in a sleep state during the attack. I suspect his EEG would, at that point, have been more like a waking EEG.

The patient was readily hypnotized. Because of the connection between sleep and the attacks, I trained J.B. to go into an active hypnosis. A sleep induction was too likely to trigger an attack.

Following up on an old idea that sleepwalking is the motoric equivalent of dreaming, my first efforts in treating J.B. were to suggest that he would dream whatever he was reenacting, and no longer have to get up and move. This was unsuccessful and, in fact, not even fragments of dreams could be produced. I decided to attempt an indirect age regression. I emphasized to J.B. that he would remain hypnotized at all times and would at no time go to sleep. I then told him that, when I gave him the signal to do so, he would have a dream-like experience that would cease instantly if I squeezed his right shoulder in a certain way that I demonstrated. I also told him that as the experience evolved, he would describe it to me. It was next specified that the dream-like experience would be of being in the jungles in Vietnam with his platoon. I again reiterated that no matter how dream-like the experience was, he would at no time fall asleep. I also made it clear that he would not be dreaming as a person does when he is asleep. The signal to have the dream experience was given. Not only did J.B. find himself in the jungles as described, but he spontaneously went back to the ambush, which he was able to describe in the first person in some detail with a show of only moderate emotions. Although J.B. usually had spontaneous posthypnotic amnesia, I still made sure that he would have amnesia for the experience by suggesting it. The session was repeated a number of times on successive days; then it was suggested that he might begin to have similar dreams in his sleep at night. At this point, I had to go out of town for about a week, and on my return, I was advised that J.B. had left the hospital AMA, leaving no forwarding address. I never saw J.B. again, but about a year later he visited the psychiatrist under whose charge he had been and reported that he was totally free of his former problem and had been so for some time. I can only surmise that J.B.'s experience in hypnosis was able to desensitize him. Had he remained in treatment, I might have gone on eventually to a full age regression.

Case of C.E.

This is the case of a 25-year-old married Caucasian female, with one male child, who had asked to be admitted by Agnew State Hospital (California) in early 1957 for psychiatric treatment. She had presented herself with a long list of symptoms that she had had for many years and that had been getting progressively worse since her marriage seven years earlier. These symptoms included recurrent attacks of shaking, dizziness, fainting and blackouts, headaches, enuresis, spasms, nausea and vomiting, nervousness, and a lump on her back. The sound of sirens was also particularly disturbing for her, and she was said to have had a phobia for ambulances and hearses. C.E. also had a nearly complete amnesia with regard to the events that had occurred during the first five-and-a-half years of her life. This included not being able to recall what her father looked like. The one memory she had of that time was of seeing her father at the hospital shortly before his death, lying pale and weak in his bed. She had been admitted with the diagnosis of psychoneurosis, probably an anxiety neurosis, with depression and psychosomatic complaints. It was also noted that she had a marked tendency to "blow up," but not to the point of being labeled an explosive personality.

The patient had a five-and-a-half year old boy. Her marriage had never been satisfactory, and there had been a seven-month separation, during which she had filed for divorce. There had been a reconciliation, but the marital relationship did not appear to be much improved at the time I entered the case. She described her husband as being insensitive, uncaring, and taking no notice of her. She cared for her son, but appeared to be overly punitive of him and treated him harshly at times.

The patient had one slightly older and one slightly younger sister and a younger brother. She also had a number of half-siblings, several of whom were illegitimate children of her mother. Of the four children, she was the only one that looked like her mother.

Her mother had been a very poor housekeeper and was sick much of the time, with the result that the patient was, as a child, responsible for doing many household chores, including taking care of her younger siblings. She seemed to have considered this to be her duty.

The patient's father, who was a well-driller and maintenance man, had unexpectedly died from a perforated ulcer at age 32, when she was five-and-a-half years old. Shortly after the death, she and her sisters were boarded for awhile in a convent that served as a school for Indians (the children had Indian blood), then came back to live with the mother, and eventually went to live with relatives, among whom they were divided. C.E. lived with her paternal aunt, her aunt's husband, and their son (her cousin), who was three years her senior. This happened somewhere between the ages of 7 and 10.

During the first 7 to 10 years of her life, the patient had grown up in a small Oklahoma community in an economically impoverished environment. She lived in the poor section of town in a rather rough neighborhood where street gangs roamed. Her relatives on her father's side were appreciably better off economically, and may have paid to send the children to the convent. Shortly afterward, the patient had moved in with her relatives, who had resettled in California and into a more salubrious environment.

The patient was apparently a difficult child to raise. She was stubborn and rebellious. Her relationship to her father was rather stormy. She had considerable difficulty with her aunt, who did not approve of her; she was very demanding of her and used her as a maid. Further, the aunt appears to have abused her. She got along well with her uncle, but had a difficult time with her cousin. She had two other aunts, with whom she appeared to have a good relationship. At the time of her admission, C.E. was also having difficulties in relating to both her mother-in-law and her sister-in-law. She also had always related poorly to her younger sister.

The patient's married sex life had been of poor quality and had continued to be so when she was home on weekend passes. Growing up, she had been involved in a great deal of sexual experimentation with other children. Her mother had been quite promiscuous after her husband's death, and C.E. had been exposed, for awhile, to considerable sexual activity in the home. There is a possibility that some of her mother's male friends may have attempted to have relations with her. She claimed that a 32-year-old man had once made sexual advances toward her when she was seven. Her male cousin had persistently made sexual advances toward her from the time she had come to live with her relatives to the time she had married at age 18.

Much of this data was pieced together from information obtained over a period of five months in interviews with the patient and in one interview with her paternal aunt. There were many confused statements and inconsistencies in some of the statements made by C.E. during the first two months after her admission to the hospital. At first, C.E. tended to be circumstantial and vague, especially about her feelings. Also, because of her amnesia, C.E.'s accounts about her early childhood (before age six) were largely secondhand; they were based upon what she had heard her paternal aunt say. Overall, the above is, nevertheless, a fairly accurate account.

This case was part of a sample of individuals believed to suffer from double-anniversary reactions. They were being studied as part of a project by Josephine Hilgard, M.D., a psychiatrist and psychoanalyst (and wife of my associate, Ernest R. Hilgard, Ph.D.). The patient was not undergoing psychotherapy with Hilgard; all therapy was being done by the hospital staff and, to some degree, by a social worker attached to the project. In fact, C.E. had never met Hilgard; all pertinent personal data was collected entirely by the social worker.

I will explain, since this is not a widely known syndrome, that the double-anniversary reaction consists of the following: an individual, permanently separated at a young age from a parent who usually died or had to be institutionalized, develops, in turn, a serious illness when he/she reaches the approximate age that the parent was when the separation took place; furthermore, there is a child who is the same age as he/she was at the time. Thus, the "double" qualification. In C.E.'s case, she had been about five-and-a-half years old when her father, who was 32, had died of a perforated ulcer, and she had a son five-and-a-half years old. Additionally, shortly after her father's death, she had been boarded in a convent by her twenty-nine year old mother, and then had gone to live with her paternal aunt and her husband. She had never seen her mother again. From the standpoint of a traumatic separation, there were thus two possible bases for the reaction.

Hilgard's reason for bringing me into the case was the possibility that I might be able to lift the patient's childhood amnesia by using hypnotic techniques. This might uncover data useful to her study. This amnesia was most likely linked with her father's death and her own symptoms. I felt that merely lifting the amnesia outside of a therapeutic context was not to C.E.'s best interest, and could easily be anti-therapeutic. On the other hand, it seemed a reasonable step to undertake as part of her therapy. I therefore agreed to attempt it, but I also stipulated that this would have to be done within a psychotherapeutic framework, and that I would have to be free to proceed as I saw fit. With this understood, my work with the patient began.

This case was, incidentally, my first clinical case, as well as my first use of hypnotism as a primary mode of treatment. It was Josephine Hilgard's first exposure to a hypnopsychotherapy.

I began to work with C.E. three months after her admission. Until then, she had had weekly sessions with the social worker. These were continued, and usually came the day after my sessions with her. At that point, there had been no progress in her condition. I saw the patient for a total of 15 sessions. There were two the first week. Thereafter, they were weekly, except toward the end, when two were done in one day. Most sessions ran an hour, but a number ran two hours and longer.

With the exception of a few sessions, Hilgard and I jointly saw the patient; I conducted the hypnotherapy, and she usually took notes. On occasions, Hilgard would ask some questions or interject comments. The sessions were usually followed by a short discussion period between the two of us.

The detailed collected data, of which the above history is a summary, constitutes a fascinating document that contains a great deal of material pertinent to the etiology of C.E.'s symptoms. It is also of interest from a psychoanalytic standpoint. Very little of this material was, however, pertinent to her treatment, for reasons that will become clear.

One aspect of the patient, also revealed by her history, was that she was basically an angry woman who usually felt obliged to contain her anger. The data suggested that her inability to express anger was associated with at least some of her somatic problems, especially the dizziness and fainting spells. To some extent, the patient seemed to recognize this, but it was my impression that many of the attacks had occurred when the patient was not aware of it. In contrast, there seemed to have been a great deal of acting out her part as a child. Exploring her inability to express anger and giving her some means of expressing it seemed to be another indicated step in her therapy.

I believe it will be instructive to briefly review each of the sessions.

Session 1. The first session was primarily aimed at getting acquainted with C.E., preparing her for work with hypnotism, and getting some idea of her hypnotizability. For this purpose, I began with the Postural Sway Test, to which C.E. gave an extremely strong and quasi-immediate response and showed evidence of entering a state of hypnosis without eye closure or sleep signs taking place. I conducted her to a chair and asked her to sit down and close her eyes. A successful Eye Catalepsy Test followed, and I then used a Visual Fixation Induction with suggestions of sleep. Five minutes later, the patient was showing all of the typical outward signs of being asleep, and she passed the Arm Rigidity Test when administered. I gave her the posthypnotic suggestion that she would reenter a hypnotic state whenever I said the word "sleep" and snapped my fingers. The patient was then to return to her normal state. She did so slowly and with some apparent difficulty. Having opened her eyes, she appeared somewhat disoriented, and she expressed her surprise at having gone to sleep. She also spontaneously gave evidence of the presence of a non-suggested amnesia.

I decided to follow this initial success with a Hand Levitation Induction, but could not obtain a hand or arm movement. However, within two minutes of fixating a spot on the wall, she was back into another hypnotic state. While the patient was in this state, I explained to her that she was in a sleep different from natural sleep; one in which she would be able to do various things, such as have dreams and communicate with Dr. Hilgard and me. The session was then brought to a close.

I will make several comments regarding the above. I did not have a broad basis for estimating C.E.'s hypnotizability, but she had shown a spontaneous posthypnotic amnesia, and this was a strong indicator that she was probably capable of developing a somnambulistic state. Her response to the Postural Sway suggestions and to the Visual Fixation Technique supported this hypothesis. I did not test the posthypnotic suggestion for reinduction I had given her. I cannot say for certain why I did not. Frequently, if I have some doubts about how effective it will be, I postpone such a suggestion until the next session. This is because it will become better incorporated, and because some type of consolidation will take place between the current and the next session. It is also my practice to introduce, early in my work with subjects, signals for reinduction for future use. I do not test them right away when I feel fairly certain they will be effective. This was my expectation in the case of C.E. It is also my practice to introduce the subject or patient to more than one induction procedure, especially to one active form and one passive form; this is why I attempted to do a Hand Levitation Test. It could have waited until the next session, but I had the time, so I did it then. I did not feel that its failure was of great concern or significance at the time. Indeed, it was not a total failure because the patient reported experiencing unusual feelings in her hand. Finally, I find it useful to educate my patients regarding what to expect of hypnosis in both their normal state and when they are hypnotized. Doing so in the hypnotic state allows me to capitalize on their increased suggestibility, and thus give them indirect suggestions regarding their future behavior.

Session 2. Hypnosis was reinduced, using, among other methods, the command "sleep" combined with the finger snap. This session (as well as the third and fourth ones) was partially devoted to helping the patient rapidly attain a deep hypnosis, partly by means of repeated dehypnotization and rehypnotization (Fractionation Technique). Various suggestibility tests that have been described in Volume 1 were administered. C.E. passed the majority of these tests; she would have easily scored maximum on the Stanford Scales forms A or B had these been available at that time, and she would have been considered a "deep" subject. A portion of the session (as was the case with most others) was also devoted to working with the patient in her normal state. In the session with the social worker, which followed this one, the patient stated that since starting her work with me, she had become much more relaxed.

Session 3. This session was partly a continuation of the previous one, but in it I also began to explore her ability to dream. Dreaming was introduced and used extensively in the therapy, partly because I was then convinced, as I still am, that dreams represent a powerful means of exploration that allow the therapist to get in touch with unconscious material in a relatively non-traumatic way for the patient. They often provide repeatable experiences that can be used for desensitization. I also viewed dreams evoked by suggestion as an excellent way for patients to work through conflictual material and release suppressed emotional energy. In C.E.'s case, I was also aware that she claimed to have very few dreams, and that she had a great deal of difficulty expressing anger through means other than her symptoms. It seemed to me that guiding her toward dreaming might offer her relief in this area. I also saw dreaming as a potential and non-traumatic way of recovering some of the lost memories; it would also be a good preparation to an eventual age regression to the time of her father's death. I was able to use dreams with C.E. in all of these ways.

Session 4. This session was a mixture of work in and out of hypnosis and a continuation of the work done in the previous sessions. Nothing remarkable occurred. It was also agreed with the patient that we would work with her another two months, after which she was to be discharged.

Session 5. The patient was asked to have dreams relating to various childhood incidents. These were short, fragmentary, and generally not particularly revealing. I was not aiming for more than this; my intent was mainly to explore what C.E. was capable of doing and also to guide her in this direction.

Session 6. The patient reported to the social worker that she had had two dizzy spells during the week, but that this occurrence had bothered her less than usual. The session began with an exploration in her normal state of what anger meant to her. She said that she was afraid of getting angry because of what she might do to others, and she therefore held her anger in.

She stated that if she let go, she would "beat'em to a pulp." She had been particularly frightened about hurting her child, on whom she had, at times, abusively taken out the anger she felt toward others. Her history showed that she had not, invariably, been unable to express her anger, but that she had often expressed it ineffectively. Also, more often than not, she had been the victim of angry attacks by others; she had accepted these passively, even when they were brutal. For example, when she was 18, her paternal aunt had angrily knocked her down over a small incident and "stomped on my head." The patient had apparently made no attempt to defend herself. As the picture evolved, it became clear that C.E. had often felt anger at her mother and her sisters; there was strong sibling rivalry. She also felt unwanted and discriminated against; she was blamed for what others had done, both at home and when she was living with her aunt and uncle.

What was left of the session was briefly used to introduce the patient to age regressions. A regression was used successfully to explore an incident in which, in anger, she had thrown a rock toward her mother.

In ending the session, I instructed the hypnotized patient that, during the week, she would have many thoughts about her childhood; she would be able to remember many forgotten events. Some would be happy ones, others would be about angry moments. It was also suggested that she would have a dream about being angry, and that she would be able to tell us about the dream during the next session. The dream would have something to do with her current problems and what anger meant to her, particularly why she feared to be angry. It was added that she would not understand what the dream meant, but that later she would be helped to understand it.

Session 7. Until now, C.E.'s condition had shown no significant change. The week that followed the fifth session was marked by a substantial increase in "black outs."

The patient reported having had two dreams: one that she remembered and one that she could not, and that had to be recovered under hypnosis. Both were explored at some length. In the first dream, the patient recalled, in some detail, an incident that had taken place when she was 17 in which, contrary to the way she had invariably presented herself as being a victim, she recognized that she had been the agent provocateur.

Session 8. In sharp contrast to the previous week, the one that followed this session was noted by the social worker as showing a definite improvement in the patient's overall condition. C.E. felt more relaxed and was relatively free of fainting spells and dizziness, and she was less concerned about them when they occurred. She was relating better to her husband, and she had been able to be more assertive toward him.

The session began with C.E. saying, "I haven't had any trouble at all this week." She then reported having had two dreams, the second coming right after the other. The first of these appears to have been a transference dream, and needs no further discussion. In the second dream, the patient found herself able to reverse roles with her aunt. Her memory of the dream was fragmentary. Reporting it, she said, "I was with my Aunt. A puzzle had been dropped on the floor. She told me to pick it up, and I wondered why I should be the one to do it, so I said I wouldn't. She picked up a stick to spank me, but I didn't let her. I thought, 'Why should I let her do the switching?' I used the switch on her." Commenting spontaneously on the dream, the patient added, "A dream is the only place you can hurt people and yet not hurt them." This was said with pleasure. She went on, "This was the first time in my dream [meaning in any dream] I ever got back at her . . . I feel pretty good about that dream . . . I don't know what her reaction would be, but I'd like to say it . . . she would be stunned. Guess she thought I was scared of her, but I wasn't. I was afraid of what I would do to her."

A little later, C.E. informed me that she had never previously dreamed about her aunt. Her aunt, she added, did not like her mother and had gotten even with her by beating the patient. She remarked that her aunt had been no better than her mother, in that she, too, had been promiscuous while being separated from her husband when C.E. was 14.

Even later, the patient was regressed to the time of her dream and allowed to relive it. This permitted us to obtain missing details, such as that in the dream, it was her male cousin who had thrown the puzzle to the floor in anger over her being better at it. In the dream, her Aunt had managed to hit her twice before she had snatched the stick away and used it on her tormentor.

I ended the session by telling C.E. that during the week, she would have dreams relating to forgotten things from her childhood that have bothered her. She was also told that she would be able to talk more freely about matters that might be embarrassing, painful, fearful, or just silly. Her ability to assert herself about making decisions and carrying them out would improve, especially when she was home on weekends. She would take more initiative in matters important to her, such as her child and her home.

The dream about the aunt was clearly a cathartic dream in which the patient was able to express her anger at being unfairly hurt. In the dream she could also retaliate, and discovered that this could be done without inflicting irreparable damage. In talking to the social worker the next day, C.E. said that her dream action had been something she had always wanted to do. She had felt 100% better after it was over. The patient then spoke enthusiastically about her dream experiences in general. They were being very helpful by letting her have experiences that she could never allow herself to have. The experiences she referred to included such things as dancing and skiing. Another detail that emerged from the exploration of the dream was the patient's ambivalence toward her slightly older male cousin, with whom she had lived. This was related to an earlier dream, in which her cousin had placed a dead snake around her neck. There were clear indications that there had probably been sexual feelings involved in their relationship, on her part as well as his.

Session 9. Additional details from the social worker's session of the week included remarks made by the patient indicating that her sex life had greatly improved. She was also experiencing more freedom to talk about her feelings with the social worker.

As the session began, the patient stated that the ward psychiatrist, under whose care she was, had told her that if she continued to progress as she had, she could be discharged in about a month. She was greatly pleased by this. She had now had two "good" weeks, with no fainting spells. She continued to feel calmer, and attributed this to the hypnosis and to being able to talk about many feelings. She felt that she had been able to get a lot of things "off her chest" that had been building up for a long time. She said, "I'm able to empty a lot now." She then remarked that she had had more dreams and that she had never dreamed as much in her entire life.

Work was done with the dream material she reported, and also with some that were induced in the session. These were largely unpleasant dreams of being pursued, attacked, and threatened with knives, but with no ill outcomes. In one of the dreams, she disarmed her assailant, using ju jitsu, and took possession of the knife. During the session, when told to dream about something unpleasant, she again dreamed of her cousin placing the snake around her neck. In associating to the dream material, she was able to recall a number of frightening incidents that had happened to her around the age of seven, and, in particular, of an attempted molestation by a neighbor. I ended the session by giving the hypnotized patient ego-strengthening suggestions as well as suggestions that she would recover more and more of her childhood memories and be able to talk about them with her therapists.

It is clear that fear of aggression from and toward others was a most important issue for the patient. There was also increasing indications that the sexual aspect of aggression was an important feature. In the past, she had felt impotent in controlling aggression, and was very fearful of the outcome. Now we saw evidence that she perceived that the outcome did not have to be disastrous, and that she was beginning to feel capable of controlling aggression. Taking the knife away from her assailant reminded us of her taking the stick away from her aunt in the dream of the last session. Her dream experience of learning and using ju jitsu could be interpreted as expressing a recognition that she is learning new, more satisfactory ways of dealing with aggression.

Session 10. The patient reported that she had two attacks of dizziness during the week.

Part of this session was spent talking about a dream the patient had in which her sister had hit her on the head with a hammer. She then recalled an incident in which she had thrown a brick at her mother when threatened by her with a spanking for fighting with her brother over the ownership of a dog. Most of the session, however, was used to get C.E. to recall what her father had looked like. Direct suggestions to see her father failed, and I decided to induce a regression dream that would take the patient back to a time prior to her father's death. The particular aim was to have her describe him. It was suggested that she would have a dream in which she was back to a time when she was playing in the backyard while her father was working there. (This was suggested on the assumption that this would most likely have actually taken place at one time or another.) She had no difficulty going back to such an instance, but in this experience, her father was watering flowers and had his back turned toward her. She was allowed to live through some of this experience in the hope that at some point her father would face her, and she would see his face. When this did not happen, I decided to force the issue, and told her that her father was turning around and looking at her. When I asked her what he looked like from the front, C.E. stated that he did not have a face! This situation remained in spite of my suggestions that features were now appearing on the face. Taking this as a warning that C.E. was not yet ready for it, I did not push the matter, and I terminated the session by only giving her suggestions of continuing improvement and that soon she would be able to see her father as she had known him when a child.

Following this session, there was a meeting to discuss the case. It included Hilgard, the social worker assigned to C.E., a psychiatric social worker also attached to the project, and myself. All participants had a psychoanalytic orientation, and the discussion was largely within this framework. There was general agreement that in spite of the patient being a highly hypnotizable person, we were, at best, tapping preconscious material, and this raised questions about the nature of the powerful repression surrounding her life when her father had been alive. The only breakthrough the amnesic barrier had been of when she had last seen him in the hospital when he was dying.

There were many speculations. The consensus was that there might have been an incestuous relationship or a sexual approach made by her father. A fair amount of data, some of which I have not detailed, could be found in the material obtained in the sessions and in the interviews in support of this hypothesis. I will not go further into the matter, since, as we shall see, this did not affect the way the remainder of the therapy proceeded; a rather different answer eventually evolved.

It was also considered that possibly the patient was not as deeply hypnotized as I believed she was, and that some of her productions were role-playing.

If so, everyone agreed that her responses had nevertheless had abreactive value. Someone also asked whether it might not be useful to further relieve the patient of the responsibility for what she remembered. Less responsibility would presumably mean less guilt.

Session 11. With the patient in her normal state, this session was partly devoted to reviewing and discussing various topics relevant to her past and future and her ways of dealing with life situations. Her discharge plans were also discussed briefly. It is not clear from my notes why this was done at that time. It is not uncommon for me to use sessions at intervals in the course of a therapy to review what has been accomplished and what remains to be done. The patient's attitude was rather passive throughout this part of the session.

During the remainder of the session, C.E. reported that she had had two dreams. In one, she was a child who had lost a baseball and had looked for it at night with a flashlight borrowed from a man. In the other, she was drowning in a creek. The patient later related the latter dream to a real incident in which she had nearly drowned trying to get her younger sister out of a pond in which she had fallen while skating.

What was left of the session was used to try a different approach to lifting the amnesia surrounding her life with her father. C.E. was hypnotized. Following a hunch that anger might be a factor involved in the amnesia, I asked her to dream about a little girl who is angry at her father. She dreamed about herself at the age of five; her father told her to do the dishes, but she refused and walked away. Then she was told to come back. She also refused to do this, and was spanked by her father. Through all this, the father remained an amorphous figure.

Still trying to find a way to get around the repression, I decided to try another approach. I asked C.E. to create in her imagination a five year old girl and describe her to me. She had no problem doing this, and described the child as blond, blue-eyed, rather tall and slender, and wearing a pink dress and black patent leather shoes. Her name, she said, was Betty. I told C.E. that we would talk later about Betty, and I terminated the session. Incidentally, the patient, as a child, had dark hair and brown eyes.

My expectation was that the patient would unconsciously identify with the imagined child. It would then be possible to deal with some of the repressed material more easily because this would place a psychological distance between her and the events that I hoped the imagined child could experience.

Session 12. The patient reported that she had two "passout spells" during the week while at the hospital. However, one of these spells was really an episode of dizziness. The patient also had been nauseated for about two days. Neither incident seemed related to the previous session.

Knowing that the patient's younger sister was named Betty, I asked her to describe her. As I expected, the description was that of the previously imagined child. C.E. had no recollection of having described her in the previous session.

The patient was hypnotized and told to see Betty again. Asked whom she reminded C.E. of, she replied, "My sister." She added, on further questioning, that she thought the child was her sister. In answer to the question of why she had chosen her in response to my instruction, she said, "She was a very pretty little girl . . . Because I wasn't." We talked a little more about her sister and her feelings toward her, then I told the patient that the Betty she now saw was actually not her sister, but was just a little girl named Betty, and that because she existed only in her imagination, she could do anything, good or bad, without there being consequences. "Anything can happen in a dream." I added, "She can grow up or she can be younger. Because it's a dream, no one is responsible for what happens in it. While you dream, you will forget who you are, and you will only think of Betty. Betty can do anything, anything can happen to Betty. No harm can happen because it is all a dream. What happens to Betty happens only to Betty."

As will be obvious to the reader, I was still hoping that C.E. would identify with Betty, and that because of the context in which the Betty experience was being placed, she would be able to allow Betty to have the experiences she had so strongly repressed. I deliberately retained Betty as she was first created because she is also a daughter of the patient's father, and I felt that this would promote a fusion of C.E. and Betty. I also felt that the choice of Betty, rather than her older sister or some unrelated child, must have had a special significance.

Having thus set the stage, I went on to suggest, in a non-specific way, a number of events in which Betty was involved, some involving good experiences, others bad ones. I will not report on all of these, but only on those that I consider significant. One suggested experience was that of Betty doing something with her (Betty's) father. This could be real or imaginary. C.E. saw Betty and her father working together in a garden. They were planting flowers. Betty was five or six. Her father told her to be careful not to walk on the flowers that had been planted. Betty was happy because she liked planting flowers. At this point, I asked what Betty's father looked like. "He is tall, has blond, no, light brown hair, and hazel eyes. He is young." More followed regarding something else Betty did with her father, but that was not particularly significant.

The particular significance is that C.E. had finally been able to describe her father as he did look.

Session 13. Between the last session and the present one, an important development had taken place. The aunt and uncle who raised C.E. from the time she was about seven were interviewed by the social worker. They revealed that C.E.'s father was either sitting or lying down by his three daughters on their bed before they went to sleep when he had his fatal ulcer attack. The aunt described her brother as handsome, big, broad-shouldered, slim hips, 6 ft. 1 in., with wavy light brown hair, brown eyes, and weighing about 185 lbs. None of this was repeated to C.E.; however, she was shown a black-and-white picture of her father that the aunt had brought with her. She showed no signs of recognition. Much additional and useful background material was, of course, also obtained.

This session was the first of two sessions that we had with C.E. that day. This one was in the morning. C.E. mentioned that she knew that her aunt, uncle, and husband had been interviewed. She said that she had asked the social worker some questions regarding what had been said, but had been told that the material was confidential. It is interesting that she made no mention of seeing her father's picture, and this was not mentioned by us.

C.E. was to be discharged at the end of the week (three days later), and there were a number of things that needed to be discussed that were not directly relevant to the work that I had been doing with her. After this discussion took place, the rest of the morning session centered around issues relating to her discipline as a child and her role in the discipline of her son.

Session 14. This was the afternoon session. By now it had become clear that her amnesia prior to age 6 centered around memories relating to her father. Until now, very little basis had been found for it. The information obtained from the aunt pointed to the strong possibility that something had happened in the bedroom that had made the ulcer attack particularly traumatic for C.E. Granted, he had died from it, and she had been with him when he was suddenly taken ill, but this did not seem to be sufficient cause for her to become amnesic for all events leading to and including this. With only one more session available to me, I decided to go specifically after this information. I hypnotized C.E. and had her dream that Betty had gone to bed and that her father had come into the room to keep her company until she fell asleep. I then added that anything can happen in a dream and that no one can get hurt, because it is a dream. This resulted in an innocuous dream of the father telling a bedtime story.

I again told C.E. that she would dream about Betty, but that this time I would tell her about some of the things that were happening. Furthermore, since it was her dream, she would fit these things into it, adding or subtracting details that her mind would provide. I now said that Betty had two sisters, and that all three were in the same bed but not ready to sleep yet. I then described the father coming into the room to quiet them down, and then lying next to them. Next, he was described as feeling ill, with a pain that grew progressively worse. Until then, C.E. had not particularly reacted. Suddenly she said quite distinctly, as if questioning someone, "You say it is bedtime?"

To my inquiry as to what was going on, she said, "We are playing games . . . They're supposed to be in bed, but they're not. He puts them in there, but they're not staying."

This is about all that I could get from her. Several more similar attempts were made, but she was not able to go beyond the sisters playing or quarreling and the father coming in to restore order and quiet the children. The dreams never evolved to the point of the father lying next to his daughters. On two occasions, I asked C.E. whether she remembered my telling her the father would lie down and become ill; she answered, "no." This was evidence of significant denial. In any case, I did not force this issue. In terminating the session, I suggested that no matter how painful it might be, she would have a dream during the night of the kind I had suggested in this session. She was also instructed to remember the dream after waking, to tell the social worker about it, and to report it to us in the next, and final session.

Session 15. This session was two days after the last one. The patient reported that she generally felt good since our last session; that is, until last night. She had a headache and felt tired during the day and felt faint while eating supper. That night, she had a comical dream in which she had laughed. We did not discuss the dream, and I went ahead and hypnotized her.

I now said to her, "That part of you that normally thinks or acts is asleep . . . that part which judges right or wrong is asleep . . . the other part is able to think . . . Because right or wrong have no meaning, then nothing can be right or wrong . . . That part of you that is normally awake is now asleep . . . the other part which knows right or wrong is gone . . . When I count three, you will find yourself like a watcher, watching . . . That part of you to which I am talking now will see a man and a woman . . . a man and a woman you do not know. They will be sitting down to eat their dinner. You are curious to see what will happen."

My intent was, as in previous sessions, to get C.E. to see, if not relive, the bedroom scene in which her father had become sick. Before doing so, I wanted her first to practice her role as a watcher; then I would bring her gradually up to watch the fatal scene. There were a number of other similar exercises. In the next one, she watched and listened through a peephole while a woman was putting a small girl to bed. Again, she watched through a peephole while a small girl was playing in a garden with a doll that she was disciplining. Presently, the child's father appeared, and she went to meet him. None of the material injected by C.E. appeared to have any connection to her past.

For the next episode, C.E. was instructed to see a room with three small girls that had gone to bed. She was only to watch and report what she saw. She gave a description of the three girls that roughly matched what we knew she and her sisters had looked like. She stated that they were respectively nine, seven, and five years of age, which was not altogether right. The girls were giggling, laughing, and playing. The father stepped in and was described as having brown hair and wearing khakis. (According to the aunt, C.E.'s father usually wore khakis.) He told the girls to go to sleep and that if he had to come in one more time, he would spank them. The father then returned to the living room where his wife was and complained of a bad headache. She gave him an aspirin. He then complained of a pain in the back; she made him lie down. The pain became worse, and a doctor was called. He examined the father briefly, then gave him some pills and gave the man a shot. The physician left, and the wife went to bed.

I started again with C.E. watching three little girls that had gone to bed but were playing instead of going to sleep. She saw the father come in and tell them to quiet down. He had a headache and did not feel well. He reclined next to the girls and began telling them the story of the three little pigs. At this point, at my request, C.E. described the girls and the father. The description matched previous descriptions. She added that the father was about 28 and very attractive. Apparently, at least two of the girls finally went to sleep, and the third one, who did not, tried to wake them up. The father became angry and told her that he would spank her if she didn't stop. At this point, he experienced a bad pain in his stomach and told the girl to get her mother. "The pain is awfully bad," he said, and a doctor was called. He diagnosed the problem as appendicitis, and the father was taken to the hospital. The problem was then diagnosed as a bad ulcer. "Where is the little girl who went to get the mother?" . . . "She's beside her Dad. She doesn't feel good. She feels bad . . . she thinks she did her Dad ill." C.E. said that an operation was performed, but the father died. Still speaking of the same little girl, she said, "She doesn't feel good. She's crying." "Does she still feel she hurt him?" I asked her. "Yes . . . because she would not go to sleep, that made him sick. Because she wouldn't mind him."

The patient was instructed to go into a deep sleep, then asked what the name of the child was. "C . . ." she answered, naming herself.

The patient was then told, "This little girl whose name is C . . . was misbehaving, but she didn't really hurt her father. It just happened. She wasn't responsible for it. Anyone could have been naughty . . . What was C . . . thinking of just before her father felt sick?" . . . "She thought maybe her Dad didn't like her . . . she was sad . . . and angry, too . . . she wished there was something she could do to make her father like her better . . . She didn't mind him like she was supposed to." When asked why she was not minding him, she answered, "She thought she'd get more attention that way." . . . "Who got the attention?" . . . "Betty . . . that made C . . . sad and mad. She felt like taking it out on Betty. Nothing she could do against her father, except not to mind him."

With a slight variation, I had C.E. go again through the above experience, with essentially the same responses. With this over and the session coming to an end, I reaffirmed that the little girl did not need to consider herself responsible for her father's death. I pointed out that whatever ill feelings she might have had toward her father, mother, or sisters could not make bad things happen to them. She was no more responsible for her father's illness than she was for the passing of the days and nights. The patient was then told that I would awaken her and that she would remember everything we had talked about today: what she had seen and heard, her sisters, herself, and her father. She would remember what her father had looked like, as well as other things. I added suggestions that she would keep improving after her discharge from the hospital, and that she would be able to handle whatever came her way.

This hypnotic session had lasted over two hours. C.E. came out of the hypnotic state slowly and with some difficulty. Her immediate comment was, "I was asleep . . . Oh." She was quiet for a few moments, then . . . "I'm awake now . . . I feel like I really slept. I feel really rested." Asked if she remembered anything about her sleep, she said, "I described what my father looked like . . . It's like the picture my aunt's got . . ." Regarding the incident in the room, she stated, "My aunt told me . . . It seemed like it was happening all over again . . . It seemed awful real." Regarding the way she had felt, she said, "Yes . . . I guess that's the way I must have felt as a kid. It seemed so real. Aunt told me that if it hadn't been for me and my mother, he wouldn't have gotten sick. Yes, I felt that way." The patient, who now looked more sober, was asked how she felt. "Relaxed, better . . . It feels like an awful load off my mind."

Epilogue. The patient was discharged the next day. She came back to the hospital a week later to see the social worker, as had been planned. She indicated that she was feeling well and that she had been quite at ease since she had been at home. There had been no further dizzy spells or other symptoms. She and her husband seemed to be getting along much better, and they had been working together in fixing up a rather dilapidated house that the husband had purchased while she was in the hospital. She appeared to be enjoying this.

She then recounted her last hypnotherapy session, and said that she finally remembered what her father had looked like. She described him and said that she no longer had any problem recalling him. She had no idea what had suddenly made it possible for her to remember how he had looked, but that after the last session, it had been possible. The only other thing she could remember about the session was that I had told her about the situation of a man who had three daughters and had asked her to describe them. She remarked that this was a situation that was comparable to her family; she had described the girls, and then, all of a sudden, it was possible for her to describe the man, too. She had no recall of how or why this had happened. She made no mention of illness or death. The interview elicited that, overall, there had been changes for the better in how the patient related to others.

It was left up to the patient to get in touch with the social worker if she wanted to do so. She did not do this, but about a year later the social worker and the patient met accidentally. The patient looked very well. She had moved into her new house, was pregnant, and was looking forward to the new child.

Further Discussion

Looking back upon this case, which was my first hypnotherapy case, I have asked myself whether I would proceed much differently today. I have decided that basically, I would not. I would not use the Postural Sway Test at the beginning, and probably not as many, if any tests of hypnotizability. I would insist on having contact with the hospital staff that worked with the patient, and I would request that I be allowed to participate in any case conference in which she was the subject matter. In the very last session, I would allow the patient to choose how much of the recovered material and of the session she would remember, and would allow her to retain nothing if this was her choice. (This may seem a peculiar step in this case, since lifting the amnesia was considered very desirable. There is, of course, a great deal of difference between an amnesia that originates in a conflict and one that does not, which is the case here. This situation is closely related to the discussion in Volume 1 of the need to distinguish amnesia as a repression phenomenon from hypnotically induced amnesias.)

There are a number of other questions one can ask. Was remembering the details of the onset of C.E.'s father's final illness crucial to the outcome of her therapy? Was remembering what her father looked like equally crucial? Was the amnesia totally lifted? To answer the last question first, we never did find out. There was no time to check this out. Regarding the first two questions, there certainly was a powerful repression centering on this event, and from this standpoint alone, one is tempted to think that lifting the amnesia partly or fully was crucial. On the other hand, the patient had certainly been showing steady progress prior to the recovery of the memories, and, possibly, would have continued to do so had we failed in this. There is no question in my mind that, quite apart from the incident of her father's death, C.E. had severe problems relating to others and with expressing anger, and this last, of course, was what I had focused on initially. This was as much a part of her therapy as was the recovery of forgotten traumatic incidents. There was a clear connection in her mind between being angry and the death of her father, and putting her guilt at rest in this matter was essential.

One can also ask how real the recovery was of the presumed lost memories. We know that she had been told by her aunt about the episode surrounding her father's collapse. She probably also had been shown her father's picture at earlier dates. My belief is that she repressed this information as soon as it became available. It is noteworthy that she had acknowledged seeing the picture of her father only after the final session.

The question had been raised earlier about whether C.E. role-played rather than had genuine experiences. It seems unlikely that she could have done it this well week after week for two months, both with us and with the social worker. Unless we take the position that her entire illness was role-played, we have her progress as evidence of the efficaciousness and, most likely, reality of the hypnotic work. It is doubtful that even a consummate actor would have been able to carry out such a charade so completely and convincingly. Finally, there is no question regarding the reality of many of the historically important elements.

Readers who have a psychoanalytic leaning or training will undoubtedly see in the above material many implications that were never touched upon in the course of therapy. One cannot help but wonder, for example, what erotic elements and fantasies may have been present in the father sharing the bed of the three daughters; not just that one, fatal time, but also at other times. What was the true nature of C.E.'s jealousy of Betty? C.E. was said to be the only one of the three daughters to be like her mother. Were C.E.'s constant battles with her father just a manifestation of being a difficult child? We also have the incident in which she reported an attempted molestation by a man of age 32 (her father's age at his time of death), which may have actually taken place, may have been a screen-memory, or, perhaps, a fantasy about her father. Sexuality was an element that frequently came up in her memories and dreams, and there is a great deal of behavior described that has both an element of masochism and of sadism. Intriguing, too, is that prior to entering the hospital, the patient and her husband had been sharing a house with her sister-in-law and her boy-friend, which was a very unsatisfactory situation for the patient, who wanted a home of her own. Her husband did not seem to care, but eventually did go ahead and purchase a house in very poor condition. She then proceeded to help him put it into shape for when she would leave the hospital. Keeping in mind the Freudian symbolism of houses, is this a remarkable acting out by the patient of her becoming better integrated and getting herself in better mental and emotional shape? It is similar to a recapitulation of the therapy. I will not pursue these aspects because, whatever the case, the therapy was not guided by them, nor was their analysis used. But, one might ask, might it not have been useful to explore these matters with the patient? I doubt it. It would certainly have taken up time that was better spent in the way I have described. Also, a psychoanalytic approach would have taken longer than the two months allotted to us.

Mine was a rather permissive therapeutic approach. Would one more authoritarian have brought about results quicker? The lifting of the amnesia could possibly have been brought about earlier had I been more forceful. I think its therapeutic value would have been diminished; there would not have been any overall gain as far as the length of treatment was concerned.

The lifting of the amnesia brings to mind an interesting question. It took place in the final session and that could be significant. This lifting of the amnesia seems suspiciously fortuitous. Would this have happened had more sessions been planned? That we had reached the final session did create an element of pressure to which the patient may have responded. It was essentially now or never! On the other hand, by then we were moving rapidly toward this resolution and, had more sessions been possible, the amnesia would probably have been lifted shortly.

A final question that should be asked is how the therapy or therapies that she was receiving from the hospital staff were related to the outcome. It is not possible to say. Although this could be a mere coincidence, the patient did not start showing progress until I began to work with her. However, I do feel that the sessions C.E. had with the social worker, who was a skilled therapist, complemented my work with her rather well and made a definite therapeutic contribution. They were an extension and an integral part of the hypnotherapy. As I have pointed out several times in earlier portions of this volume, hypnotherapy should be seen, in general, as consisting of the use of hypnotic techniques used in conjunction with non-hypnotic procedures. In the absence of the social worker, I would have had to do what she did in addition to the hypnotic work.

I have discussed this case in detail because it demonstrates that the use of hypnotic techniques is not a haphazard process, nor can it be accomplished in one session. There can be a great deal of repetitiveness, as this case demonstrates. Many different things can be and are done with hypnosis, and frequently, a procedure must be used several times before it works. Patients must be carefully prepared for what is to come, and one needs to explore gently what each technique can or cannot do. Changes that are brought about may be subtle and gradual. With the help of appropriate suggestions, there can be much therapeutic work in force between therapy sessions. This case also shows the usefulness of hypnotic procedures in dealing with multiple causations. In this case, dream work was used extensively to deal both with the patient's problems with anger and with her amnesia. Indirectly, her entire symptomatology and inadequate life style became included and altered for the better.

6

Semi-Clinical and Non-Clinical Applications of Traditional and Semi-Traditional Hypnotism

INTRODUCTION

HYPNOTISM IN FORENSICS

HYPNOTISM IN SPORTS

HYPNOTISM IN EDUCATION

HYPNOTISM IN PHYSICAL THERAPY AND
REHABILITATION

A SELECTED AND ANNOTATED BIBLIOGRAPHY
ON THE APPLICATIONS OF TRADITIONAL AND
SEMI-TRADITIONAL HYPNOTISM

INTRODUCTION

In recent years, hypnotism has intermittently received publicity about its use in police investigations and in athletics. Other areas of attempted applications include physical therapy, physical rehabilitation, and education.

HYPNOTISM IN FORENSICS

In 1889, Liégeois, a French professor of law, published the first comprehensive work of hypnotism as related to jurisprudence and the law. A great portion of the work dealt with the history and nature of hypnotism, and the remainder mainly discussed the possibility of crimes being committed through the use of hypnotism. A number of famous early European cases that had been tried in his time were reviewed in detail. Since then, there have been a number of rather spectacular cases tried in European courts. The issue has been, in each case, the culpability of the alleged hypnotist and, in some cases, of the culprit who had allegedly been "hypnotized." In the United States, there have been a number of criminal cases in which the claim was made that certain crimes had occurred while the defendant was in a spontaneous, accidental, or self-induced hypnotic state, with the intimation that, if this were the case, they were not responsible for their acts. Assuming that these individuals were truly in some altered state of mind, I question whether it was a hypnotic state. This presents some controversial issues, some of which have been discussed in Volume 1, and I shall not attempt to pursue the matter any further. I will discuss, instead, attempts that have been made in criminal investigations to use hypnotism to uncover crucial evidence. Many courts of law do not accept such evidence. Also, the use of hypnotism on potential witnesses has raised serious questions regarding their reliability with regard to other, subsequent, testimonies that they might be called upon to make.

The most common use of hypnotism has been to uncover and recover details missing from testimonies by witnesses and victims. In some cases, it has also been used on a suspect, with his consent, to obtain additional details that he claimed not to remember, or to establish that he had acted unknowingly. These uses have been much acclaimed by some of the police officials who used them. However, the use of hypnotic techniques by police personnel is often similar to their occasional use of psychics.

The widespread belief that a person testifying under hypnosis can tell nothing but the truth is pure fiction. There are presumably *drastic* ways of insuring truth under hypnosis, but none have actually been satisfactorily checked out. Speaking from personal experience in working with police officials over many years, the recovery of missing information through hypermnesia and age regressions is rarely successful, and most often it is highly distorted and contaminated by confabulatory material. Such uses of hypnotism are often associated with some profound and irrational misconceptions about what hypnotism can do. It is quite common for the hypnotist to try indirectly to improve the witnesses original sensory experiences. For example, in a case of rape that I was consulted about by the defendant's attorney, the victim had awakened in her bed just prior to being overpowered. The only light in her room was moonlight reflected through her open window. Her assailant's face had remained in darkness at all times. Subsequently, she was hypnotized by one of the detectives assigned to the case who had taken a workshop in hypnotism for police investigators. He suggested to her, under hypnosis, that her unconscious would dispel the shadows over the assailant's face, and she would then be able to see it clearly. He pressed for this effect until, eventually, the woman declared that she could see the face as clearly that of a Negro. She was then told that she would be shown various pictures, and that when she saw her assailant, she would immediately recognize him. She was later shown a collection of pictures of possible suspects, one of whom she identified. He was a local man, and he was apprehended. He was booked and charges were pressed on no more than this identification. It is quite unreasonable to think that the subject's perception could be improved in the above situation. The only visual data that could have been recorded was the image formed on the victim's retina at the time. This, in turn, was the distribution of light, which was essentially none, reflected by her assailant's face. An original insufficiency in lighting that prevents details from being imaged cannot be changed by any amount of suggestion. Granted, image processing techniques exist that can do much in cleaning up poor pictures; but it is rather unlikely that the average man or woman would have the inner or innate knowledge and understanding to do this at some level of mental functioning, even assuming the necessary neural/mental processes were available. This was actually the explanation the hypnotist used in the above case to support the results of his hypnotic work.

This is not to say that under certain conditions, forgotten, even unnoticed, but *registered* details are not recoverable under hypnosis. They probably are, but this is a different matter and a limited one. Although this needs to be confirmed, it might be possible, under hypnosis, to have a person reexperience a past event in slow motion, possibly using time distortion, and thus recover details perceptually missed because of the speed with which an event took place.

A serious problem, exemplified by the above case, is that the witness or victim may be subtly influenced in subsequently making a questionable identification. There is a good chance that given a posthypnotic suggestion they will recognize an alleged criminal from pictures or in a lineup, this can compel them to make some kind of identification. At a level below consciousness, subtle alterations of the presumably recovered material may take place and lead to a pseudo-memory, and then on to a false positive recognition that is firmly believed by the subject to be veridical. There is little doubt that a police investigator's preconceived ideas and expectations can subtly influence the subject. Without extensive research work being done in this area (and none has been done), the use of hypnosis in police investigations is of questionable usefulness.

I also have some serious doubts regarding the utility, and especially the validity, of results obtained using hypnotism in determining the culpability or innocence of individuals who have allegedly committed crimes during a "blackout."

Any professional person interested in working with law enforcement agencies should be forewarned that it can be time consuming; he may find himself repeatedly called upon to testify long after a case seems to be closed. I once worked with potential witnesses in the case of a mass murder. Ten years after it was supposed to have been terminated, I was still being contacted by various interested parties because of attempts by the attorney of the defendant, who had been found guilty, to appeal the verdict.

Readers interested in this type of application should read Orne (1979), also Coons' (1988) very recent article on a forensic misuse of hypnotism. Highly relevant material can also be found in two of the issues of the *International Journal of Clinical Hypnosis*. These are volume 27, no. 4, 1979 and volume 32, no. 3, 1984.

HYPNOTISM IN SPORTS

There have been reports of spectacularly successful uses of hypnotism in sports. When carefully examined, they are found to be quite vague and always very poorly documented. Furthermore, one would expect that there would be some failures, but none ever seem to be on record. I have been more impressed by the success of the hypnotist selling his dubious bill of goods to coaches and team managers than by the subsequent alleged superior performance of the athletes. My own experience with this has been limited to working with one golfer, with equivocal results. From this one experience, I decided that any practitioner attempting to do this kind of work should have some first-hand knowledge of the sport.

I am willing, however, to speculate about the potential uses of hypnotism in this area. It is reasonable to expect that the creation and reinforcement of appropriate motivation could be aided by suggestion. Appropriate changes in attitude is another logical approach. Suggesting greater exertion, greater endurance, and the disregard of discomfort and even pain is certainly a possibility. Suggesting greater strength and stamina is unlikely to have direct effects because these are purely somatic matters. It may, however, possibly help indirectly. Hypnotic suggestions can be expected to be helpful in insuring proper eating, sleeping, and other relevant behavioral factors.

Another potential area of application is that of visualized practice. Once the athlete has had an opportunity to learn the correct or effective way of performing, he may be given the task, in hypnosis, of visualizing himself going through the proper motions again and again. There is a possibility that appropriate time distortion can make this even more effective. The athlete should not only see himself performing, but should feel himself doing so as much as possible. Experiencing kinesthetically and proprioceptively may be more important than doing so visually. Watching, while in hypnosis, demonstration and replay films or videos in normal and slow motion, listening to analyses of plays, and so on, with appropriate suggestions, could be helpful. Many of these methods are said to be effective in the absence of hypnosis, and their effects should be reinforced by hypnosis. This approach, and variations of it, are unlikely to have anything to do with or to be able to make use of recently *hypothesized* holographic-like processes taking place in the brain. I mention this because of recent efforts by a certain firm to convince the public that they have training video tapes that make use of the holographic hypothesis and are capable of producing miraculous effects. Even if this hypothesis was an unquestionably demonstrated fact, its application in this manner, if possible, would most likely be far in the future.

Group hypnotism with teams probably has limited value for the same reasons given in the case of group hypnotherapy.

HYPNOTISM IN EDUCATION

There is very little of definite value available in this field. There have been secondhand reports of a wide use of "suggestology" and hypnotism in the Soviet Union and satellite countries for specialized and general education. Some of the techniques that have been described as used in classes and on an individual basis are, to say the least, bizarre, and the results poorly, if at all, documented.

So-called sleep learning is often confused with learning in hypnosis. There is a difference between the two, at least methodologically. As far as sleep learning is concerned, available research data do not support its vaunted effectiveness. Many past reports of success have been made by professional actors and public speakers who are already adept at memorizing. If, in their case, sleep learning has indeed been effective, this effectiveness may be related to their already existing mnesic abilities. With regard to learning under hypnosis the documentation is very poor, even at the research level. Research data that do exist tend to indicate that, with the exception of specific age regressions and inductions of hypermnesia, a general everyday marked improvement in memorization or recall ability is not possible. Nor, in general, are learning and problem-solving abilities directly amenable to marked improvement through hypnotic suggestions. I say this even though there are several firms in the United States that widely advertise entire courses, taught on cassettes, that use self-hypnosis, which they also teach (or induce). These will somehow magically inculcate the purchaser, in short time and without any effort, practice, or experience, with the equivalent of many semesters of college level training in innumerable fields of learning. Their commercial success demonstrates evidence of the gullibility and ignorance of the American public rather than of the possibility of near-instant hypnotic learning.

There is essentially nothing available on the use of hypnotism applied to learning disabilities. Most applications have focused on normal individuals encountering problems in the course of furthering their education or studying to meet a new job requirement. For example, I was once consulted by a woman having difficulty memorizing a protocol that she would have to use as the manager of a beauty salon. Another time, it was an individual who wanted to qualify for a position in the postal service and who was having difficulties memorizing part of a city map. A typical problem encountered in colleges and professional schools is individuals who panic in examinations and literally "go blank." I have worked with a number of medical students, and have found that a few sessions of hypnotism can be quite effective with these individuals. It can also be effectively used in removing bad study habits and replacing them with better ones. However, my experience in doing this kind of work has shown me that, sometimes, much work in educational counseling and guidance has to be done conjointly in the normal state. Sometimes the problem is one in which a student has been poorly advised about his curriculum, and is either overloaded with courses or taking courses he is poorly prepared for. In such cases, the solution is a situational one that has little to do with hypnotism. There are also cases in which the problem is with conflicts or with characterological factors. In such cases, nothing less than extensive psychotherapy will suffice. The woman studying for the position of manager (that I just mentioned) was such a case. It was clear that she was experiencing a severe conflict regarding the position. Furthermore, this conflict was a reflection of a much deeper emotional problem.

HYPNOTISM IN PHYSICAL THERAPY AND REHABILITATION

The main use of hypnotism in this area is to facilitate the processes involved. It is employed largely in a supportive role. The suggestions that need to be used vary considerably. They include suggestions aimed at neutralizing pain and discomfort associated with exercises and prosthetic devices, improving coordination, instilling positive attitudes, accepting the infirmities, improving morale and self-perception, and diminishing self-consciousness. Many patients who lose a major bodily function go through a grief reaction not unlike that observed with the loss of a loved one. Hypnotism is useful in helping the patient to deal with it.

A SELECTED AND ANNOTATED BIBLIOGRAPHY ON THE APPLICATIONS OF TRADITIONAL AND SEMI-TRADITIONAL HYPNOTISM

Crassilneck, H. B., & Hall, J. A. (1975). *Clinical hypnosis: Principles and applications.* New York: Grune & Stratton.

(This is a good survey of and reference source for the main clinical applications of hypnotism. There are no details regarding specific procedures.)

Hartland, J. (1971). *Medical and dental hypnosis and its clinical applications.* London: Bailliere Tindal.

(This has an excellent coverage of the various clinical applications; it contains considerable details of specific applications. Many of the suggestions to be used are given verbatim.)

Kroger, W. S. (1963). *Clinical and experimental hypnosis in medicine, dentistry and psychology.* Philadelphia: Lippincott.

(The title is deceiving because the work has little to do with research. It does have a good coverage of clinical applications with verbatim models included.)

Ritterman, M. (1983). *Using hypnosis in family therapy.*

(Although this work is oriented toward strategic therapy, and thus toward the non-traditional approach to hypnotism, I list it here because semi-traditional techniques seem applicable in its context.)

Schneck, J. K. (1965). *Principles and practice of hypnoanalysis.* Springfield: C. C. Thomas.

(This is one of the few works available on the use of hypnotism in a psychoanalytic context, and is recommended reading.)

Wester, W. C., II, & Smith, A. H., Jr. (Eds.) (1984). *Clinical hypnosis. A multidisciplinary approach.* Philadelphia: Lippincott.

───── (1987). *Clinical hypnosis. A case management approach.* Cincinnati: Behavior Science Center.

(The above two books are excellent collections of long articles by several authorities. They give a wide coverage of the clinical and non-clinical applications of hypnotism with detailed accounts of specific uses, including verbatim material. These books favor a client-centered approach and lean toward non-traditional methods.)

Wolberg, L. R. (1945). *Hypnoanalysis.* New York: Grune & Stratton.

(This is a detailed verbatim account of the hypnoanalysis of a patient done in a psychoanalytic context; it is an excellent work.)

───── (1948). *Medical hypnosis.* Volumes I and II. New York: Grune & Stratton.

(The title of this work is deceiving because its two volumes are entirely devoted to psychotherapy. This otherwise excellent work offers a detailed survey of the applications of hypnotism in the context of various psychotherapeutic approaches. The first volume discusses the applications in general terms; the second volume presents a variety of detailed cases with verbatim accounts of the therapy. This work is highly recommended.)

7

The Ericksonian Approach to Hypnotism: The Erickson/Rossi Interpretation

ERICKSONIAN CONSCIOUS/UNCONSCIOUS DICHOTOMY
LEFT/RIGHT BRAIN FUNCTIONS AND HYPNOTISM
ERICKSONIAN HYPNOTHERAPY AND STRATEGIC THERAPY
FINAL CONSIDERATIONS
AN ADDENDUM: MIND-BODY HEALING
SELECTED BIBLIOGRAPHY ON THE ERICKSONIAN APPROACH

INTRODUCTION

One aim of this chapter is to present the essentials of Ericksonian hypnotism or, more accurately, my understanding of Milton H. Erickson's way of practicing hypnotism and of his thoughts on the subject. I have also related this to traditional and semi-traditional hypnotism, to the extent that this can be done. Establishing whether there is or is not a relationship and, if there is, to what extent and its nature is of scientific importance. As I have explained in Volume 1, if eventually there is to be a true science of hypnotism, one cannot have two totally unrelated objects of discourse called by the same name of "hypnotism," even with qualifications such as "traditional" and "Ericksonian." For a sharing of the same label "hypnotism," *there has to be a sharing of some basic common feature or features.* Furthermore, it cannot be just a sharing of a superficial resemblance, but must be related to the identification or definition of the objects in question. Short of this, the use of the term needs to be abandoned in one case or the other. The rule of historical precedence for scientific nosology clearly indicates that, in the present case, it is Ericksonian "hypnotism" that would have to be renamed, were we to find no satisfactory common ground. As we shall see, the Ericksonian distinction between "therapeutic hypnosis," "hypnosis," and "laboratory hypnosis" is a very superficial one, and there is sufficient ground for continuing to associate the label "hypnotism" with at least *some* of Erickson's work with patients and demonstration subjects. Those who have already read Volume 1 will find that procedurally, semi-traditional hypnotism is transitional between traditional and Ericksonian hypnotism and, therefore, is a good introduction to Ericksonian hypnotism.

This chapter is more than just a presentation of Erickson's modus operandi and thinking; it also contains a critical examination of it, as well as the interpretations that others have made of Erickson's various procedures and some of the concepts that have been associated with them. As we saw in Volume 1, there are still many unsettled questions and much that is taken for granted in the areas of traditional and semi-traditional hypnotism. Although traditional hypnotism has been greatly written about, argued about, and fairly extensively studied in the laboratory in its nearly 150 years of existence, much of the practice of traditional hypnotism remains based more on tradition and experience than on well-established scientific principles and concepts. One could hardly expect that Ericksonian hypnotism, the specifics of which have been set down only in the last decade, would be in better shape, especially since, in contrast to traditional hypnotism, hardly any specific research has been done in the area of Ericksonian practices and concepts. Of course, there is a common ground for the two approaches to hypnotism, and it can be reasonably assumed that many of the conclusions drawn from research specifically done in the context of traditional hypnotism carry over into the Ericksonian context. This is particularly true for the various phenomena, examined in Volume 1, that one can bring about by means of suggestions given within the hypnotic state. On the other hand, for reasons that will become clear later, this is less likely to be the case when one considers such issues as the distribution of hypnotizability and susceptibility and what factors produce greater or lesser hypnotizability and susceptibility. The lack of pertinent research data may be related to Ericksonian hypnotism *calling for a highly individualized and flexible approach* to the induction of hypnosis and to the production of hypnotic phenomena. This makes accepted research methodology often difficult to apply in its context. Still, as we shall see, there are many aspects of Ericksonian hypnotism that could and should be researched. In the meantime, what one does is done simply because it *seems* to work, and this is even more the case with Ericksonian hypnotism than it is with traditional and semi-traditional hypnotism. Why and how it works can only be conjectured; *how well* it works is for the most part undetermined. For example, consider Erickson's use in a Hand Levitation Induction of the largely rhetorical question, "I wonder which one of your hands will rise first?" According to Erickson, there is an additional hidden message in this question because it carries the implication, *"One of your hands will rise,"* which constitutes a powerful *indirect* suggestion. But is this really more effective than to give the *direct* suggestion, "One of your hands is going to rise," or even, "Your left (right) hand will rise?" This could be easily tested, but it has never been done. Hypnotists apparently prefer to act on faith rather than on facts. I must admit that I use this in doing Hand Levitation Inductions, but not as an act of faith. I use it because it does seem to help in certain cases, and there is nothing lost in doing it. At worse, there is no gain. I have chosen this particular example for an additional reason. It is said to be especially effective because it is, or creates, a potent "double bind." This topic was briefly discussed in Volume 1 and will be much more extensively examined further on. I will now limit myself to pointing out that a careful examination of the situation raises serious questions as to whether or not there really is a double bind. Since at present no good test for the existence of a double bind is available, the issue must remain an undecided one.

The study, thus the description and discussion of Erickson's hypnotic techniques and approaches, is complicated because so much of his hypnotic work was inextricably enmeshed in psychotherapeutic procedures *that are not necessarily hypnotic in themselves,* and it is difficult to separate the one from the other. In some cases, it is impossible because, in essence, his therapeutic strategies are frequently indistinguishable from his hypnotic strategies, and I am not sure that Erickson himself always worked with a clear distinction between the two constantly in mind, or even if he cared to make one. In any case, I think it is important to realize that much of what is called Ericksonian hypnotism most likely contains elements *that have nothing to do directly with hypnotism,* but are used in a supportive manner or as adjuvants. Consider the use of anecdotes and storytelling to illustrate, make a point, or elicit a useful association. I would seriously question that, in general, anecdotes and stories have anything to do with hypnotism, even when they make a profound and lasting impression. Are there any good reasons for thinking, when told in a hypnotic setting, that they function any differently than outside such a setting? It is important to distinguish carefully between two alternatives: do they have a specific "hypnotic" action, or is their normal action possibly rendered more effective for some purposes by the setting? I do not know the answer, and I do not know that anyone else does. Perhaps I can make one of the issues involved clearer by going to a simpler situation. A person in his normal state of mind, when asked to think of eating a favorite food, will often begin to salivate. One may explain this effect as the result of an association, or of a conditioned response having been set off. Few, if any, would say that this is a suggested or a hypnotic effect. Some hypnotized individuals will salivate when given a direct suggestion to do so, and some will not, and of these, many will if told to hallucinate eating something. Are there any reasons to believe that this effect has something to do with suggestions or hypnosis, or that it is different from the case of the normal individual, especially if, instead of hallucinating, the hypnotized subject is told to imagine eating, or even to think about it? I consider the answer to this question an important one because, in Ericksonian language, this is a "utilization" technique. Utilization is considered a major feature of Ericksonian hypnotism, which has even been said to be a utilization theory of hypnosis. It is also said that to do the above is to suggest salivation indirectly; Ericksonian hypnotism is also said to be the use of indirect suggestion par excellence. These are some of the questions we shall have to examine seriously as we look at what constitutes

Ericksonian hypnotism, what makes it "hypnotism," and what makes it different from traditional or even semi-traditional hypnotism.

Let us return to anecdotes and stories. The parallel with the salivation example should be clear. But what do we say about a carefully planned anecdote or story that is presumably used to bring about a hypnotic state, or that is used to bring about a complex hypnotic behavior? Here, indeed, we touch upon a highly characteristic feature of Ericksonian hypnotism. While such an approach leads to some rather spectacular demonstrations, whether or not it is generally, or in particular, more effective than traditional and semi-traditional approaches remains to be firmly established. It is relatively easy to come up with a list of reasons why one would expect anecdotes and stories to be especially effective in certain situations involving the use of hypnotism. However, these reasons usually amount to nothing more than untested or poorly tested hypotheses that are too often mistaken as established facts. We shall later see what some of these hypotheses are. In the meantime, I will agree that, for the most part, they are sufficiently reasonable to validate the use of anecdotes and stories in hypnotic and hypnotherapeutic work. But their use is based on hypotheses, not hard data.

One element that should be kept in mind when reading accounts of Erickson's remarkable cases and demonstrations is that people came to Erickson, more often than not, seeking to be hypnotized, if not directly, then at least indirectly. As his reputation grew and tales were told about his abilities, many people that came in contact with him, especially in seminars and workshops, most likely developed an expectation that they might be hypnotized at almost any time by him by a mere glance, a word, or a gesture, and probably would not know that this was happening until it had happened. Others most likely expected that this would happen by something unusual Erickson would do. Erickson was very much aware of this and capitalized on it. One needs only to read a record of what occurred in a seminar with Erickson such as the one Zeig (1980) has published to see evidence of this. The quotes below from Erickson, Hershman, and Secter (1961, p. 125) are offered as more direct evidence. Erickson had, somewhat earlier, done a spectacular induction, so it seemed, by simply first asking the subject, after she had joined him on the stage, whether she was wide awake or not, then persistently questioning the subject's certainty that she was not in a hypnotic state. This, I might add, was a favorite technique used by Erickson in demonstrations. Referring to the induction, a seminarian later asked,

QUESTION: There was no induction?

ERICKSON: She was already in a trance, a light one. Coming up on the stage, she came for a definite purpose. She was going to assist. Therefore she was in the proper mental set, the physical set, the psychological frame of reference.

Erickson's further explanation of how the questioning worked was that it had created doubts in the subject's mind regarding her actual state of mind. She was not as yet aware that she was already in a hypnotic state. The questioning placed her in the position either to come out of the trance (awaken) or to remain in it, and even to go into it more deeply. By volunteering, the subject had already made a commitment to enter hypnosis; therefore, there was no question as to what her choice would be.

Erickson was usually not so open about the matter, and he allowed his audience to perceive a magic that was not there. I am not faulting Erickson for this. No questions were asked, and he did not volunteer information. Clearly, when asked, he responded with the truth. Nor am I detracting from the reality of the effects he produced. I think, however, that one needs to be aware of the kinds of factors that may have been at work in Erickson's case. Furthermore, while there are many accounts of spectacular rapid results obtained by Erickson, there are also many accounts that show Erickson arriving at much less spectacular effects and taking an appreciably much longer time to do so. Some of the books by Erickson and Rossi (1976, 1979, 1981) have some good examples of this. To set the record straight, the 1976 volume was co-authored with Erickson by Ernest and Sheila Rossi. The latter, however, served primarily as subject and had very little input, if any, with regard to the technical discussions in the book. References made to Rossi in the present chapter are to Ernest Rossi. Also, when referring to all three volumes at once, I have only mentioned one Rossi as co-author for the sake of simplicity.

Erickson is no longer with us, and it remains to be seen whether Ericksonian hypnotism in the hands of his students will retain its reputation of effectiveness. Some of his students appear to have acquired a certain reputation, but none, to my knowledge, have come near to attaining Erickson's reputation for effectiveness and for spectacular achievements. Is the fate of Ericksonian hypnotism to be the same as that of Transactional Analysis, Gestalt Therapy, and the many other therapies that evolved some years ago and that were to revolutionize mental health? Only time will tell. In the meantime, one might also consider that there are traditional and semi-traditional hypnotherapists who, in their own ways, have acquired a high reputation in professional circles as very effective hypnotherapists; indeed, their reputations have extended well beyond the cities and states where their offices or clinics are located. I will not say that they have equaled Erickson, but they are the equal of many of his successors, and have even surpassed them in reputation.

Finally, nothing less than a full, detailed study of the available transcriptions of recorded work done by Erickson with subjects and patients can give the full flavor of his approach. Even these transcriptions are deficient in that a great deal of non-verbal material of importance is lost. The best I can do, in a text such as this, is to describe some of the more basic features of Ericksonian hypnotism and to provide a reasonable number of examples.

MILTON H. ERICKSON: SOME RECOLLECTIONS IN APPRAISAL OF THE MAN AND HIS CONTRIBUTIONS

I personally knew MHE, as he was often referred to by friends, students, and colleagues, from 1956 until his death in 1980. While I did not spend time studying under him intensively, I had a great many personal contacts with him over those years and both extensively and intensively studied his writings. I was present at many of his famous demonstrations given at the height of his career at various workshops, seminars, and at private sessions. He was a good and respected friend and colleague whose respect I am proud to have earned.

As has often been pointed out by others, Erickson was not interested in theorizing. He was essentially a very practical, highly intuitive man who was concerned with obtaining results whether or not he had an explanation for his methods. I am convinced that many of the explanations that have been ascribed to him in later years were developed retrospectively by him, quite late in his life, because of the pressure put upon him by many of us to explain what and why he had done certain things. I question whether, when he acted in certain ways or said certain things, he always clearly had these explanations in mind, or even knew what they were immediately after his actions took place. There was a great deal of ad libbing on his part. This is not to say, however, that if this was the case, these explanations were less correct. I also suspect that some of the thoughts that have been ascribed to him by various writers have perhaps been, at times, more those of the writers than those of Erickson. MHE had a peculiarly frustrating habit of rarely giving straight answers to questions asked of him, and he often left it up to his interlocutor to make the final interpretation. Often he would not give a "yes" or "no" answer, but would make a comment that might or might not be directly related to the question.

While today MHE is best known as a (hypno)psychotherapist *sans pareille,* he also made important research contributions, prior to 1940, that I consider outstanding. He gained his initial reputation in the field of hypnotism for this research and not for his concurrent psychotherapeutic work. Modern researchers have discounted much of his research on the basis that he had little use for statistically based experimental designs or complex statistical analyses of his data. Erickson believed that it was better to work intensively and in-depth on a problem with a few very "good" subjects than to work more superficially with a large sample of individuals of widely ranging hypnotic abilities. He was a very creative and meticulous worker who believed that the proper "hypnotic" preparation of each subject was extremely important in obtaining veridical data. To do so usually precluded using the kinds of controls that have been so characteristic of modern behavioral research, and for this reason, among others, Erickson has been accused, at times, of being a "credulous" researcher. He was anything but credulous (Weitzenhoffer, 1963, 1964). He had certain convictions about hypnotism and hypnotic phenomena, but who among the most respected of researchers does not? One of Erickson's strengths as a researcher was his ability to utilize naturally occurring controls and turning a hypnotism session that was not directly planned into an impromptu research situation. For example, on one occasion, while he was giving a general informal demonstration of hypnotic behavior to some students and colleagues, he found that he had an unexpected visitor: a psychiatrist who had a good knowledge of hypnotic behavior. It occurred to him that this would be an excellent opportunity to study how well a hypnotized person could behave like a normal person if instructed to do so. Would his visitor still detect who was hypnotized among those present? Another example of his use of naturalistic experimental situations is exemplified in his famous published study on the experimental production of Freud's "everyday psychopathology."

A great deal of myth has arisen centering on Erickson and his work. That this happened was no fault of his. Tales have been told about him that could have been obtained only second- or even third-hand, and whose accuracy needs to be questioned. In some cases, their authors admit that they received the information from others; other authors, who should admit this, do not. I mention this because certain events that have been related in this manner have, indeed, been incorrectly told. One possible reason for the misinformation regarding MHE is because he told allegorical stories. This was one of his ways of explaining and teaching. Some of the stories were told in the first person as things he had done or experienced. I strongly suspect that not all of these accounts were fully based on actuality. Perhaps this is immaterial, since they did effectively make their point. However, failure to recognize this possibility only furthers the myths. Since it is not possible to know, in many of these accounts, what was fiction and what was not, little can be done to rectify matters except to keep the above in mind.

I would not want to give the impression that MHE did not consciously and deliberately develop strategies in his work with patients and experimental subjects at the time he worked with them. Frequently, he would spend *many hours* working these out in detail *before* doing the actual work. His famous treatment (Erickson, 1944) of a case of *ejaculation praecox* is a good example of this. One of the more remarkable instances in which Erickson developed a strategy on the spur of the moment was one I witnessed in 1958. For several days, I had met in Philadelphia with MHE, Jay Haley, and the late Bernard E. Gorton, M.D., as part of a project aimed at better understanding Erickson's methods and ideas. The plan was to eventually publish the results. One evening, MHE agreed to give a demonstration. A small number of local professionals were invited. One of the visitors presented a young woman, whom I shall call Joan, to be the subject. After introductions were made, MHE began to work with Joan. She readily developed a hypnotic state, but seemed unable to produce much phenomena. Undaunted, and knowing that she was usually a "good" subject, Erickson continued to work with her in a conversational manner. While he was doing this, I observed him nonchalantly picking up a sheet of paper that was lying near him on a coffee table. While still talking to the subject, and without looking at the paper, he rolled it into a cylinder, as if absent-mindedly playing with it. He then let it unroll, and then once again made a cylinder out of it. Holding it in his right hand near the middle, he had one end point toward the subject; then he rotated it counterclockwise so that this end now pointed toward his left, and he slowly introduced one finger of his left hand into that end, withdrew it, and then allowed the paper to unroll and fall to the floor. He appeared to have lost interest in it. With this last act, the subject's inability to perform vanished, and Erickson proceeded to give a noteworthy demonstration. When I questioned Erickson about the above incident, he explained what had happened. He had recognized Joan as a former medical student or intern who had attended a lecture and demonstration of his a year or so earlier and who had participated as a subject. Although nothing had been said about this earlier encounter during the introductions, Joan must have remembered it, too. On that first encounter, MHE had noticed that Joan had an engagement ring; she was no longer wearing it on this second meeting, nor was she wearing a wedding band. He hypothesized that Joan's relative refractoriness was due to resistance caused by anxiety that the failure of her engagement would somehow be revealed during the session. Erickson had therefore cleverly communicated to her non-verbally while conversing with her that he remembered the ring, was aware there was no ring now, and that he was not interested in pursuing the matter. With this reassurance, Joan's resistance had vanished.

MHE's skill as a hypnotist has taken on a legendary turn. He was once known in some circles as "Mr. Hypnosis." Was he really that good, and uniquely so? I think it is important, first, to separate his accomplishments as a hypnotherapist from those as a demonstrator of hypnotic phenomena. Since I witnessed only a very small number of brief therapies performed by him, and never had access to follow-up data on them, I cannot be a judge of that part of his work. On several occasions, I did have serious questions about whether or not the patient had been hypnotized, and I had the impression that very little had been therapeutically accomplished during the session. Then, after subsequently learning how MHE operated as a therapist, I decided that I could have been greatly mistaken. One needs to keep in mind that MHE often used informal, indirect methods of induction, and he often worked with patients in and out of hypnosis, in the same session, while using indirect suggestions. Such a procedure made it very hard for an observer to know exactly what was happening from moment to moment. Besides doing hypnotherapy, Erickson also conducted therapy not intended to involve any hypnotism. If hypnosis was induced in such cases, it may have been without his knowledge or intention. From Erickson's viewpoint, it was therapeutically immaterial whether or not the patient was hypnotized; I suspect that there were times when he could not have subsequently told an observer whether and when the patient had been in hypnosis, simply because this had been of no concern to him. Was there a certain irresponsibility in this? Erickson felt that any hypnosis occurring spontaneously during a therapy session would be self-terminating at its conclusion, and it could only be a help during therapy. Also, Erickson was generally careful to make sure that his patients were returned to a normal state before they left his consulting room. In later years, as MHE came to rely more and more heavily on the use of indirect suggestions, he began to view all of his therapy sessions as involving hypnosis, for he came to adopt a position in which responding to an indirect suggestion was equivalent to being in a "trance." Finally, in evaluating MHE as a hypnotherapist, one should not overlook the fact that he had some equally famous predecessors. I have often heard it said that he was the world's foremost hypnotherapist. This may have been true, but it is hard to prove when confronted by the reported tremendous success of such nineteenth-century European hypnotism clinics as those of Liébeault and Bernheim in France and of van Rentergheem in Holland, to only name two. Had these men been contemporaries of Erickson, they might have seriously contested the above title.

From the account I have given of the Philadelphia ring incident, which is only one of several of this type that I could recount, it is obvious that MHE was a master hypnotist—or perhaps it would be more accurate to say a master communicator. One of his most masterful demonstrations was one that he did in Mexico in which he, who could not speak Spanish, hypnotized a nurse, who could not speak English. He nevertheless produced a glove anesthesia in her hand. Was it the hypnotist or the communicator who succeeded? Perhaps the two functions are inseparable. In any case, his mastery is clearly demonstrated by his research and clinical articles. On the other hand, some of the remarkable things he did were not done uniquely by him, as the legend would make it seem. For example, his famous induction of hypnosis with a hand shake had been repeatedly done many years earlier by the stage hypnotist Ralph Slater. Slater had become quite famous for this during the 1940s, and I would be surprised to learn that Erickson did not know about this. Slater never explained how he did it, and it has often been proposed that, like other stage hypnotists, he used appropriately prepared subjects planted in the audience, as I explained in Volume 1. Or, perhaps Slater was as astute as Erickson, and he independently used the same technique. Be that as it may, Slater kept his technique a secret, but Erickson carefully detailed his technique (Erickson & Rossi, 1981) which is one that certainly does not require a previously prepared subject.

In evaluating Erickson as a master hypnotist (and therapist), one should also keep in mind that he eventually acquired much prestige as such. Laboratory research has failed to support the hypothesis that prestige and expectation are important determinants of success with hypnotism. Perhaps I am merely reflecting a personal bias and that false ideas die hard, but I have never been fully satisfied with these studies. For one thing, laboratory studies have never duplicated the kind of prestige situations that have existed in the case of such men as Erickson or Slater, or, even much earlier, of Liébeault, Bernheim, and van Rentergheem. Also, there were times when Erickson became somewhat of a showman. There is a natural tendency to do this when giving public demonstrations, even to professionals, and this may come more naturally to someone who is adept in suggestion techniques and is constantly using them. By Erickson's own admission, he often selected subjects from his audience on the basis of signs that indicated they would be "good" subjects. There is nothing wrong in doing so. If I want to be certain that I can demonstrate certain phenomena, I will most certainly try to use a good subject, especially one that I know will exhibit the phenomena in question. The audience should also know this. Many of those who watched Erickson were not aware of this, and they were left with a false impression of his abilities. Based on my observation of Erickson at work, I have concluded that he gave the impression, perhaps unwittingly, that he had accomplished much more than he had. Some of the techniques he used have been described in Volume 1 in my discussion of stage hypnotism. I say this with no intimation of right or wrong. Much was expected of MHE at his demonstrations, and he was certainly human. Above all, he was a clinician; he remained so even in demonstrations, and he had a primary concern for the well-being of his subjects and for meeting their needs. Frequently, his subjects volunteered for personal reasons. It was as much for his subjects as for the show that he turned apparent failures into apparent successes. I say, "apparent" because what was not a success from my viewpoint may have been one for MHE. Almost *any* response he observed when giving a suggestion was thought by him to be a success, especially in a clinical situation. Vague evidence of a hallucination or a rudiment of a regression were accepted by him with the same enthusiasm as a much more complete response would have been. Hypermnesia, rather than the age regression that he sought, was satisfactory. He never considered the possibility that the overt

movements of a presumably hallucinating subject might be purely suggested motoric effects. His testing of induced analgesia and anesthesia in
demonstrations was a particularly weak test. That he knew better is clearly
indicated by his reported research and some of his clinical work. A factor
that greatly influenced Erickson during the 1950s and 1960s was his strong
need to convince the many hesitant, skeptical, and even antagonistic members of the medical and dental professions that hypnotism could be successfully used by any professional. He could best do this by being liberal in his
criteria of success.

I have no doubt that MHE used the word "hypnosis" and its derivatives to
denote essentially the same phenomenology as has been generally described
for the last 150 years. His early writings, his founding of the American Society
of Clinical Hypnosis, his editorship of its official publication, and his many
demonstrations of hypnotic phenomenology all support the above statement.
This needs to be said, because there is an undercurrent of belief that
"Ericksonian hypnotism" is somehow something else. If it were, then there
would be no further point in discussing it any further in this work, and one
ought then to raise serious scientific questions as to whether Ericksonian
methods should continue to be associated with "hypnotism." Obviously, I
think otherwise, and view it as a particular approach. I will clarify my reasons
in subsequent pages.

OVERVIEW AND GENERAL CONSIDERATIONS

The simplest way of defining Ericksonian hypnotism is to say that it is the way
Milton H. Erickson *practiced* and *perceived* hypnotism. There is no evidence
that Erickson induced or used a state different from the one we have called
"hypnosis" in Volume 1 and he appears to have used the term suggestion in
the same way that we have been defining it. Furthermore, contrary to the
impression that has been given by various writers, the Ericksonian approach
was not one that used *only* indirect forms of suggestion; nor was it a strictly
permissive one. It was, rather, one in which he was at times authoritarian and
in which he also used direct suggestions. The permissiveness was frequently
more apparent than real, as when Erickson would say to a subject, "I wonder
which hand will rise first, your right one . . . or your left one? . . ." There
may have been a choice of hand, but no question, at least in his mind, that a
hand would rise! Erickson maintained that the type of statement exemplified
in the above and variations of it actually *leave no choice* to the subject, who
has no alternative but to respond!

"Utilization" has often been viewed as a key concept in defining Ericksonian hypnotism. This view is also only a part of a far more complex whole.

Still, while it does not fully define Ericksonian hypnosis, the utilization of the subject's potentials for response is a dominant feature. It was not a missing element in the work of earlier hypnotists, but Erickson was probably the first to recognize it explicitly for what it was, and certainly he employed it more extensively and more methodically than any one before him. Ericksonian hypnotism is a philosophy and *general* approach to influencing others as much as it is hypnotism per se. One can certainly analyze in various ways what Erickson did and abstract certain elements and procedures that seem specific to his way of viewing and doing things. Erickson, Rossi, and Rossi (1976) and Erickson and Rossi (1979, 1981) have done this, as have Bandler and Grinder (1975) and Grinder, Delozier, and Bandler (1977), but they have left us with unanswered questions, such as specifically when and how to make use of these features. *This still remains up to the hypnotist or therapist to decide,* and his success in doing so is a function of acumen, sensitivity, creativity, problem solving ability, memory for details, and experience, just to name a few factors and attributes that lie beyond the results of such analyses. The engagement ring incident I described earlier is illustrative of this.

One of the best statements Erickson made of his conception of hypnotism and hypnotherapy is found in one of his early articles (Erickson, 1948). He uses the term "trance" synonymously with hypnosis, and has this to say about it:

> As for the trance state this should be regarded as a special, unique, but wholly normal psychological state. It resembles sleep only superficially, and it is characterized by various physiological concomitants, and by a functioning of the personality at a level of awareness other than the ordinary or usual state of awareness. For convenience in conceptualizing, this special state, or level of awareness has been termed unconscious or subconscious. (p. 573)

Erickson believed it was important to differentiate between trance and trance induction. The latter is preparing, teaching, and enabling the patient to develop a trance state, or, as Erickson states:

> To continue the process of inducing a trance should be regarded as a method of teaching the patient a new manner of learning something, and thereby enabling him to discover unrealized capacities to learn, and to act in new ways which may be applied to other and different things. The importance of trance induction as an educational procedure in acquainting the patient with his latent abilities has been greatly disregarded. (p. 572)

Regarding the importance of making this differentiation, Erickson adds:

> Both the therapist and the patient need to make this differentiation, the former in order to guide the patient's behavior more effectively, the latter in order to learn to distinguish between his conscious and his unconscious behavior patterns. During trance induction, the patient's behavior is comprised of both conscious and unconscious patterns, while the behavior of the trance state should be primarily of unconscious origin. (p. 573)

Erickson points out that failure on the part of the patient to understand this distinction will lead the patient to make use of *both* conscious and unconscious behavior in the trance instead of relying *mainly* or solely on unconscious behavior patterns.

For Erickson, the ideal trance is a condition in which all behavior is determined from within and outside of the patient's conscious mind. Although this does not come out clearly in his 1948 article, it seems, from some of his other writings, that Erickson felt traditional hypnosis, as exemplified by stage and laboratory uses of it, is characterized by (a) usually being a mixture of conscious and unconscious behavior and by (b) not giving the subject an opportunity to use "inner processes of a disorganizing, reorganizing, reassociating and projecting of inner real experiences" in the production of desired effects. Erickson also sees this as a failure of the traditional uses of hypnotism for therapy. It was probably this consideration that led Erickson, in later years, to specifically speak of the "therapeutic trance" in many of his writings.

Although Erickson fails to give a precise definition of what he understands by "suggestion" in his 1948 article, he does make an effort to clarify his distinction between "direct" and "indirect" suggestions. According to him, a direct suggestion explicitly calls for the desired response. An indirect suggestion calls for and initiates a train of mental activity as expressed under (b) above. While this train of activity is not the desired response, it is conducive to it as an end point. To clarify this point, Erickson uses the example of producing an anesthesia by suggestion. The direct approach might attempt to produce a glove anesthesia by suggesting that either there will be an absence of sensations, or there will be an experience of numbness in the hand. In contrast, the indirect approach may ask the subject to recall the feeling of numbness that he experienced after being given a local anesthetic. An even more indirect way is to suggest to the patient that she will develop the anesthesia in terms of her own experiences when her body was without sensory meaning for her. According to Erickson, this more indirect approach will often work when the direct and less indirect approaches fail. Erickson may not have been the sole originator of the indirect approach to the production of analgesia.

Erickson's special interest in indirect suggestions appears to have been motivated by his search for ways of overcoming the frequent refractoriness of patients to direct suggestions and traditional trance inductions. That is, he sought to increase the percentage of success beyond the accepted limits of the time. Erickson viewed refractoriness, which he usually referred to as "resistance," as being largely of conscious origin because it is an interference, by conscious habitual sets, biases, and learned limitations, with the production of the desired effects. He felt that the way to confront this problem was to bypass and/or to decommission, or, as he was much later to say, to "depotentiate" the conscious. With this in mind, he went on to develop a multitude of forms of indirect suggestion.

Erickson (1948) has this to say about hypnotherapy:

> The role in hypnotic psychotherapy of this special state of awareness is that of permitting and enabling the patient to react, uninfluenced by his conscious mind, to his past experiential life and to a new order of experience which is about to occur as he participates in the therapeutic procedure. This participation in therapy by the patient constitutes the primary requisite for effective results. (p. 573)

Erickson's views and use of the unconscious and of trance in relation to hypnosis is also a mark of Ericksonian hypnotism. Erickson was definitely familiar with the Freudian concept of the unconscious, and in his earlier writings, he seems to have had it in mind when speaking of the unconscious and of unconscious actions. In later years, however, he came to view the unconscious as a mental entity more like Morton Prince's concept of the subconscious: as a second source, or center, of intelligent activity lying outside of an individual's normal consciousness, presumably coexisting with it, and capable of acting independently and unknown to it. Just what he did with the Freudian unconscious, if he still recognized it, is not clear. He certainly still seemed to recognize most, if not all, of the dynamisms of psychoanalysis as being present. One of his last public statements regarding this matter is reported by Zeig (1980, p. 33). Erickson stated at a seminar:

> . . . I emphasize a state of conscious awareness and a state of unconscious awareness. For convenience sake I speak about the conscious mind and the unconscious mind . . . Now the conscious mind is your state of immediate awareness.

Erickson then points out the multiplicity of things his audience is aware of and makes the further point that conscious awareness is a state of divided attention. He adds:

> The unconscious mind is made up of all your learnings over a lifetime, many of which you have completely forgotten, but which serve you in your automatic

functioning. Now a great deal of your behavior is the automatic functioning of these forgotten memories.

On the basis of other writings and personal talks with Erickson, my impression is that, for Erickson, the unconscious eventually becomes, the totality of all actual and potential non-conscious mental activities an individual is capable of, including activities ascribed to the Freudian unconscious. His concept of the unconscious included *all* native as well as acquired processes that come under nervous, and possibly hormonal, control, no matter how remote and tenuous or indirect this is. I make these last points because Erickson definitely believed in the possibility of producing tissue and other changes through accessing the unconscious, and he often spoke of the unconscious' ability to make use of all "learnings." He viewed the unconscious as a totality having the ability to act autonomously and intelligently in at least a problem solving or goal directed manner. This is not obvious in the above quotes, but was indicated more than once during the above mentioned seminar. Whether or not Erickson was aware of some of the serious implications such an idea had for the concept of conscious functioning is unclear; if he was, he never gave any indications.

Erickson's concept of trance, or hypnosis, is intimately related to that of the unconscious. Again, in his earlier years, Erickson subscribed to the traditional concept, and especially to Bernheim's view, of hypnosis. (This can be found in Volume 1.) It was in the early 1950s that he increasingly began to identify the occurrence of hypnosis with *any elicitation of unconscious activity in response to a communication.* With this change, he also began to speak about "trance," while prior to this, he spoke only of "hypnosis." Zeig (1980, p. 39) quotes him as saying, "Hypnosis is the ceasing to use your conscious awareness; in hypnosis you begin to use your unconscious awareness." Hypnotizing thus became simply a matter of promoting and eliciting unconscious behavior, and one obvious method of doing so was by interfering with conscious control, or as he later would say, by "depotentiating" the conscious. Another obvious way was to bypass the conscious; this is the foundation on which lies his indirect methods of suggestion. Finally, speaking directly to the unconscious in the presence of the conscious was still another alternative. This led him to the use of storytelling, metaphors, and the interspersal technique. Contrary to popular belief and to what some writers have implied, storytelling and the use of metaphors did not originally dominate his work.

Erickson often said that he did not believe there was a clear connection between suggestibility and the presence of a trance; hypersuggestibility was not a characteristic of it. More specifically, this was his position with regard to what he referred to as the "therapeutic" trance, which he felt should be distinguished from the "laboratory" trance (traditional hypnosis). *Yet* he made frequent references to the subject's or patient's "heightened receptivity" when in trance, and with Rossi, as well as elsewhere, states (Erickson & Rossi, 1981, p. 41), "The heightened receptivity is essentially what we mean by the term hypnosis." This type of statement, and his constant alternations between speaking of trance and speaking of hypnotic phenomena, with no clear distinction made between them, seems to me to represent his ambivalence toward using the language of traditional and semi-traditional hypnotism, rather than a fundamental difference in the subject matter. For Erickson, the importance of the trance was that its induction went along with a progressive decrease in participation by the conscious and a progressive increase in participation by the unconscious. An induction is simply a process whereby there is progressive decrease in voluntary behavior with an offsetting progressive increase in automatic behavior until, at least theoretically, *all* behavior becomes automatic.

According to Erickson, Rossi, and Rossi (1976), and as viewed by Erickson, the trance is an inner directed state; a restricted focus on a few inner realities, an active unconscious learning, a highly motivated state, and an altered state of functioning. Erickson's distinction between therapeutic and laboratory trances seems to be largely founded upon his view that the laboratory imposes severe restrictions on the manifestations of the trance state, whereas Ericksonian hypnotism and hypnotherapy allows full freedom of expression, and therefore is not a fundamental distinction.

Since Erickson did not consider suggestibility to be an essential aspect of trance, his assessment of the presence of trance and of its depth depended on his observation of various clinical symptoms. Table 7.1 contains a list of those he accepted.

The list includes many of the traditional symptoms listed in Volume 1. I have marked with asterisks those symptoms that Erickson used most, and double asterisks indicate the greatest use.

Obviously, Erickson viewed trance as a broader entity than traditional hypnosis. Erickson has also broadened the concept of suggestion to cover any communication that elicits unconscious processes. The traditional concept comes under this. One of the problems in determining what constitutes a suggestion and what does not when going over Erickson's sessions is that the suggestions proper become lost in the overall interaction and conversation because of his extensive use of indirectness. Erickson's divergence from traditional hypnotism is in his extensive reliance on clinical signs *to the exclusion of hypersuggestibility.* If we can agree, as proposed in Volume 1, that there is a large class of trance states of which traditional hypnosis is merely one member, then we can perhaps say that Erickson sometimes produced a trance (hypnosis) identifiable with traditional hypnosis, and at

TABLE 7.1.   Clinical Symptoms Used by Erickson to Assess the Presence of Trance

Autonomous ideation	*Economy of movement
Objective and impersonal ideation	*Facial features ironed out
Pupillary changes	Feeling distant
**Balanced tonicity	Slowing pulse
Response attentiveness	Slowing respiration
Lack of body movement	Feeling good after trance
Comfort, relaxation	Sensory, muscular, and body changes
**Eye changes and closure	*Time lag in motor and conceptual
Retardation of swallowing and blinking	behavior
reflexes	*Slowing and loss of blink reflex
Spontaneous hypnotic phenomena	Literalism
Amnesia, regression, anesthesia,	Changed voice quality
catalepsy, time distortion, etc.	Lack of startle response

* Symptoms used frequently by Erickson.
** Symptoms used most by Erickson.

other times he may have produced one or more other members of the trance class. Erickson unfortunately confounded the conditions by speaking of all of them as if they were one and the same trance or hypnotic state. More accurately speaking, it would appear that there may be at least one trance state that ought to be specifically called "Ericksonian hypnosis" (or possibly the "Erickson effect"), which is not to be confused with traditional hypnosis, which can also be produced by the procedures used by Erickson.

The traditional concept of suggestion views it as strictly eliciting a reflex-like action. Erickson goes a step beyond this and includes action elicited through the cooperation of an intelligent unconscious.

On the other hand, as points of similarity between Ericksonian, traditional, and semi-traditional hypnosis, one might note that for Erickson, the trance arises in the context of a dyadic interpersonal relationship in which there is still a director and a directee. Permissive as he is, the relationship still maintains the characteristic dominance/submission, the one down complementary relationship (Haley, 1958), aspect of traditional hypnotism. Rapport remains an essential aspect of it. With few exceptions, the induced trance is initiated by Erickson and terminated by him. The aim remains that of having maximal production of automatic behavior. The range of effects that can be elicited remains essentially the same.

A trance state can be *shaped* by the situation in which it is produced and used. In the case of hypnosis, the very manner in which the hypnotist goes about producing the state and utilizing it is to be suspected of strongly shaping the form under which the state appears. To what extent is this applicable to Ericksonian hypnotism? I am not ready to say, but I feel this possibility needs to be given serious attention. Should it hold true, we may again have to speak of one fundamental state taking on multiple forms.

Erickson, in a very *distinctive* way, often made *explicit* statements to the subject regarding the *existence* of a conscious-like unconscious in him, and he instructed the subject *to allow* his unconscious to function *without participation by his conscious.* Statements to this effect were frequently made quite early in his interaction with the subject, as well as later in it. As in the case of Hilgard's "hidden observer" discussed in Volume 1, there are strong possibilities that such instructions set the stage for the appearance of a suggested, artificial "unconscious" that functions very much like the suggested secondary personalities also discussed in Volume 1.

Traditional and semi-traditional hypnotism make use of such instructions to the subject, such as saying, "Allow whatever happens to take place," "Do not try to interfere," and "Do nothing else but listen to my voice." Is there not an implication that something other than the subject's consciousness is going to control behavior, even though it is not referred to specifically by name? Is this basically different from what Erickson does? In fact, is it not, essentially, an indirect way of communicating the idea that a directing conscious-like unconscious will come into existence? The differences between Ericksonian and traditional hypnotism may not be as great as one might at first think. Still, until it can be shown that these two ways of dealing with the same thing are equivalent, it would seem prudent to consider the two approaches as distinct.

I would like to add three historical notes to this. First, it is my impression that Erickson's shift in the 1950s to the use of the term "trance" in preference to "hypnosis" may have been largely guided by his desire to get greater acceptance of hypnosis by professionals and the lay public. "Hypnosis" had unfortunate connotations that "trance" did not have. Then, too, as part of the effort to make hypnosis more acceptable, there was a tendency among professionals using hypnosis to tell others that becoming completely involved ("entranced") in a movie or story, going into a so-called "brown study," and "losing track of time" were evidence that trance was a natural everyday phenomenon. How many who stated this believed it and how many did not is not clear. While I did not believe it, I did find it useful to make an analogy between hypnosis and such states in developing the text for the Stanford Scales of Hypnotic Susceptibility.

The second historical note pertains to the increasing practice of directly questioning and instructing the "unconscious" in hypnotic work. This began to happen about that same time, and it became widely disseminated and used. This was a direct outgrowth of Erickson's teachings. Others then independently developed the technique and used it with an increasing lack of discrimination and understanding in what they were doing (Weitzenhoffer, 1960a, 1960b).

Finally, Erickson's belief that one could simultaneously communicate with the subject on at least two levels, conscious and unconscious, may have grown out of early research work he had done with automatic writing. He had found by accident that, when hypnotized, a subject could frequently, if not always, decipher the otherwise cryptic automatic writing of another subject. This went along with the then current and still ongoing idea that the unconscious communicates in a language of its own.

Today, most of Erickson's fine research contributions are all but forgotten, and he is best known for his techniques of induction and of indirect suggestion as he used them in psychotherapy. As with traditional and semi-traditional techniques, Erickson's way of proceeding was *entirely* oriented toward eliciting *a maximum of non-voluntary* or, as he preferred to say, unconscious behavior. Shifting the patient from conscious to maximum unconscious participation was his main goal in any induction. To this end *he developed a multitude of approaches.* In their book *Hypnotic Realities,* (Erickson, Rossi, & Rossi, 1976) as well as in an article (Erickson & Rossi, 1976, 1976a) a table is provided that outlines, summarizes, and classifies various techniques and procedures used by Erickson and that indicates their basic effects. While I believe this breakdown oversimplifies matters in some instances, and it does not always assign procedures to the right subheading, on the whole it is a useful table. I have reproduced it as Table 7.2. I will use it as a guide in discussing various aspects of Ericksonian hypnotism in the pages that follow. There have been other attempts at this type of classification, and my choice of the Erickson/Rossi classification is not an intimation that they are any less accurate or useful. An excellent overview of them can be found in an article by O'Hanlon (1985), and also in his more recent book (1987).

Unlike learning the techniques and procedures of traditional and semi-traditional hypnotism, learning those of Ericksonian hypnotism is much more than a matter of memorizing model procedures that can usually be applied with a minimum of modifications to the situation at hand. This is because, from the very start of the production of effects, the Ericksonian approach is based on an ever changing moment-to-moment interaction between subject and hypnotist that depends on the ongoing and changing perceptions of the situation by both the subject and the hypnotist. To some degree, these are also factors in semi-traditional hypnotism, but not nearly to the extent that it is in Ericksonian hypnotism. Additionally, much of Erickson's approach is highly permissive and indirect. For this reason, it calls for much more variability in wording, and it makes extensive use of non-verbal communication. There is a definite pattern to Erickson's work with *any given* individual, but it changes from subject to subject, and, like all patterns, it can best and sometimes only be seen when the totality of the elements involved is available. Therefore, it usually has to be viewed retrospectively. For this reason, the ideal method for studying and learning the

TABLE 7.2. The Microdynamics of Trance Induction and Suggestion

(1) Fixation of Attention	(2) Depotentiating Consciousness	(3) Unconscious Search	(4) Unconscious Processes	(5) Hypnotic Response
		Indirect forms of suggestion:		"New" datum or behavioral response experienced as hypnotic or happening all by itself
1. Stories that motivate interest, fascination, etc.	1. Shock, surprise, the unrealistic and unusual	1. Allusions, puns, jokes	1. Summation of: a. Interspersed suggestions b. Literal associations c. Individual associations d. Multiple meaning of words	
2. Standard eye fixation	2. Shifting frames of reference; displacing doubt resistance and failure	2. Metaphor, analogy folk language	2. Autonomous, sensory and perceptual processes	
3. Pantomime approaches	3. Distraction	3. Implication	3. Freudian primary processes	
4. Imagination and visualization approaches	4. Dissociation and disequilibrium	4. Implied directive	4. Personality mechanisms of defense	
5. Hand levitation	5. Cognitive overloading	5. Double binds	5. Ziegarnik effect	
6. Relaxation and all forms of inner sensory, perceptual or emotional experience	6. Confusion nonsequitors	6. Words initiating exploratory sets	6. Etc.	
7. Etc.	7. Paradox	7. Questions and tasks requiring unconscious search		
	8. Conditioning via voice dynamics, etc.	8. Pause with therapist attitude of expectancy		
	9. Structured amnesias	9. Open-ended suggestions		
	10. Etc.	10. Covering all possibilities of response		
		11. Compound statements		
		12. Etc.		

Source: Erickson & Rossi, 1976. "Two Level Communication and the Microdynamics of Trance and Suggestion," *American Journal of Clinical Hypnosis, 18,* 3, 153–171. Reprinted by permission of *American Journal of Clinical Hypnosis.*

Ericksonian approach *is to have access to the complete text* of sessions held by Erickson, including details of movements, pauses, inflections, and many other pertinent aspects of communication. A number of fully described sessions, with commentaries, by Erickson himself are available in print and have already been referred to (Erickson, 1944; Erickson, Haley, & Weakland, 1959; Erickson & Rossi, 1976). They should be carefully studied because they contain the exemplification of the essence of Erickson's approach to suggestion and the induction of hypnosis.

Erickson has also written many highly pertinent articles that, while less detailed with regard to procedures, are nevertheless highly edifying and useful. These have been collected by Haley (1967). Other full sessions with commentaries are to be found in such works as those of Erickson, Rossi, and Rossi (1976) and Erickson and Rossi (1979, 1981), of Bandler and Grinder (1975b), of Grinder, Delozier, and Bandler (1977), and of Zeig (1980). One should keep in mind that the commentaries in the case of Bandler and Grinder are not Erickson's.

A word of caution: I have serious doubts that works written by Erickson in collaboration with others from 1975 on are strictly representative of his thoughts. This is particularly true for those he co-authored with Rossi. This seems to have been recognized by O'Hanlon (1985), who attributes the analysis and models presented in the three volumes by Erickson and Rossi solely to Rossi. When I last saw Erickson in his home in 1975, he had become physically very weak, was easily fatigued, and most of the time he could barely speak above a whisper. My efforts at the time to enter into a dialogue with him regarding some of the material that was to appear in his and Rossi's 1976 book met with failure. Erickson was willing, but not up to doing this. For this reason, I doubt very much that, prior to publication, he had either the strength or inclination to go over the material he co-authored with Rossi, and certainly not carefully. At least, we do have verbatim reports of answers and comments made by Erickson, and it is, perhaps, important to note that frequently Erickson does not affirm the correctness of some of Rossi's statements to him. This may be an indication that he agreed, or it may mean that he disagreed and chose to ignore them because he had already made his point. Additionally, Erickson was not a theoretician, and in his later years, he much preferred to leave it to others to make hypotheses and interpretations. In his hypnotic and, especially, in his therapeutic work, Erickson seems to have functioned as much in terms *of what he felt* as he did in terms of what he reasoned would work in a situation. My experience with him was that when pressed for explanations, Erickson could usually produce reasons for his actions, but this was always retrospectively. Still, there is no question that he also let himself be guided by logic and intuition as, for example, in the case of the engagement ring that I mentioned earlier. Also, in earlier days, he would spend considerable time formulating his approach to cases prior to the sessions he had with his patients. There is less evidence that he did this as extensively in later years. I definitely know of a number of inductions that he performed at workshops and at impromptu gatherings *without* preparation or preknowledge regarding the subject.

Works such as those of Grinder and Bandler and of Erickson and Rossi are still useful to read. They contain much relevant material, even though they present what are probably adulterated versions of Erickson's thoughts. In particular, they contain complete verbatim reports of extensive and complete sessions held by Erickson, and this material can be studied independently of the authors' comments. Finally, Rossi, Bandler, and Grinder have done some serious thinking in their efforts to understand Erickson; they have ideas that merit attention. Distancing also often makes it possible for an observer to see things that the person involved in a process cannot see.

In the pages that follow, I shall both present and critically examine various techniques and procedures used by Erickson. Table 7.2 will serve as a guide. How the techniques and procedures all fit together can, of course, best be seen in the detailed sessions given verbatim, with their analyses, in the works that are cited in this chapter. It is not possible to cover all of Erickson's procedures in detail in less than a large volume. On the other hand, for purposes of the present work, I do not feel that such a detailed presentation is necessary.

According to the annotated examples of inductions that have been published elsewhere, it seems that almost every sentence and word has a special significance and purpose. Because each induction also has to be tailored to the subject, it may appear to readers that performing Ericksonian hypnotism is a formidable enterprise, particularly since some of the procedures call for definite skills. I doubt, indeed, that many who attempt to practice this form of hypnotism follow Erickson exactly. However, the examples in question represent *a highly selective* sampling. In the larger picture, Erickson *also* used semi-traditional direct approaches alone or in combination with indirect procedures. As indicated by Table 7.2, one has a choice of a great many indirect procedures; one is not obligated to use any single one. In the remainder of this chapter, I will discuss those aspects of Ericksonian hypnotism that I feel need special attention for one reason or another. Readers who have mastered the material of Volume 1, have read this chapter, and, especially, have studied a few of the detailed inductions by Erickson that have been published should not find it difficult to begin to use Ericksonian methods, if they wish to do so, without having to attend workshops or courses on the subject.

THE DYNAMICS OF TRANCE INDUCTION

Erickson's approach to the use of suggestion and to hypnotism *makes no* specific effort to separate non-hypnotic from hypnotic suggestions. Like the hypnotists of old, he makes no distinction and treats them as one and the same. His interest was always in what can be accomplished with hypnotized individuals. Erickson hinted of his awareness that suggestion has existence apart from hypnosis, but his work has always been within the framework of inducing and utilizing hypnosis, whether through suggestion or other means; the distinction we have made elsewhere between the two therefore has little application in his work. His lack of concern for the distinction may also reflect that the definition of a suggestion given in Volume 1, which I believe is essentially what he understood the term to mean, is equally applicable to the hypnotized and to the normal subject.

Erickson, Rossi, and Rossi (1976) view four processes as contributing to the production of hypnosis, or the trance. These processes are fixation of attention, the depotentiation of consciousness, eliciting an unconscious search, and stimulating existing unconscious processes. These four processes are listed in Table 7.2. This table, which describes the "microdynamics" of trance induction, gives the impression that a sequence of processes takes place when an induction is performed. Although some inductions can occur in the steps as described, Erickson, Rossi, and Rossi (1976) make it amply clear that these processes usually function simultaneously, collapsed, so to speak, into a single process. Furthermore, in many cases, one can begin with any one of these processes. These authors claim that, basically, once any one of the conditions given as the heading for the first three columns (1, 2, or 3) has been set into motion, the processes of the last two columns (4 and 5) are automatically carried out. There is even an intimation in the above work that the processes of the remaining first three columns may themselves also be automatically activated at times. Presumably, the more the first three types of processes can be set independently into motion, the more effectively the last two processes will be brought about. There appears, incidentally, to be no particular significance to the use of the term "microdynamics" by Erickson and Rossi beyond their intent to indicate that their aim is to examine the dynamics of trance induction and suggestion in relatively fine details.

Sequence or no sequence, Table 7.2 is a fairly complete compilation of procedures and processes that Erickson and Rossi consider to be conducive to effective trance induction and suggestion. The first two columns can be viewed as listing steps that can be taken to *prepare* the subject for the production of the effects defining the next two columns.

Some of the procedures listed in a given column are complex procedures that can contain features belonging to other columns. This is particularly true, for example, of the Eye Fixation and the Hand Levitation procedures listed in column 1. They have elements that belong equally well in columns 2 and 3. It is understandable, in the light of this remark and material to follow, that working with either of these procedures would not only lead to fixation of attention, but would also depotentiate consciousness and initiate an unconscious search. Readers may find it useful, at this point, to review the material of Volume 1 on these two methods of induction.

Looking a little more specifically at the five processes that head the columns of Table 7.2, the following can be said:

Fixation of Attention

This consists of a shift in awareness. According to Erickson, Rossi, and Rossi (1976), the aim of this step is to focus the subject's attention inward on a few inner realities. They claim this facilitates the "depotentiation" of consciousness. Erickson also states, "all hypnosis is a loss of the multiplicity of the foci of attention," and also, "hypnosis is a lack of response to irrelevant stimuli." Are we to understand by this that Erickson, like Braid, views hypnosis (or is it trance) as nothing more than a state of concentrated attention on one thing? If so, what is the function of the four other steps? Erickson makes it very clear that *he does not* ascribe to Braid's concept of monoideism, but he does not clarify the matter further. As mentioned earlier, trance induction seems to have generally been for Erickson a much more comprehensive procedure than it is in traditional and semi-traditional hypnotism, which formally separate trance induction from trance utilization. In the Ericksonian scheme, the two are merged into one. In the resulting single process, there is no specific point at which one can say, "now the subject has just become hypnotized (entranced), and we shall begin next to produce hypnotic (trance) phenomena." Furthermore, in this, perhaps, lies the significance of Erickson often specifying that he is speaking of a "therapeutic" trance. Many things he does in the context of trance induction appear to have little to do directly with the production of hypnosis or hypnotic effects *per se*. Rather, they are oriented toward bringing about changes in his patients that he thinks are desirable for their therapy. For example, quite independently of hypnosis, he sees the breaking down of habitual modes of dealing with reality as an important first therapeutic step. It also happens to be useful in the production of a trance state or effect, so he incorporates it, as well, into his overall trance induction. For Erickson, trance is usually a broader concept than traditional hypnosis. Yet, Erickson also specifically refers at times to "hypnosis," as in the earlier quotes. Is this a reversion to old habits, or is it deliberate and thus significant? When giving demonstrations, Erickson would frequently point out the instant at which he perceived that a subject had entered the trance state. At such times, he was using the term "trance" in a more restrictive sense that is synonymous with traditional hypnosis. One can only conjecture, because Erickson does not say anything more about this. In any case, the reason for four additional steps is that they are needed for the full induction of hypnosis because trance is possibly more than the traditional state of hypnosis. Assuming for a moment that traditional hypnosis was nothing more than a state of monoideism, in the Ericksonian scheme it would represent but a step in the creation of a more complex condition. The remainder of the steps would then serve to shape the hypnosis into the final trance form. Erickson also speaks of deepening the trance, and the four other steps might also be seen as deepening procedures. These steps do further the development of the subject's automatic (unconscious) participation, and this is nothing more than a deepening of the trance in the Ericksonian scheme.

Starting with Braid, fixation of attention has continued through the years to be considered an important, if not essential, initial step. Ericksonian, traditional, and semi-traditional hypnotism seem to be in full agreement in this respect. Where they differ is partly in their interpretation of what fixation does, but they differ more in the way of bringing it about. In traditional and semi-traditional hypnotism, the subject is usually directly requested, prior to starting an induction or giving a suggestion, to "pay close attention," or "pay attention," to the hypnotist's words, to an object (target, hand, etc.), a sensation, and so on. In Ericksonian hypnotism, where indirectness is the rule, such statements as the above are abandoned, and devices that will indirectly generate an attentive response, or set, are often used instead. The various procedures for fixation of attention used by Erickson are listed in column 1 of Table 7.2. They include the use of traditional techniques of induction, and thus of direct requests. With one exception, the list is self-explanatory. For readers not familiar with Erickson's work, I will explain that the pantomime approach is a strictly non-verbal way of inducing trance and trance phenomena. It originated on the occasion that Erickson, who could not speak Spanish, was asked to do this with a Mexican subject, who could not speak English.

It should be clear to those familiar with the contents of Volume 1 that many of the procedures used to produce fixation of attention do much more than this, and that their action also comes under other headings of Table 7.2. The stated fact that fixation of attention causes or facilitates "depotentiation" is a good example of this. Erickson, Rossi, and Rossi (1976) do recognize this fact, and they also recognize that, frequently, *a procedure will have multiple effects,* just as specific statements may serve several functions.

The Depotentiation of Consciousness

This process is associated by Erickson, Rossi, and Rossi (1976) with the concepts of "conscious sets" and "habitual frames of reference." They leave it up to the reader to determine what they mean by these expressions. Rossi, being a psychologist, perhaps meant the psychological meaning of set and, therefore, that "conscious set" refers to a readiness to respond in a certain way or selectively to certain stimuli. Whether the qualification "conscious" used in this connection is significant is not clear. Nor is it clear just what is meant by "frame of reference." It may refer to a person's habitual way of perceiving events and carrying out actions. The authors do explain very briefly that depotentiation is an alteration in, or a breaking down of, an individual's habitual patterns of functioning. This involves an elimination of the influence and even a breakdown of habitual frames of reference that limit what consciousness can accomplish. Usual patterns of awareness are also removed. A great deal of guessing has to be made regarding what this all means. Basically, it all seems to add up to a statement that the subject becomes unable to use his conscious mind in the usual, normal ways and/or is no longer able to control consciously activities normally under its aegis. But depotentiation is not just an incapacitation of normal conscious functioning; it is a mental condition that leaves an individual open to a reorganization of his mental processes, particularly to the instillation and installation of new sets and new frames of reference with which he can presently operate. As a consequence, new associations and new ways of functioning become possible. In particular, Erickson sees depotentiation as facilitating creativity and problem solving and, therefore, as allowing an individual in therapy to find appropriate solutions to life problems previously not available to him. Erickson sees much of the work of the therapist as enabling the patient to find such solutions on his own. Finally, as used by Erickson and Rossi, "depotentiation" seems, at times, to be essentially synonymous with the elicitation of automatic behavior. Perhaps this is because the extent to which this can be elicited depends upon the extent to which volitional activity can be kept out of the action. The concept of depotentiating consciousness is uniquely used by Ericksonian hypnotism. However, one can see a forerunner of it in Janet's (1889) use of distraction to facilitate the giving of suggestion, and one early hypothesis regarding the function of induced sleep can be related to it.

The procedures listed in column 2 do not all use the same principle of action. Some, like cognitive overloading, or those that shock or confuse, clearly seem to function by taxing the coping power of the conscious mind. Others are really nothing more than statements aimed at eliciting automatic responses. "Not doing, not knowing," "losing abilities," conditioning, and the "double bind," to be taken up in a section of its own, are all examples. As we have seen in Volume 1, eliciting a maximum of automatic behavior is essentially what traditional and semi-traditional hypnotism are also about. The main difference between this and Ericksonian hypnotism is, again, in the indirect character of the procedures just mentioned. For example, the subject might be told in the traditional situation, "You cannot keep your eyes open any longer," but in the Ericksonian approach he might be told, "It will be interesting to experience that moment when you can no longer keep your eyes open." I must admit that I do not see there is a great deal of difference in these two statements. Incidentally, this is an example of "losing ability." An example of "not knowing" is, "You don't need to know where your hands are." The direct form would be "You will have no awareness of where your hands are." Some procedures, like the "negative" and "doubt," are actually quite involved procedures that utilize intonation and inflection as a means of conveying a message other than the one contained in the words that are used. For example, "You understand, don't you?" can be turned from an affirmation to the negation, "You really don't understand," with the proper use of doubt in one's voice. Similarly, firmly saying, "Won't you?" can be made to reaffirm doing an act just requested, or can reverse the effect if said with a doubting tone. This then has the equivalence of a second indirect message, "Do not do it." At least, this is what Erickson and Rossi claim. In the latter case, however, by the authors' own admission, it is far from clear what kind of action is really involved.

One question about many of the above procedures is how or why they depotentiate. The explanations that Erickson and Rossi give, when they give one, are frequently very weak and often highly conjectural. Sometimes no explanation is available, and one is told that this is just the way it is, as in the case of "losing abilities." One explanation that is often alluded to by Erickson is that these procedures create a situation in which the patient or subject finds it much easier to go along with whatever comes up next, rather than to try and unravel the meanings and implications of the messages he has just received. Erickson has maintained that the extensive use of confusion creates an intense need in the subject for anything that will bring surcease from his state of confusion. Thus, the patient becomes open to any meaningfully stated demand, be it direct or indirect, coming from the hypnotist.

Erickson and Rossi's discussion of depotentiation also presents a major conceptual problem. Earlier, I raised the issue of whether or not some significance needed to be attached to the use of the qualification "conscious" in relation to sets and habitual frames of reference. Sets, and, in general, anything that is habitual, is usually viewed in psychology as being something that lies outside of awareness and conscious action. True, one can sometimes become aware of their existence, but their influence is something that is generally considered to take place outside of consciousness and volition. In the absence of any clarification regarding this choice of words, one might consider that "conscious" is not particularly meaningful, and that it even creates a contradiction.

The concept of depotentiation of consciousness seems a useful one that can, perhaps, be reduced and greatly simplified to the statement that it is any process that prevents consciousness from taking part in or interfering with the production of automatic behavior. This should include decomissioning consciousness as well as bypassing it.

Unconscious Search

According to Erickson, Rossi, and Rossi (1976, p. 228), when sets and frames of references break down or are eliminated, there occurs "an automatic search at unconscious levels for new associations to restructure a more stable frame of reference through the summation of unconscious processes." In brief, the patient's mind becomes open to inputs that will satisfy this search. This would then seem to constitute an ideal time for the hypnotist or therapist to make selected material available to the unconscious. In particular, this would be the time to make communications regarding effects that one wishes to see occur at an automatic level. Within the framework of traditional and semi-traditional hypnotism, this would be a time of maximal suggestibility. However, the situation is rendered somewhat ambiguous by Erickson and Rossi also stating (1975, p. 170), "All approaches listed in column 3 are communication devices that initiate a search for new combinations of associations and mental processes that can present consciousness with results in everyday life as well as in hypnosis." This seems to be saying that the new procedures are aimed at initiating what is already initiated! Rather than try to elucidate something that probably cannot be elucidated, I will merely briefly discuss the main procedures that are listed here and let the reader come to his own conclusion regarding their purpose and mode of action.

Multilevel Communication

This would be better spoken of as dual-level communication, and is based on the idea that one can communicate simultaneously with the conscious and the unsconsicous. Erickson and Rossi (1976) conjecture that the context of a communication addresses the first of these, and the words themselves address the second. Allusions, puns, jokes, metaphors, analogies, and folk language presumably function in this manner. The trick for the hypnotist, then, is to present in one of these forms of communication whatever message he wishes to communicate to the unconscious, this message being, as we shall see, the suggestion proper. To a large degree, this has to be individualized, so that one cannot say that there are standard metaphors, analogies, and so forth, to be used with all subjects.

The issue of communication at an unconscious level plays a central part in Erickson's work. It is, indeed, much of its essence. Erickson relies very much upon the idea that certain manners of speaking activate automatic processes and actions. He perceives much of his approach as aimed at communicating at two levels: with the conscious and with the unconscious. This concept of two-level communication is compatible with the linguistic concept of "surface" and "deep" structures to which Rossi makes allusions. However, since this linguistic concept remains to this day rather hypothetical, it cannot be used as evidence of the correctness of Erickson's view. It seems reasonable that the process of communication should activate non-conscious processes, and psychology has long recognized this. One can also appeal to reasonable psychological and neurophysiological mechanisms for support. Reasonableness, however, is not proof. Our best evidence remains the reports of subjects and reasonable inferences that can be made from their overt behavior.

Implication

This is treated by Erickson and Rossi as a separate topic, although, as we shall soon see, it involves a double message. Frequently, Erickson would initially say to a subject, "Which of these chairs would you like to sit on?" This implies that sitting down will take place. Erickson saw this type of statement, then, as containing an indirect command, instruction, or request to sit down. If the person does sit down in one of the chairs, rather than comment on the matter or state that he would prefer to remain standing or sit on the floor or choose another chair, Erickson sees this sitting down as an automatic response to a directly unstated proposition. Indeed, inquiry into the matter, when this happens, does usually show that the person did automatically (non-voluntarily) sit down with, at most, only making a conscious or semi-conscious decision regarding which chair to sit in. A more complicated example given by Erickson and Rossi is Erickson saying, "Your unconscious can try anything it wishes." Here, Erickson explains, the word "try" implies the action actually cannot be performed, and that there is a second message that says, "your unconscious cannot act as it wishes." In this particular example, Erickson immediately follows the above sentence with, "Your unconscious isn't going to do anything of importance." This, he states, implies that now the unconscious will do exactly the opposite. Erickson sees a further implication in this combination of sentences: the subject's unconscious will do whatever he subsequently suggests (presumably because the subject will view it as being important).

Another good example of the use of implication by Erickson is that of his saying to a rebellious teenager at the very start of his treatment, "I don't know how your behavior will change." A variation on this he could have used would have been, "I don't know when your behavior will change." The implication is that there will be a behavior change, and therein lies the indirect suggestion for the behavior to change. According to Erickson, this brief assertion actually has another important feature. By saying that he does not know when the change will occur, he disarms the patient's resistance by creating a momentary "acceptance set."

It is easy to see an implication where there is none. For example, Rossi and Erickson (1976, p. 60) give the following as an example of a suggestion by implication: "If you sit down, then you can go into a trance." The "If . . . then . . ." is, of course, as the authors say, the traditional form taken by logical implication. But it is also what is known in linguistics as the "conditional" form, which is something different. Going into a trance is made contingent upon sitting down. One way to distinguish the one from the other is to see if a logical conclusion is being derived. This is not the case in the above example. The more likely explanation of why this kind of assertion works when it does is, as the authors themselves next point out, that by setting a condition (such as of sitting down) that is most likely acceptable to the subject, a "yes set" is produced that then facilitates the actual suggestion of going into a trance. In brief, implication has probably little to do with the results. I say "probably" because, as the authors also repeatedly point out through the book, the subject's perception of what is being said is as important, if not more, than the operator's perception of the same. Thus, there is always the possibility that the patient may have perceived the above, not as a conditional, but as an implication, as Erickson and Rossi did.

Another example of a questionable implication, (found in the 1976 work on p. 12) is, "I can tell your unconscious mind that you are an excellent hypnotic subject." According to the authors, this is supposed to imply, "I don't have to convince your conscious." I find it very difficult to derive this implication from the above statement, even when looking at the total context in which it was made and at all of the interchanges that have preceded it. Another example (p. 29) we might look at is, ". . . while you listen and then beginning to drift away. Your eyes can now close and you will note that the drifting can occur more rapidly." Erickson makes the point that "more rapidly" implies that drifting will occur. But note that Erickson has *already* told the subject to "drift away." I am inclined to view this as only reinforcement of the first suggestion of drifting. However, in this case there may conjointly be an implication at work. It is that drifting must have *occurred,* since something cannot become more rapid unless it is already in progress. The action can perhaps then be equally understood as being a subtle form of pacing.

The subject matter of implication is a complex one. Implication should not be translated to mean necessarily logical implication. Rossi speaks at times of logical implication and at other times of "psychological" implication, without elucidation. It needs to be recognized, without going into details, that philosophers, logicians, and semanticists distinguish between *material* and *strict* implication, the latter being also called *entailment.* In the first case, the meaning of the words involved is not of concern, but the opposite is true for the second case. The picture is rather more complicated than this, and I would refer the reader interested in pursuing the matter further to such a work as that of Lyons (1977). In the present context, implication should, at the very least, really read "entailment." Keep in mind that tone of voice, inflection, and other audible features of speech play important parts in determining the meaning of words and sentences. Compare "your hand feels very heavy, try to lift it," to "your hand feels heavy, *try* to lift it," in which "try" is stated strongly and incisively. Following a negative such as "you cannot lift your hand," "try" carries the same message, and doubly so if also emphasized. Certain linguistic features, such as a word being in a question or in an affirmation, makes a difference regarding what it imparts. Compare "lift your hand" to "can you lift your hand?" following the above negative. Erickson was very adept at using such devices, as well as various non-verbal cues, in making his communications. This is not always well indicated in some of the transcripts analyzed by Rossi.

Implied Directive

This is closely related to implication. Let us begin with an example. Erickson says to a subject, "As soon as you know that you are in a trance, your right hand will descend to your thigh." The implied directive, which is the suggestion proper, is "go into a trance." This is *preceded* by a statement *which states a condition,* in this case a time, and *is followed* by a statement for an action that *constitutes a signal* that the suggestion has been carried out. Another good example (1986, p. 187) is the following: "And when you have completed, really looking at her, you will awaken and tell us only those things that you are willing to share." The implied directive is of awakening. In brief, the patient or subject is not directly told to do something, but what will be done is implied in the overall text. This can probably also be seen as a form of imbedded command. Presumably, the same processes that make implications work in general also function here.

As with implications, some of Erickson and Rossi's examples are questionably implied directive, as thus defined. For example, Erickson says to the patient, "I want you to feel naked from the waist up." He pauses, then adds, "Do you want R to look at you?" It is difficult to see an implied directive in this. For one thing, the communication is not tripartite, and this is a feature that Erickson and Rossi clearly consider to be characteristic of implied directives. They interpret the above example as being an implied directive because, they argue, the question requires that the experience *has* taken place. But if it has already taken place there is no further need for a directive! Furthermore, it seems to be to the very point, in the definition of the implied directive, that, when the directive is given, the effect has not yet occurred. Equally, and possibly more to the point, one could hardly have more of a *direct* suggestion of feeling naked than in this example. With the proper inflection and intonation, one could make the question one that reaffirms the suggestion and even confirms it in a leading way. Otherwise, it is a nice indirect test of whether or not it has taken place.

The reason that Erickson and Rossi (really Rossi) speak of an implied directive will not be clear to many readers. One has to read a paper presented by Erickson and Rossi at a scientific meeting in 1976 (published later by Rossi, 1980), in order to clearly understand. What evolves from this paper is that such an assertion as, "As soon as you know that you are in a trance, your right hand will go up," is viewed by Rossi as being equivalent, first, to, "Any time after this, if you know you are in a trance, then your right hand will go up." Alternatively, he also proposes that the original statement can be replaced by, "Your right hand will go up as soon as you know you are in a trance," which he then claims is equivalent to, "Your right hand will go up only when you know you are in a trance." But this, he further argues, is equivalent to, "Your right hand will go up only if you know you are in a trance." In this way, he believes he has demonstrated that the original statement can be reduced to a logical implication in which the direction (thus the use of "directive") to raise a hand is implied.

There are a number of problems with the above reasoning and manipulations. In the logical analysis of propositions and their relations to each other, it is permissible to make such changes in wording as the above provided that there is equivalence. But this is hardly the case for "as soon as" and "any time after this." The first designates a specific point in time, but the other designates an indefinite temporal point. Likewise, "as soon as" is not the counterpart of "only if," because the first expression allows the occurrence of other events to be associated with the hand movement.

Thus, from the standpoint of the logical manipulation of propositions, Rossi fails to demonstrate that the original assertion is a logical implication or that it contains one. However, this is really all beside the point, because, in the first place, *one is not dealing with logical propositions in the above.* Although Rossi does mention that besides logical implication, one must consider "psychological" implication, he fails to recognize that logic is related to what Reichenbach (1947) has called the "cognitive" use of language. There is also an "instrumental" use. These uses are differentiated one from the other in that the "truth" and "falseness" of every proposition must be considered in the cognitive use (logic), whereas this consideration is irrelevant in the instrumental use. When we say to someone, "As soon as you know you are in a trance, your hand will go up," it is meaningless to say that either part of this assertion is true or false. Even if it was worded, "If you know you are in a trance, then your hand will go up," or some variation of this, being true or false is not applicable to either half of the assertion. If the reader is still unclear about this issue, let him consider the following counterparts: "As soon as the temperature on the thermometer registers 1200 degrees, press the red button with your finger," and "If the temperature on the thermometer registers 1200 degrees, then press the red button with your finger." It should be clear that logic is in no way involved here. These are just instructions to be followed regardless of why. Now it is true that if, at any given time, the red button is pushed or not pushed, certain logical inferences can or cannot be made regarding what happened to the temperature. But this is another, and altogether different, situation, because now one is dealing with observable data and "false" and "true" are applicable qualifiers.

This is not to say that there are no situations in Erickson's work that justify the use of "implied directive" in their connection, but those examples that are discussed by Erickson and Rossi do not.

Compound Statement

This appears, from the examples that are given, to consist of two statements joined by the conjunction "and." The first statement always seems to be a "truism" (a statement of indubitable fact), and the second is the suggestion proper. However, there are indications from some of the examples that are given that the first statement could be the suggestion and the second one a reinforcing statement or even a second suggestion. A typical compound suggestion would be, "You are sitting down listening to me, and you can now go into a trance." There is little to add to the discussion of this topic. "Truisms" are viewed by Erickson as foolproof suggestions; their use here is, therefore, particularly indicated. On the other hand, there are no reasons to think that other kinds of suggestions would not be equally effective in this position.

We shall later be discussing another kind of compounding of sentences in which the conjunction "or" is used. For reasons to be seen, Erickson and Rossi prefer to discuss this matter under another heading. Although they do not realize it, the justification for their doing so is actually because "or" can be used in an *exclusive* and an *inclusive* sense. In the exclusive sense, "A or B" is to be interpreted as meaning, "Either A or B, but not both." In the inclusive sense, "A or B", is to be interpreted as, "Either A or B, or both." When thus interpreted, "A or B" comes under the present heading. In general, people understand the use of "or" in the exclusive sense, and this justifies, to some extent, Erickson and Rossi not considering the use of "or" under the present heading. For this reason, too, I use the expression "and/or" when I want to insure that the inclusive sense will be understood. It would be an easy matter to check out the extent to which "or" is interpreted one way or the other in normal conversation.

Open-Ended Suggestion

Erickson and Rossi (1976, p. 27) say (in reference to Erickson), "he *offers* suggestions in an open-ended manner that admits any possibilities of response as acceptable. Suggestions are offered in such a manner that any response the patient makes can be accepted as a valid hypnotic phenomenon." On page 76, they add, "There is thus no possibility of a patient failing on a suggestion since all the responses are defined as admissible hypnotic phenomena." A further advantage of this is that "since anything the patients do is defined as an adequate hypnotic response, they cannot resist or withdraw from the situation." Finally, a last objective that the therapist/hypnotist can attain is to have an opportunity to explore the patient's response tendencies for future use. Most examples of this approach tend to be rather involved, and usually consist of conversationally mentioning many possible experiences that the subject could have or responses that he could give. This is frequently stated indirectly in terms of the behavior that other individuals might have if hypnotized. Much less involved suggestions of this type include statements such as, "You can have all sorts of experiences," and "You will have only those experiences that you are ready to have." As Erickson once said to me as a further comment, "Of course, the subject is bound to do or experience something new sooner or later." "If one waits long enough," he might have added. Indeed, it does not have to be much; it could be merely an involuntary twitch, a shift of the body, or a new noise.

This approach gives me an uncomfortable feeling that a deception of both subject and hypnotist is being carried out. Can one truly say that a response, overt or covert, that has no other relevance to the "suggestion" than it coincidentally happens in its context, is a suggested effect? Surely the sound of an unexpected commotion in the hallway can hardly be thus classified, even though it is a new experience for the subject. Can we interpret, with certainty, that a sudden muscular twitch, a sigh, or a slumping of the body is a bona fide suggested response and not just some natural incident? Even the subject becoming drowsy and having hypnagogic experiences under these circumstances cannot be ascribed with certainty to the use of such an open-ended suggestion. I am not questioning the possible utility of such a procedure, nor that some of the subject's experiences and actions occurring in its context may not indeed be appropriate suggested effects. The situation is not unlike one discussed in Volume 1, in which intended suggestions are mixed with instructions calling for the subject to do something that will naturally and artificially produce an effect similar to the suggested one. There is justification for letting the subject perceive something that is not a suggested effect as being one, but there is no justification for the hypnotist also misperceiving the situation.

Covering All Possibilities of Response

This has a strong resemblance to the use of the open-ended suggestion. A restricted set of possible responses is offered to the subject. The use of the conjunction "or" is characteristic in this approach. The subject is given a large choice of *specified* responses. The Hand Levitation Induction described in Volume 1 offers an excellent example of this. "You may experience a warmth in your hand, or possibly a feeling of coolness, or maybe an itch, or perhaps something else I have not mentioned . . . ." The reader might, at this point, review this material and see what other features exemplify this approach. It is of some interest that the above also contains an open-ended suggestion segment. Although Erickson and Rossi do not speak of this form as being a "compounded" suggestion, it should be included under that heading. It is, of course, entirely possible that some of the suggested effects will occur spontaneously, and, therefore, will not be a direct effect of some of the elementary intended suggestions that make it up. In this case, the latter may simply serve to pace the subject. The major difference between the open-ended case and the present one is that an attempt is made to relate specific effects that occur to specific contents of the suggestion. The above example is fairly direct. The same can be done in a more indirect manner. Also, in its most direct form, this type of suggestion basically constitutes a permissive approach. Its primary virtues seem to be that it minimizes failures and allows the hypnotist to explore the subject's potentialities for responses at the same time that it provides him with responses that can be elaborated and used to lead into other responses.

Pause with Attitude of Expectancy

This is very cursorily treated by Erickson and Rossi. The principle involved seems to be that, having given a suggestion, a pause conveying expectancy supposedly constitutes an affirmation that the suggested effect is going to take place. It's effect is an additional message that says, "I'm waiting . . . now do it."

The remaining entries in column 3 will be considered elsewhere. "Intercontextual cues" will be discussed under "interspersed" suggestion, of which they are a special aspect. The use of questions will be discussed under the "double bind." "Ideomotor signaling" will be separately discussed, too.

Unconscious Processes

It is far from clear just what makes the subject matter of column 4 a distinct step in the dynamic sequence that Erickson and Rossi have attempted to outline. It seems to be a collection of processes that is likely also to be active or potentially available in all of the prior steps (columns 1 through 3).

Some of the items listed in column 4, such as defense mechanisms, are preexisting non-conscious processes that have been inferred to develop in everyone and to be present through life. Others, like the Zeigarnik Effect, are special processes or mechanisms that have been inferred to develop in individuals under certain conditions. An individual might come to a hypnotism session with a Zeigarnik Effect already active, or one might be put into action in the course of working with the patient or subject. These are nonconscious processes that are neither trance nor suggestion phenomena in themselves, but that can potentially be utilized in the production of the latter. They essentially have a position similar to any of the existing physiological mechanisms that an individual has at the time he is hypnotized or is given a suggestion. The same remarks probably apply to what the authors refer to as autonomous, sensory, and perceptual processes. Admittedly, this is largely a guess, because one has to guess what, in the first place, the authors are talking about. Presumably, the idea is that at this point in the dynamics being outlined by Erickson and Rossi, the hypnotist is in a position to make the most use of such processes.

Literal and Individual Associations

The only additional information that one can find is the following (1976, p. 226): "Erickson has devised a number of other techniques to activate the individual, literal, and unconscious associations in words, phrases, or sentences buried within a more general context." It is anybody's guess as to what this is about. The statement is puzzling, if in no other way than that it is hard to conceive of associations, be they "individual," "literal," or of other kinds, as being anything but unconscious processes in the first place, so that to speak of "unconscious" associations seems rather meaningless and certainly redundant. Be that as it may, the use of "interspersed" suggestions seems to be an application of the above.

Multiple Meanings

The use of multiple meanings of words is closely related to the use of puns and jokes, and it also plays an important part in the "interspersal" technique. Erickson makes the point that many words have homonyms, or, more specifically, homophones, and that, as a result, one can, at least theoretically, convey one message under the guise of conveying another. For example, consider the word "change." One can make change, meaning convert money of one denomination into money of another denomination, or return the difference between the price of a purchased good and the amount received. On the other hand, one can change something, meaning alter it, and one can, in particular, change an attitude or a habit. Erickson was firmly convinced that by carefully using a word like "change" with other selected ones in, for example, a story about someone making change (in the monetary sense), and by emphasizing these words, one could convey a special message to the subject or patient about making a change (alteration) in some aspects of himself. A very simple abbreviated example of this would be to start a conversation about a transaction, allowing one to say somewhere in it, ". . . and *you* know he gave me the right *change* this time." The two emphasized words become, according to Erickson, a message to the patient's unconscious, and thus an indirect suggestion about making a change. Or, one might even say something like, ". . . and I told him I am going to show you how *you can make the right change* every time *you need to* . . . ."

In the trance induction of Sue, that has been described by Erickson, Haley, and Weakland (1959), Erickson says to Sue, ". . . I'll tell you when to go to sleep Sue, but *you won't know it.* I'll tell you when to go to sleep, but you won't *know* it. But you'll go to sleep." Erickson subsequently explains that "you won't know it" is a double statement. The first time it means, "you will not be aware of my telling you to go to sleep." The second time it means, "but nevertheless you will know I told you so." Unfortunately, Erickson does not further explicate the matter. My interpretation is that the second statement *implies* that, since the conscious has already been excluded, the knowing will occur at the level of the unconscious, and that the latter will execute the suggestion to sleep. One interesting and significant feature of the exchange that went on between Erickson and his co-authors at this juncture is *their misperception* of what Erickson had said, and the possibility of another, potential way in which the above segment could have been an effective suggestion. What Haley heard in the second "you won't know" statement is the homophone "no," which he then interprets as Erickson indirectly saying, "you won't 'no' my command," that is, you will not reject my command, or refuse to carry it out. This alternative is most certainly a possibility, and for all one knows, this is exactly the way Sue understood the second message, even though this was not Erickson's intent. This incident once again shows the problems inherent in knowing what really goes on in this type of situation.

Interspersal Technique

This is the imbedding (interspersing) of suggestions within and throughout a wider text, most of which is simply intended to be a diversion (distraction). This can, of course, be done without clever uses of words. Not just words, but entire sentences can be imbedded within phrases. These imbedded suggestions seem to be what the authors refer to as *intercontextual* cues and suggestions. The basic idea, as we shall shortly see, is to imbed the suggestions at various strategic points within a communication ostensibly concerned with other matters. The imbedding may be whole or piecemeal. One technique of activation referred to appears to be the use of anything that will make chosen words and sentences stand out in a text. Changes in intonation, special inflections, pauses, changes in the body posture of the hypnotist, touching the subject in a specific way, making a noise, and interjecting an unrelated comment, all done at the appropriate time and place, are methods that Erickson has been known to use for this purpose. Another method is that of making deliberate errors, such as saying "suntower" for "sunflower." In my experience, I have found that the larger context in which the imbedding is done can be used as more than a diversion to work with the patient on his problem at a conscious level.

To conclude this section, I will briefly describe Erickson's use of interspersed non-verbal material in a demonstration I witnessed. Erickson's demonstration with Ruth (described in Erickson and Rossi, 1981) that I had organized on the Stanford campus was followed that evening by some further impromptu demonstrations in a private home. After doing a number of things with a subject (a guest whom we shall call G.B.), Erickson had him hallucinate being in a row boat on a calm lake. There ensued a conversation that had little to do with the state of the lake, but while holding this conversation, Erickson began to rock his body backward, forward, and sideways, moving it much as it would have moved had the boat been rocked by waves. The movements were at first small, then later they became broader. It was not too long before G.B. remarked that the water was getting a little choppy. In no time, without ever saying a word about it, he had G.B. hallucinating that the boat was being rocked by large waves and that the fair weather had changed to stormy. Erickson then terminated the experience, as he realized that G.B. was showing incipient signs of becoming seasick!

Column 5 is fairly self-explanatory, and I shall not elaborate on it.

Miscellaneous

There are a number of procedures that Erickson and Rossi talk about in their books, but which they have not allocated to any of the five columns. I will now describe and comment on some of these.

Yes Set

This is the idea that if a person is placed in a situation in which he repeatedly and in fairly quick succession agrees to a series of statements made by the therapist or hypnotist, he will develop a tendency to continue to do so even with regard to something he might not have agreed to otherwise. Erickson and Rossi feel that this prepares the patient to accept suggestions. As we saw, this is a principle that has been applied in traditional and semi-traditional hypnotism, too. Getting the subject to respond positively to requests, commands, or instruction creates, perhaps through conditioning, a set to continue perseveratively to give positive responses. The principle has been widely used, even though never adequately substantiated. In any case, with this in mind, Erickson would make a number of statements to the subject that literally call for a "yes" answer or its equivalent. He might thus successively and correctly say to the patient, "your name is _____," "you are _____ years old," "we are at _____," and so on. The answers need not be overt verbal ones. That is, they can merely be covert assents as one will supposedly make to a statement of fact such as a "truism."

According to Erickson, asking a subject a dozen or so casual questions and making remarks that require obvious "yes" answers can create a positive momentum, so that when the subject is finally asked something like, "Are you ready to go into a trance now?" he will agree and do so.

Conditioning

This is actually used by Erickson in a much more straightforward way than has been hypothesized in previous examples. He believes, for example, that a conditioned response was produced in the following example described by Erickson and Rossi (1976, p. 235). Having noticed that the subject's eye blink reflex has begun to slow down, he warns the subject, without explaining why, that he is going to say "odd" and "even" for awhile. He then proceeds to say "odd" whenever the blinking is slow, and "even" when it is fast, and he continues doing this for about six blinks. This, Erickson believes, sets up a conditioned slow-blink response to the word "odd." Having judged that he has succeeded in doing so, he can then merely say "odd" between blinks to cause an increasingly slow blink to occur that eventually becomes indistinguishable from an eye closure. Having reached this point, he could have shifted to an acceptance of the eye closure (pacing) and then induced some further related effect. Because eye closure, or even slowing of the blink reflex, is never mentioned in the above procedure, this is viewed by Erickson as an indirect suggestion of these effects. To the extent that one can argue that the word "odd" has come to denote "you will next blink less quickly" outside the subject's conscious understanding, and that it does have an effect at an automatic level, this procedure meets essential criteria for being indirect. It is also a suggestion within the general framework of a suggestion as a communication that evokes a non-voluntary response reflecting the primary ideational content of the communication.

Truism

This is a statement whose truth cannot be argued. It can be about the world at large, or more specifically about the patient, as in, "Everyone has abilities," and "Your eyes are open" (if they are). But frequently, with Erickson, they are statements about behavior that the subject has so often experienced that he cannot deny it. For example, one might say to a patient, ". . . and then there have been those times when you discovered that you can easily forget that dream when you awaken . . . ," or, "You know how on many occasions you have nodded your head to say 'yes'." Erickson usually talks thus when he intends to produce by suggestion a related effect. In the case of the first example, this could be an amnesia. In the case of the second example, it could be an automatic (ideomotor) nodding of the head. The wording of the first example contains an additional feature of interest. It could have served its purpose, too, by having been worded, ". . . that you could easily forget . . . ." But by using the above form instead, a more direct and forceful suggestion of amnesia is given, but still in an indirect manner. According to Erickson, a truism stated before a suggestion proper can create an acceptance set for it. If it comes after the suggestion, it can reinforce it.

In keeping with their position (Erickson & Rossi, 1976, p. 7) that "suggestions are statements that the patient cannot possibly argue with," Erickson and Rossi classify truisms as "suggestions." I must seriously question the validity of these two assertions, but will leave the discussion of the matter to later, when I will discuss Erickson's concept of suggestion in detail. On the other hand, the recommendation he makes that suggestions are always given in a form that the patient can easily accept is a sound one.

Some examples of truisms that Erickson and Rossi use are questionable. For example, "Sooner or later, your hand is going to lift" is viewed by them to be a truism utilizing time. While I would agree that this is a suggestion, this does not automatically make it a truism, even if we accept for the moment that all truisms are suggestions, because the converse does not hold. Even Erickson and Rossi would agree to that. There is no certainty that the hand will ever rise except in some very remote sense that indeed sometime, somewhere, in the course of everyday life, the subject must eventually raise that hand. This is overstretching the concept of truism. But that this is indeed what they have in mind seems indicated by the following passage from Erickson and Rossi (1976, p. 22): "He [Erickson] would never say, 'Your headache is gone,' because it might not be, and the patient would, with some justice, begin to experience a loss of belief." Instead, Erickson turns the direct suggestion into a truism by saying, "The headache is going to leave shortly." He then adds that actually this could be a matter of seconds, minutes, hours, or even days, but sooner or later it is bound to happen in the natural course of events! That is, unless there is a pathological condition making this impossible. As a side note, for my part, were I the patient, I would not consider hours, and especially days, to fall under "shortly!"

There is a certain reasonableness in Erickson's concern in the patient losing belief. However, as pointed out in Volume 1, the effects of belief on the efficiency of suggestions remains a grey area. It is common to find subjects who do poorly on a suggestion, but who then go on and do very well on another of equal or even greater difficulty. For example, I have frequently known subjects who can hallucinate certain tastes and not others, regardless of the order in which I try them. This type of observation goes against the idea that failed suggestions have adverse effects.

Apposition of Opposites

This procedure is said to be a favorite of Erickson's. It refers to a juxtaposition of opposites. An example Erickson and Rossi (1976) give is, "You can forget to remember or remember to forget." Forgetting and remembering are obviously opposites. This form is often found in examples of Erickson's use of confusion, and it probably works through creating confusion that depotentiates the conscious. Also, according to Erickson and Rossi, this example is a "double bind," and its effectiveness may derive from that. Rossi, however, is inclined to believe that some kind of hypothetical neurological balance mechanism is elicited and, therefore, that the above statement elicits a non-voluntary response. Consequently, it has to be a suggestion, and it also brings the trance about, or at least facilitates it; that, at least, seems to be their argument.

Contingent Suggestions

Potential readers of the writings of Erickson and Rossi should be aware that these authors seem to confuse the above situations with this one, which they also mention independently elsewhere in their texts. These are the same kind of statements as were discussed under this heading and that of chaining in Volume 1. One suggested effect is made contingent upon the occurrence of another one. "As your hand lifts, your eyes will begin to feel heavy," and, "As your hands become warmer, your forehead can become cooler" are typical examples. According to the two authors, these statements are also examples of the apposition of opposites. I suppose "heavy" might be considered the opposite of "lift" because of its implication, by association, of a potential downward movement of the eyelids. Of course, "cooler" and "warmer" are obvious opposites. I suspect that Rossi would argue this point by conceding that these statements are, indeed, contingent suggestions, but would add that, *in addition,* they are applications of the apposition of opposites. Perhaps they are. Anything is possible with this vague idea and principle.

Ratification

This is verification of the trance and is another important concept in Ericksonian hypnotism. This is the act of providing the subject and, to some extent, the hypnotist with evidence that a trance is present or has been present. This is not usually a problem with a good subject, but can be with an individual who is skeptical, resistant, or not very responsive at the beginning. Erickson feels that it is important to provide such individuals with as much evidence as possible that they have appropriately responded to the induction. This is not just a matter of satisfying the subject, but is a facilitating step in any induction. The authors explain that in the trance, the observer function of the patient's ego is usually more or less active. As a consequence, the patient may be unwilling to believe that he was in a trance, and this may interfere with further work. Ratification demonstrates to the patient that the trance and non-trance state are different. As stated in Volume 1, belief in the success of a procedure seems to engender further success. As then proposed, this effect is possibly the result of a conditioning-like process leading to generalization of responsiveness (receptivity). Then, too, there may be some individuals who have a need for this kind of feedback and who cooperate better when they get it.

There are any number of ways in which ratification can be accomplished. Having the subject describe his sensations and experiences after termination of a trance, or at various critical stages in the induction, is one way. As noted in Volume 1, subjects frequently do not volunteer such information, and in this case, the hypnotist needs to resort to asking specific questions. In this process, the subject becomes more aware of unusual experiences and changes that the hypnotist can point out to the subject as being signs of trance. If there are other observers, this step can be done indirectly through the simple expedient of talking to them instead of to the subject. In the absence of an observer, I have found that a good way of doing this is to have a tape recorder and to dictate or pretend to dictate appropriate comments to it. Effects I have in mind are blurring of vision, a feeling of lightness, of numbness, of relaxation, of drowsiness, and other experiences of this type listed in Volume 1. For the hypnotist, any of the clinical signs of hypnosis, listed in Volume 1 and in this chapter, that he observes can serve for his own ratification, but can also be used to ratify the trance for the subject by mentioning them to him or to others who are present. A trance sign that Erickson seemed to like particularly is an alteration in time perception, as when, on being "awakened," the subject grossly underestimates or overestimates the duration of the trance, or even of some event during trance. The subject's experience with such induced effects as a hand levitation, a catalepsy of the hand, or the Hands Together Suggestion can be very rich in material that can be used for ratification. Any feeling of apartness from the hands or arms can generally be taken as evidence of *dissociation.* The same is true when there is a loss of feeling with regard to these members. Reorientation of the body, stretching, shifting of the body, adjusting the feet, and so forth, on "awakening" from a trance, are considered by Erickson to be good signs of a trance having occurred. When inducing the Hand/Arm Catalepsy, Erickson was always careful to place the arm at an odd angle. If the angle was preserved by the subject, he considered this to be a good indicator of trance. For reasons to be discussed, I do not feel that one can always consider this to indicate a trance, but would certainly consider it to indicate that an effective suggestion had occurred.

Redintegration

I prefer to call this reintegration. It is briefly discussed by Erickson, Rossi, and Rossi (1976), although not by name. As explained in Volume 1, this is an effect nicely demonstrated when a person, who has already experienced being in a hypnotic state, is asked to silently review the steps previously gone through. Frequently, one finds the subject becoming hypnotized while doing so. I first learned about this from Erickson in 1960. At that time, he spoke of it as a "redintegration" of past behavior. This can also be seen as a case of utilization. It can also be viewed in the context of a conditioning effect. Erickson described to me an application that he had made of this effect. As he talked to a patient in preparation to inducing a hypnotic state, Erickson would nonchalantly move a paper weight in sight of the patient from one position to another. After the patient had closed his eyes, he would put the paper weight back in its original position. Thereafter, according to Erickson, moving the paper weight as he had previously done frequently acted as a signal for the subject to enter a hypnotic state. This is about as indirect a posthypnotic suggestion as one can think of. Similarly, if the subject is sitting in a different chair than the one in which he was initially hypnotized, asking him to change to the latter can act as a cue for a reinduction of hypnosis, or will at least facilitate it. Erickson would sometimes state that the very act of coming for a session with him was sufficient to initiate the start of hypnosis as the patient entered his office.

Being aware of the possibility of this type of conditioning—associating becoming hypnotized with various cues belonging to his office and the situation—Erickson would watch for specific signs of hypnosis, as have been discussed. Having detected such indications of impending hypnosis (or of hypnosis), Erickson would then promote its further development in various ways. He might be quite direct, perhaps saying, "And now you can go into a trance." Or he might be a little less direct, and say, "Are you ready to go into a trance?" Or again, he might say, "When you are ready you can go into a trance." An even more indirect suggestion was, "As you sit in that chair, I want you to find how easy and pleasant it is to go into a trance." The reader should have no difficulties in thinking up other, even more indirect, variations of this. However, Erickson had some truly indirect ways of doing this. For example, he might simply look at the patient with expectancy, saying nothing. Or he might look at the patient, with or without expectancy, and slowly close his own eyes momentarily. Or again, he might take a deep breath and visibly relax in his chair.

Resistance

Dealing with this has been another one of Erickson's interests and concerns. Resistance takes many forms and has various origins. Although he recognized the existence of the type of resistance psychoanalysts talk about, his primary concern was with patterns of association and experience that prevent people from making use of their abilities. This kind of resistance is "an erroneous mental set that gets in the way of new experience." The techniques that Erickson uses in this context aim at "displacing" and "discharging" the resistance. Many of the examples discussed by Erickson have more to do with resistance to therapy than to hypnosis. It should be obvious that in the context of therapeutic hypnotism all resistance is dealt with regardless of what its focus is. Sometimes the procedure is short and fairly simple; sometimes it is fairly long and involved. One example given by Erickson, Rossi, and Rossi (1976, p. 221) concerns a patient who announced that he wanted hypnotherapy, but who also asserted that he could not be hypnotized. On that occasion, Erickson had three additional empty chairs in his office. Erickson began by telling the patient that there was a possibility that he could be hypnotized. He then recognized the greater possibility that he could not be hypnotized. He then said, "Now let's try this chair." Erickson continued by pointing out that even if the patient failed to become hypnotized in that chair, it was still possible that he could do so. After trying three chairs unsuccessfully, the patient became hypnotized in the fourth one. Erickson and Rossi explain that being able to fail a number of times allows the resistance to be used up and discharged. But they also recognize that there is a great deal more involved than this in the above procedure. The initial statement aims to open the door to the possibility that hypnosis can be induced. By next accepting the patient's negative attitude, Erickson believes that he establishes a beginning of rapport that favors acceptance of his initial assertion. Trying the first chair not only begins the process of discharging resistance, but also establishes, by implication, that becoming hypnotized is associated with sitting in some particular chair. The use of the word "try" is critical in establishing this implication.

Another method recommended by Erickson, Rossi, and Rossi (1976) is to start out in a conversational manner with a series of questions to the patient about matters far removed from the therapy or hypnosis session and that are most likely or are certain to evoke a "no" answer. After a half dozen or so of these questions have been asked, new questions are asked that will elicit a "yes" answer. The authors explain that all or most of the patient's negativeness gets displaced and discharged in the first half of the procedure, and that the second half creates a "yes" set. They do not explain why the first series of questions does not establish a "no" set, as one would expect, and therefore reinforce the negativism of the patient. Also, one cannot help but wonder whether something such as not liking smog (this being in an example used here) is really a counterpart of a deep-seated fear of losing control if hypnotized, as the authors assert. In any case, the technique is interesting. Erickson's approach to resistance can be very subtle. He will say to a subject, very early in the induction, something like, "You don't need to listen," and then will talk, perhaps, about the subject's mind wandering. Erickson explains that if the patient has any tendency to rebel, his rebellion can be focused into doing exactly what he has been told to do, "not to listen." It would be easier to follow Erickson's thinking if he also told us that the situation contains an initial implicit injunction to listen, to which the subject will tend to respond negatively. But why doesn't the subject respond negatively to the message of not listening *by then listening?* The answer may lie in the permissive wording Erickson uses in this instance. The subject is not told "don't listen," but that he "doesn't have" to do so. One may also wonder whether Erickson could not have, indeed, reached the same objective by using the subject's negative tendency and telling him not to listen. We shall see an example of Erickson using this very approach in a rather similar situation when we discuss double binds. There are no reasons to think that in the situation described by Erickson and Rossi (1981, p. 183) this would not have worked too, and perhaps there is no answer as to why Erickson chose to go one way here and the other way in the other situation. The 1981 volume contains other interesting examples of Erickson's handling of resistance in non-hypnotic situations. The reader may wish to examine these.

CATALEPSY

Catalepsy has a rather unique place in Ericksonian hypnotism, and Erickson and Rossi (1981) devote a full chapter to it. Catalepsy was viewed by Erickson as a sign of the presence of a trance, as a means of inducing and reinducing a trance, and as a method for deepening the trance.

In the above volume they state that it is the suspension of voluntary movement. Elsewhere, Erickson also states that it is *a condition of well-balanced tonicity.* As such, it can be limited to only certain groups of muscles, or it can involve the whole musculature. In the 1981 work, the authors also seem to consider it to be a special mental and physical state differing from the normal one while, at the same time, claiming that the occurrence of transient catalepsy is a normal everyday behavior. This last agrees with their general contention that all hypnotic phenomena are aspects or derivatives of normal behavior. As I understand catalepsy, I agree that the first description may be partly correct, but, since trance is consistent with movement (automatic as it may be), catalepsy as thus manifested can, at best, only be a temporary trance characteristic. Erickson and Rossi (1981, p. 41) explain that the receptivity that allows a part of the body to become immobilized reflects a like mental receptivity to further suggestions. They propose that, at least in some cases, the manipulation of the subject's member is associated with the subject wondering and speculating about just what is going on, and that leaves his mind open to suggestions. In other words, the procedure depotentiates the subject's consciousness. In any case, the appearance of a trance when an arm or hand catalepsy is induced has been partially documented on the basis of the coinciding appearance of other clinical signs of trance. How consistent the appearance of these other signs is remains unclear.

Catalepsy has a fairly long history; at one time it was considered to be a disorder. In the older literature it is used synonymously with so-called waxy flexibility (*flexibilitas cerea*), and has often been defined as a state of involuntary retention of position, or of limbs or other parts of the body, in positions they have been placed. It has been particularly associated with hysteria, schizophrenia, and, of course, hypnosis. Braid may have been the first one to call attention specifically to catalepsy of the arm as a symptom of hypnosis, although he did not call it by name. Charcot went much beyond considering it a symptom, making it, instead, a syndrome. For him, it was a mental and physiological state. It was one of three forms that hypnosis could take, and it affected the whole body. It was associated with a specific mental state. With Bernheim, catalepsy, as well as Charcot's other two forms of hypnosis, became reduced to being suggested effects. Since then it has been quite common for hypnotists to use the term rather loosely, and talk, for example, of the inability of some presumably hypnotized subjects to open their eyes, whether spontaneous or suggested, as an "eyelid catalepsy" or "eye catalepsy." Catalepsy has also been extended in the past by many hypnotists to *suggested* rigidities of specific members or of the whole body. Thus one hears of arm and of total body catalepsies in this sense. As demonstrated and used by Erickson, catalepsy is similar to waxy flexibility, and may be the same thing. Since Erickson nearly always, if not always, demonstrated catalepsy with a subject's hands and arms, it is not possible to know whether or not there was a general catalepsy of the body in such cases. In any case, Erickson, more often than not, spoke of specifically inducing a catalepsy "of an arm" or "of a hand," rarely of inducing a total body catalepsy. There are indications in the 1981 book by Erickson and Rossi that in his later years, Erickson may have envisaged catalepsy more and more as a generalized condition, although one that can be produced in a limited way at first and gradually extended. This observation confirms Erickson, Rossi, and Rossi's (1976) view that hypnotic phenomena can often be brought about in segments (or fragments) that are eventually united into a whole. This idea was discussed in a different context in Volume 1, and procedures for using segmentation were described at the time. According to Erickson and Rossi (1981), transitory catalepsies are a very common occurrence in daily life. If catalepsy is a symptom of trance, this claim would follow from their claim that transitory trances are a common occurrence in daily life. This is actually a poorly documented matter, and the impressive list of examples of daily life catalepsies given by the authors is strictly conjectural. There is an attempt in the work, most likely Rossi's contribution, to give catalepsy a neurophysiological and anatomic foundation. It is premature, consists mostly of generalities, and can be dispensed with.

A variety of procedures for producing, using, and testing for catalepsy, mostly of the hands and arms, are given by Erickson and Rossi. These are essentially the same procedures that were discussed in considerable detail under the heading of "hand levitation" in Volume 1, with the difference that in the case of verbal inductions, some are more spread out and indirect. If there is a special muscular tonus associated with the appearance of a trance, it is therefore masked by procedures capable of producing it through suggestion. In later years, Erickson made much more use of non-verbal inductions than of verbal inductions. Also, he spoke less and less of hand (arm) levitation, preferring the use of the term catalepsy. Erickson and Rossi tend to restrict the designation "hand levitation" to the use of verbal suggestions in causing the hand to rise, and that of "hand catalepsy" when the non-verbal technique that I described in Volume 1 is used. Is there an intrinsic difference? The mode of communication may be the only change. A major issue remains unsettled. Is there a special, characteristic tonicity associated with trance (hypnosis) not caused by suggestion?

I was introduced to the Hand Levitation Induction by Wolberg's book (1945). It was my impression that he had been the originator of the technique, an impression that was furthered by references in the literature to it being his technique of hand levitation. According to an account by Erickson (1959), he would have antedated Wolberg, and it is quite possible that Wolberg obtained the technique from Erickson and failed to mention it. As described by Wolberg, it has a definite Ericksonian flavor.

IDEOMOTOR AND IDEOSENSORY SIGNALING

Ideomotor signaling has already been discussed at some length in Volume 1. Again, from both Erickson and Rossi's (1981) work and an earlier article by Erickson (1964), Erickson appears to have been the originator of ideomotor signaling. My own introduction to it was by Leslie LeCron at a seminar in the middle 1950s. Actually, as Erickson and Rossi (1981) recognize, it could be argued that ideomotor signaling is much older; automatic writing and the movements of the dowser's pendulum and forked twig are likely examples of its applications. Indeed, if Chevreul (1854) was correct, and I have little doubt he was, the table tilting of spiritists, as well as the use of the ouija board (also known as the "planchette"), would also be earlier examples. In contrast to LeCron and others, Erickson seems to have made minimal use of ideomotor signaling as an analytical tool for accessing the "unconscious." He used it mostly as an induction and deepening technique and for trance ratification. Erickson perceived the elicitation of ideomotor signaling as synonymous with trance induction. This, however, has not been a view universally ascribed to by other users of the technique. LeCron, for example, distinguished between using finger signaling in hypnosis and in the non-hypnotic state. In any event, if ideomotor signaling is not trance inducing in its own right, it is an excellent way of initiating the process, as exemplified with the use of the Chevreul pendulum in Volume 1. I would also agree that it is an excellent way of deepening hypnosis.

One of Erickson's favorite ways of using ideomotor signaling was for the production of non-voluntary nodding and shaking of the head in response to questions. The Ruth induction (Erickson and Rossi, 1981) is one of the best demonstrations of that application. In it, Erickson gives one of his best demonstrations of his use of indirect verbal and non-verbal techniques in eliciting these responses, and later, of subtle ways to establish their validity. It is also a nice one-procedure demonstration of induction, deepening, and ratification of the trance.

Erickson and Rossi also point out that spontaneous ideomotor signaling can occur, and they give various examples from everyday life. However, they do not elaborate on their possible use in relation to the induction of trance behavior. In some of the examples of Erickson's procedures that are available in the literature, such as in the Ruth induction, one does find instances in which he makes such a use.

Erickson and Rossi also make a brief mention of what they call *ideosensory* signaling. By this they mean spontaneously occurring unusual sensations that, being covert, are usually not recognized by the therapist. These may be a feeling of warmth, a prickling, an itch, and so forth. There is a hint in this short discussion that such sensations may sometimes arise instead of the ideomotor response that one is attempting to elicit. Presumably (the authors do not actually say so), they become known when the patient makes a verbal communication regarding them or shows some overt signs that cue the therapist that something covert is happening and that leads him to inquire. Erickson and Rossi feel these spontaneous effects are often communications coming from an unconscious level.

Although Erickson has done this at times, the authors fail to mention that ideosensory signals can, of course, also be set up by means of direct and indirect suggestions. One could interpret the mention of possible warmth, prickling, and itching of the hand in the Hand Levitation Induction described in Volume 1 as being just that. Ideosensory signals can even be combined with ideomotor signaling. The subject might be told, "When you are ready to answer 'yes' or 'no' with your fingers, you will experience a warmth in your hand."

DISSOCIATION

This is another concept widely referred to by Erickson, but that he essentially never defines or clearly explains. He apparently believes that everyone will know what he means. He views dissociation as a trance characteristic, but one that is far from being universally present. For Erickson, inducing a dissociation often seems to be the same as inducing a trance. He also views its production as a way to deepen a trance. On the other hand, it seems clear from his writings that trance does not always entail a dissociation, at least not an obvious one.

As the term implies, in a dissociation there is a breaking of mental associations, or, perhaps more correctly, a disassociation. But what kinds of associations are we talking about? A very typical example of dissociation that is mentioned by Erickson is when a person develops a feeling of separateness from some part of his body, such as a hand. The subject perceives it as no longer a part of himself, but as an object. An even more complete dissociation would involve a total unawareness of possessing this hand. Dissociation seems to have the peculiar property, in this case, of the conscious being fully active, but not having access to certain information. Dissociations often occur spontaneously, or they can be induced by appropriate suggestions. Such suggestions can directly or indirectly suggest the unawareness in question. The use of "not knowing" is seen as a good indirect way of doing this. One of Erickson's favorite ways of producing dissociations consisted in telling the hypnotized subject that his head would "awaken," but the rest of his body would remain "asleep." Producing dissociation can be done very indirectly, such as when Erickson induced surgical anesthesia in a patient by suggesting she was geographically elsewhere than on the operating table. In the case in question, he had her experience herself as reclining in some other part of the operating room and watching with interest an operation being performed on "someone" lying on the operating table. Erickson explains the success of this method in producing anesthesia with the remark, "You cannot experience pain inflicted where your body is not." This is obviously a use of implication. A simpler version of the last example, and that I have seen Erickson demonstrate a number of times, consisted of his telling a hypnotized subject, whose hand was lying on his lap, to continue to watch the hand and keep looking at it as it lay on his lap. As he said this, Erickson would gently move the hand to the side in such a way as to induce catalepsy in it, if this was not already present. He would then demonstrate that the hand was now anesthetic. Erickson viewed catalepsy as always involving a dissociation, and he would routinely demonstrate the presence of anesthesia after demonstrating a catalepsy.

I am not sure that everyone would agree that all cases that Erickson considered to be dissociations were actually so. For example, Erickson reported at a seminar (Erickson, Hershman, & Secter, 1961, p. 70f) that he had once had a hypnotized subject who stated that he was experiencing being in the living room of his childhood home while at the same time being fully aware of his current surroundings. The subject argued on the basis of the latter experience that he could not be hypnotized, and he insisted that he was "wide awake." Erickson explained to his audience that this was an example of a dissociation "with a duality of conscious and unconscious functioning." I prefer to think of this case as showing an incomplete regression and falling in the same category as a subject having an incomplete hallucination, such as when a subject states that he sees a hallucinated vase but that it is lacking substance. When a subject reports that his cataleptic arm and hand no longer feel a part of him, he should also be showing, to use Erickson's words, a duality of consciousness. However, to my knowledge, Erickson never mentioned this, in discussing limb catalepsies, as examples of dissociations. In any event, Erickson's view of dissociation, especially in relation to hypnosis, is definitely different from that of Janet, and even of Hilgard. For a more complete discussion of dissociation, the reader is referred to Chapter 7 of Volume 1.

UTILIZATION

It has often been said that Ericksonian hypnotism is a *utilization* theory of hypnotism. Rossi, in particular, holds this view. Erickson (1958) originally introduced the idea under the heading of *naturalistic* techniques, saying:

> By naturalistic approach is meant the acceptance of the situation encountered and the utilization of it without endeavoring to restructure it psychologically. In so doing, the presenting behavior of the patient becomes a definite aid and an actual part in inducing a trance, rather than a possible hindrance. For lack of a more definite terminology, the method may be termed a naturalistic approach, in which an aspect of the principle of synergism is utilized. (p. 3)

The above statement also holds the essence of his preferred mode of handling resistance in general and of his approach to therapy.

In brief, Erickson believed that hypnotic suggestion is the process of eliciting and *using* a patient's own *preexisting* mental processes in ways that are outside of his normal range of voluntary control. More specifically, he saw this (Erickson & Rossi, 1975) "as evoking, mobilizing, and moving a patient's associative processes and mental skills in certain directions" to achieve various goals, particularly therapeutic ones. Even using the term "theory" in the loosest sense, this is more correctly a definition rather than a theory of suggestion. More important, is doing the above really unique to Erickson's work? One can reasonably maintain that a good portion of the process of education is predicated upon doing this type of thing. Similarly for the practice of traditional and semi-traditional hypnotism and for psychotherapy in general. What I see as unique about Ericksonian hypnotism in this respect is Erickson's specific recognition of the existence and role of these processes in the production of suggested and hypnotic phenomena, his *deliberate application* of this observation, his devising of a great many procedures aimed at evoking and directing these processes, and his highly *systematic* planned use of these processes, often stepwise, to attain specific goals. As Rossi states, (Erickson, Rossi, & Rossi, p. 302), "The effectiveness of his [Erickson's] words is in their calculated design to evoke preexisting patterns of association and natural mental processes in the patient."

The following quote, also taken from Erickson (1958), is a much better statement of his utilization principle:

> One of the most important of all considerations in inducing hypnosis is meeting adequately the patient as a personality and his needs as an individual. Too often, the effort is made to fit the patient to an accepted formal technique of suggestion, rather than adapting the technique to the patient in accord with his actual personality situation. In any such adaptation, there is an imperative need to accept and to utilize those psychological states, understandings and attitudes that the patient brings into the situation. To ignore those factors in favor of some ritual of procedure may and often does delay, impede, limit or even prevent the desired results. The acceptance and utilization of those factors, on the other hand, promotes more rapid trance induction, the development of more profound trance states, the more ready acceptance of therapy and greater ease for the handling of the total therapeutic situation. (p. 7)

In contrast, the traditional and semi-traditional hypnotist uses a relatively small number of procedures that have been found by trial and error to work, and he applies them with little thought given to the mechanisms that are being evoked or to their organization. Nor is there much concern about individual attributes of the subject. When traditional and semi-traditional hypnotists use a segmental approach to the production of an effect, they do so largely by using gross responses. In contrast (although at times he does likewise), Erickson also extensively focuses on the segmental use of elemental responses.

BINDS AND DOUBLE BINDS

Origin, Definition, and Early History of the Double Bind

The concept of the double bind was first presented in a multi-authored article (Bateson, Jackson, Haley, & Weakland, 1956) primarily concerned with a new theory of schizophrenia based on a communication model. Bateson was given credit in this article for coining the term "double bind" and for using the concept to account for the symptoms and the etiology of schizophrenia. Haley was credited for providing the hypothesis that schizophrenics have an inability to discriminate "logical types," a concept borrowed from formal logic. The double bind was seen by its creators as being an outgrowth of this hypothesis. The theory of logical types was evolved by the logician Bertrand Russell to deal with logical paradoxes that had their roots in a confusion that existed over what constitutes class membership. For purposes of this discussion, it is not necessary to know anything further about the theory of types, since an understanding of the double bind does not depend on that. As a matter of fact, the definition of the double bind provided by the authors makes no reference to logical types. Also, the theory of types is actually only very indirectly relevant to the matter at hand because the paradoxes dealt with by Bateson et al. actually have a different origin than a failure in discrimination between logical types. Many paradoxes are indeed logical in nature, but many also have their origin in meaning rather than in logic. The theory of *semantic levels,* which is the counterpart of the theory of types in the case of semantics, was developed by logicians and semanticists to resolve semantic paradoxes (often referred to as descriptive paradoxes). Such paradoxes arise out of the failure of individuals to discriminate between statements and statements *about* statements. It remained for Watzlawick, Beavin, and Jackson (1967) to clarify the picture one step further by pointing out that communications that give rise to semantic paradoxes will often lead to several response tendencies that jointly constitute a "pragmatic paradox" if they are called forth simultaneously and they are incompatible with each other. There are no reasons to think that pragmatic paradoxes cannot arise from other causes, but these writers do not discuss that aspect.

Thus far, I have used the term "paradox" on the assumption that the reader would have some idea of what I am talking about. To be more specific, and without getting involved in the technical language of formal logic and semantics, one might simply say that paradoxes are situations in which two aspects *coexist* in irreconcilable opposition. That is, the presence of the one is totally and absolutely incompatible with the presence of the other. The essence of a paradox is in this "impossible" coexistence. In theory, there can only be one of the aspects in question.

For Bateson et al., a double bind situation comes into being when an individual finds himself *compelled* to simultaneously carry out two actions that are incompatible with each other; in this way, the situation is somewhat reminiscent of a paradox. Expressed in its simplest form, it is a condition of simultaneously having *to do and not do*. As Haley (1958) states, it is a no win situation. There are many colloquial expressions denoting this situation, such as, "being between the devil and the deep blue sea," "jumping from the frying pan into the fire," "being on the horns of the dilemma," and finally, "you are damned if you do and you are damned if you don't." Also, *colloquially speaking,* this has been usually referred to as "being in a bind," and it is not at all clear why Bateson et al. chose to call it a "double" bind. If there is any special significance to this qualification, they have not indicated what it is. As far as I can see, the term "dilemma" is perfectly descriptive of and applicable to the above.

To be more specific, Bateson et al. (1956, 253f) originally defined the "schizophrenic double bind" as a situation that consists of the following features:

1. *Two or more persons.* Of these, we designate one, for purposes of our definition, as the "victim."

2. *Repeated experience.* We assume that the double bind is a recurrent theme in the experience of the victim. Our hypothesis does not invoke a single traumatic experience, but such repeated experience that the double bind structure comes to be an habitual expectation.

3. *A primary negative injunction.* This may have either of two forms: (a) Do not do so and so, or I will punish you," or (b) "If you do not do so and so, I will punish you." Here we select a context of learning based on avoidance of punishment rather than a context of reward seeking. There is perhaps no formal reason for this selection.

4. *A secondary injunction conflicting with the first at a more abstract level, and like the first enforced by punishments or signals which threaten survival.* This secondary injunction is more difficult to describe than the primary for two reasons. First, the secondary injunction is commonly communicated by nonverbal means. Second, the secondary injunction may impinge upon any element of the primary prohibition. Verbalization of the secondary injunction may, therefore, include a wide variety of forms.

5. *A tertiary negative injunction prohibiting the victim from escaping from the field.* In a formal sense it is perhaps unnecessary to list this injunction as a separate item since the reinforcement at the other two levels involves a threat to survival, and if the double binds are imposed during infancy, escape is naturally impossible. However, it seems that in some cases the escape from the field is made impossible by certain devices which are not purely negative . . .

It is made clear in the remainder of the article that the reference in the above quoted material (condition 4) to "a more abstract level" of interaction is a very important feature of the theory. To further clarify this aspect, other statements in the article show that the double bind is viewed as more than two contradictory injunctions having been given. As Haley (1958) explains in a later article, "Note that there were not merely two contradictory messages, they were two contradictory *levels* of messages," with the second one *qualifying* the first. For this reason, using a term borrowed from formal logic, the second message is said by the authors to be a "metacommunication" or a "metamessage."

It is not entirely clear from these two articles whether two levels of communication are absolutely required for a double bind to exist. There are intimations that this may be an optional feature for Bateson et al. On the other hand, for Erickson and Rossi, who refer to this feature time and time again, it would appear to be an essential requirement of their adaptation of the concept to hypnotic behavior.

According to Bateson et al., what happens under the conditions listed above is that, when in a double bind, the ability of the individual to discriminate between logical types breaks down, and this is reflected in his/her behavior as *abnormalities.* They are careful to state that *this is a hypothesis,* and this is what it remains today.

A typical schizophrenic-inducing double bind that they discuss in considerably more detail can be summed up in the following example: There is a mother who cannot tolerate intimate (loving) contact with her child. At the same time, she cannot tolerate her feelings of hostility and anxiety toward her child. She copes with this by expressing (simulating) overtly loving behavior in order to elicit loving behavior from her child, thus giving credence to her being a loving mother. This simulated loving behavior on her part *serves as a comment* (metastatement) on her hostile behavior by denying the implication of not loving. Here, then, is the second level message. If the child does not respond lovingly, she withdraws from him. Of course, she cannot help herself from also withdrawing from the child if he responds lovingly. The net result is the child receiving a double message: "love me or be rejected" and "do not love me or be rejected." He is the loser however he acts. For the child, this can be extremely threatening, especially if the mother's withdrawal involves other punishing actions. Obviously, the child is in no position to withdraw from the situation or comment, and the situation *is a repeated one.* Actually, there is still another bind (double bind?) in the above situation that is not mentioned by the authors. This is that the mother is also in a bind; she wants expressions of love from the child and she does not want them. Both are threatening and a source of anxiety. Social, religious, or other pressures may effectively prevent her from escaping the situation, which also gets repeated over and over. What seems to be missing is the metamessage.

In explanation, the somewhat peculiar term "victim" was used because Bateson et al. viewed the schizophrenic as being a victim of his/her parents. There are also other observations. When the double bind is taken out of the context of schizophrenia, punishment or threat to survival do not specifically appear to be a requirement as long as there is an equivalently *strong compelling element* in the situation to force the crucial opposing responses. Whether or not the compelling elements for the two injunctions must be the same, as it is in Bateson et al.'s examples, is not stated. One can conceive of paradoxical situations, comparable to the double bind, in which this would not be the case. The relationship does not specifically have to be that of a parent and child, but can be *any equivalently intense interpersonal relationship.*

Also, it is not obvious why the second injunction should be a metamessage. One can certainly think of situations that have all the other features of the double bind, but in which there are no metamessages, that are equally traumatic. It ought at least to be recognized that there are potential situations that are not paradoxical in the sense we have used this term; these, colloquially speaking, would also have to be called "binds" and are associated with compelling needs for action. In any case, a more concise and somewhat more general statement of the double bind as conceived by Bateson et al. might be as follows: A double bind situation exists when

1. There is an intense interpersonal relationship between at least two individuals.
2. There is a primary injunctive message to do something with compelling reasons for not doing it.
3. There is a second injunctive contradictory message (at a different level of communication?) qualifying the first one and calling for an opposite action with compelling reasons for not doing so.
4. There is no escape from the situation either physically or by being able to comment on it.
5. There is repetitive exposure to it.

While we shall not try to follow Bateson et al. in their detailed explanation of how schizophrenia develops out of double binds, since this is not pertinent to the production of hypnosis, we will look more closely at what they had to say about it in relation to hypnotism. The authors think that many of the manifestations of schizophrenia, such as hallucinations, delusions, personality changes, and so forth, can be reproduced in normal subjects through the use of hypnotism. This observation meant to them that the production of some of these phenomena, if not all, should be explainable in terms of the double bind. In support of this claim, they examined and dissected two examples to show that they involved a double bind situation.

One of these examples is Erickson's production of the hallucination of a hand moving, which the authors presumably witnessed. Erickson first produced a hand catalepsy, then said to the subject, "There is no conceivable way in which your hand can move, yet when I give the signal, it must move." The subject is said to have hallucinated the hand moving.

Bateson et al. believe that all the ingredients called for by a double bind are present in the above example. However, criterion (1) is not clearly satisfied unless one *takes for granted* that something like a rapid, intense transference occurs in such a situation. Criteria (2) and (3) are satisfied regarding contradictory injunctions, but not so clearly regarding the existence of a powerful compulsion. Possibly the authors are *assuming* the reality of the compulsion that is said in the literature to accompany hypnosis. No information is available regarding this. In any case, what the second level communication (metacommunication) is, if there is one, is anyone's guess. Criterion (4) is questionably satisfied. Can the subject really not get out of the situation? Assuming he is hypnotized, he could come out of the hypnotic state, as subjects have been known to do when placed in a conflict. Finally, there is no evidence that criterion (5) has been satisfied. Speaking from personal experience, the described effect can be produced when (5) is definitely not met. The above seems a poor example of a double bind.

Their second example, which is too complex to describe, is even less satisfactory mainly because many important details are left out. In any event, one has to question seriously whether criterion (1) was ever satisfied. Again, the question of the source and nature of the required compulsion for criteria (2) and (3) is anything but clearly established. Likewise for the second level message. There is some ambiguity whether (5) was ever satisfied. The answer depends on how one interprets the multiple exposure requirement. Only (4) seems to have been satisfied, but one still has to make some assumptions.

Perhaps one should not be surprised that Bateson et al. cannot make a better case for the double bind in relation to hypnotic phenomena, because there is a great difference between this situation and the schizophrenia-inducing one.

In any event, the creation of a Batesonian double bind does not allow one to predict directly what specific behavior will arise, but merely that it will be unusual behavior for the subject. Applied to the arm catalepsy example, it does not predict that a hallucination will necessarily be the response, only that this is one possible response. This is important.

Possibly because he became aware of some of the above difficulties, Haley (1958) subsequently published the following more general description/definition of the double bind in an article specifically about hypnotism:

> A "double bind" is present when one person communicates a message and qualifies that message with an incongruent message in a situation where the other person must respond to these contradictory messages, cannot leave the field, and cannot comment on the contradiction. (p. 52)

This definition does not say anything about the second message being a metamessage. Whether or not Haley considers this to be an optional feature, there is no question that in the discussion that follows the definition, it is indicated that this factor is clearly important.

Haley's main focus of the application of the double bind concept to hypnotic behavior is the "involuntary" character of the hypnotic behavior. For him, this is the crux of what defines suggested behavior. He views all hypnotic behavior as involving simultaneous requests to the subject that he *do* something and that he *do not do* it (that it will be automatic). This, Haley says, is a double bind that is resolved by the subject carrying out the act and subsequently saying he did not do it, that it was not done, that it was not done for the hypnotist, or that it was not done in this time and place. It is not at all clear from Haley's discussion whether or not he is taking the position that hypnotic behavior is some form of role-playing. In any event, the double bind situation as just described differs significantly from that described by Bateson et al. in that now the outcome is specifically predictable. Haley presents a good case for his position by showing how his version of the double bind applies to a number of selected examples and by ignoring many obvious hypnotic effects that are not so readily explained as, for example, the hallucination of movement in the arm catalepsy case cited earlier. In this case, Haley's model predicts that an actual arm movement will take place!

Quite apart from these considerations, and even with criteria (1) and (5) obviously eliminated by Haley's definition of the double bind, one must still question the ability of the double bind to account for hypnotic behavior, particularly since Haley seems to take the dangerous position that it can do so in *all* instances. Criterion (4) is actually rarely satisfied in his examples. The source of compulsion, if it exists, remains unclear and a hypothesis of its own. Identification of the metamessage is often difficult and even impossible.

Finally, there are alternative explanations for the behaviors he describes. Considering that Haley was the communication expert in the original group of investigators, and that he very clearly makes communication central in his theory of hypnotic behavior, one would expect him to recognize, when discussing his account of the Hand Levitation Demonstration, that to say to someone, "lift your hand," and "your hand is lifting," potentially carries two different kinds of messages. The one intimates actively, willfully doing something, whereas the other intimates the opposite. This is even more true when, as is often the case in practice, the subject is told that his hand is "floating," or that a force is acting on it. Again, either deliberately ignoring it or for lack of wide experience, Haley fails to recognize that many hypnotists do not start a Hand Levitation by saying, "I don't want you to move your hand." When this is the case, the incongruity so important for his case simply vanishes. When he discusses the Eye Catalepsy Test, he fails again to recognize that there can be an important difference for some individuals in telling them to *do* something as against *trying* to do the same. As with the Hand Levitation, Haley seems to be provincially ignorant of the many other variations of the Eye Catalepsy Test that are in use. In particular, subjects are not always first asked to squeeze their eyes together before anything else is done. In any event, there are many other test situations, such as the Hands Together Test and The Chevreul Pendulum Test, in which there are no "do" and "don't" contradictions and that Haley completely ignores.

Haley's article covers much more than the double bind; it is worth reading for the different and interesting points of view of hypnotism that it offers.

The Ericksonian Bind and Double Bind

From the very beginning, Erickson became enamored of the double bind concept. His uncritical acceptance and use of it helped greatly to make it one of the most popular and misunderstood ideas in the history of hypnotism. It seems clear that by the time Rossi began to work with Erickson, the idea was being applied rather uncritically, even by its originator, to all types of situations, including mountain climbing. Berger (1978, p. 218ff) has reported verbatim a rather revealing and telling interchange, between Bateson and a member of a symposium, that shows to what extent, even 20 years later, the whole matter of the double bind had remained a confused issue. It also shows Bateson's inability to deal with the confusion he had created. In any event, around 1973 Rossi and Erickson asked me for a critique of their proposed *Hypnotic Realities,* as well as a foreword for it. The version of the book that I saw contained a much less detailed discussion of the double bind than the final version did. In my critique, I raised some serious questions regarding the validity of their calling certain situations double binds. I also questioned the appropriateness of using the term "double bind" rather than "bind" in denoting these situations. Sometime later, I met in Phoenix with Erickson and Rossi to confer further with them on their book. At that time, Rossi assured me that they had resolved the issues I had raised. He mentioned that the resolution was to be found in recognizing that some of the messages in the double bind were being made to the "unconscious," and I must admit that I did not press for details at the time. About a year later, Erickson and Rossi (1975) offered, for the first time in an article, the classification of double binds and their distinction from binds as subsequently presented in the final version of the book. Although the authors do not say so, I feel this material evolved in answer to my comments to them. In any case, with this article and the subsequent book, the double bind takes on *still another form,* and it can hardly be said that it is any longer the "double bind" *as originally conceived by Bateson.* In fact, as we shall later see, the criteria used by Erickson and Rossi (1975) and those used by Bateson et al. appear more as being opposite than as being alike. Be that as it may, it remains to look at this last version of the double bind, which, perhaps, should be called the "Rossi/Erickson double bind" to distinguish it from the Bateson and the Haley versions, and also to recognize that, while Erickson supplied the examples, it was Rossi who analyzed and classified them.

Whereas the Bateson model can only predict a class of potential outcomes, and the Haley model only predicts that the subject will affirm the non-voluntariness of his responses, the Rossi/Erickson model focuses on the production of specific effects, be it a trance, a Hand Levitation, dissociation, or some other effect. That is, their double bind usually specifies a variety of effects to be produced, indirectly as this may be.

Furthermore, in contrast to Bateson et al. and to Haley, Erickson, Rossi, and Rossi (1976) use both the terms bind and double bind. They state (p. 62) that binds are "tactful presentations of the possible alternate forms of constructive behavior that are available to the patient in a given situation. The patient is given free, voluntary choice between them; the patient usually feels bound, however, to accept one alternative." This is certainly a far cry from anything Bateson et al. or Haley wrote about. Typical examples are, "Would you like to go into trance now or later?" and, "Would you like to go into trance standing up or sitting?" Choices do not have to be limited to two, but can be any number. Certainly *these are not* a "bind" in any colloquial sense of the word. They are, however, *permissive statements.* One may even see in them an *indirect* suggestion by implication that a trance will occur, for the choice is *how* or *when* the subject will go into a trance, not whether he will go into one. The latter is indirectly asserted to be an unquestionable verifiable eventuality. That the subject usually feels "bound" to go into a trance is, however, a gratuitous hypothesis that, at best, has been verified only in some cases. In my experience, in successful cases most subjects speak much less of feeling bound or coerced than of simply going into a hypnotic state with little or no understanding of why they did. I think one must question the reasonableness of speaking of the above examples as "binds." Assuming that it has a special effectiveness, this effectiveness could be explained in other ways. Such questions may have a distracting effect that cause the subject to focus his attention on the issue in question and allow the idea of trance to be free to act ideodynamically, or, in Erickson's terms, at an unconscious level. Or, to use still another mechanism Erickson writes about, this kind of question is of a type likely to instigate an "inner" or "unconscious search," a process he believes promotes the appearance of a trance. Another issue that needs to be considered is, of course, whether this approach really has a special effectiveness. It seems that this would be a fairly easy thing to check. To my knowledge, no one has done this. Nor has anyone even collected data on how the subject perceives the situation. I use the approach mainly for its permissiveness and indirectness, and have little reason to believe that there is much more to it than that.

"By contrast," Erickson, Rossi, and Rossi state (1976, p. 62) regarding the double bind itself, it "offers possibilities of behavior that are outside the patient's usual range of conscious choice and control." They go on to say, "The double bind arises out of the possibility of communicating at more than one level. We can (1) say something and (2) simultaneously comment on what we are saying." They refer to the first communication as being "primary" and the second one as being a "metacommunication." "A peculiar situation exists," they add (p. 63), "when what is stated in a primary communication is restructured or cast into another frame of reference in the metacommunication." To clarify this, they give the example of patients who are first "asked" to "let their hand lift," then "to experience it as lifting in an involuntary manner." They claim that the only way the patients can do this is by letting the hand move involuntarily. Getting this type of activity is Erickson's main goal because, for him, it is the essence of suggestion and of hypnotic behavior. They continue with, "We have many ways of saying or implying to patients that (1) something will happen, but (2) you won't do it with conscious intent, your unconscious will do it." They specifically refer to this as the *conscious-unconscious double bind.*

They point out that the metacommunication does not have to be in words, but can be in the form of a tone of voice or an inflection; it can be non-verbal, and it can even be in the form of hidden implications in verbal messages.

But even then, at least looking at the example they give, it is not that clear in what way there is any kind of bind, be it single or double. That they do understand the term "bind" as used in the colloquial sense is indicated by their subsequent reference to the messages being conflictual and placing the patient in a quandary. But where is the conflict in messages in the above example? Where is the quandary? The patient is first told, "let your hand lift." What does the patient understand by this? Some subjects, we can expect, will understand just this, to let the hand rise *of its own,* that is, non-voluntarily. Now this may or may not fit into their perception of how they function. If it fits, the second injunction merely supports the first, and no bind of any type exists. In many such cases, the second injunction is superfluous. If the subjects cannot conceive of their hand rising of its own, they may then try to reinterpret the perceived instruction or request and figure out something like "this is his (the hypnotist's) peculiar way of asking me to raise (voluntarily) my hand." The second statement then either confirms or disconfirms the subject's interpretation of the first message. If it confirms, it also reinforces any incipient automatic response. If there is disconfirmation, and the subject believes there has to be meaning to the hypnotist's second message, then, indeed, he may be placed in a quandary as to what to do, and he may, if anything, become confused. In this case, there may be some applicability of Erickson and Rossi's point that the "conflict is frequently enough to disrupt the patient's usual mode of functioning . . . so that more unconscious and involuntary processes are activated" (1976, p. 63). They amplify by adding, "These quandaries are indirect hypnotic forms insofar as they tend to block or disrupt the patient's habitual attitudes and frames of reference so that choice is not easily made on a conscious, voluntary level." Using another expression they have coined, the conscious is effectively "depotentiated" by the quandary. Or, using another mechanism they discuss elsewhere in the book, the quandary may elicit an "inner search" that decreases conscious contact and interaction with outer reality and constitutes the start of a "trance."

There may thus be some basis to the double bind as just discussed, but the matter is much more complex than Erickson and Rossi portray it. For one thing, as we have seen, some subjects can be expected to respond at an automatic level for quite another reason than the existence of a conflict that for them does not exist. Erickson and Rossi are careful to point out that double binds, whether unconscious or of another type, *do not always work.* The authors fail, however, to realize that intended double binds may also seem to work when actually there is really no double bind for the subject in the first place, for, as Erickson and Rossi recognize, whether or not a double bind is present is *partly a function of the subject's perception.*

Consider, for example, the following situation, which appears, on first examination, as a clear, irrefutable case of double bind. It has been cited as an example of double bind par excellence. Picture a group therapy session in which a patient announces, "My problem is that I cannot say 'no' to anyone." Thereupon, the therapist tells the patient, "I want you to go around the group. Each member will ask you to do something and you are to say 'no' to any request made of you." If ever there was a "bind" in the colloquial sense, this seems to be one. Whatever the patient does, he will have to say "no" to someone, since refusing to carry this task out is implicitly to say "no" to the therapist!

But how well are the conditions for the existence of a double bind satisfied? Some of these are satisfied, and in an unusual way. For example, the patient cannot leave the field because to do so is effectively also to say "no" to the therapist. Also, there are two contradictory injunctions, although the two injunctions do not have a common origin in the therapist. One has its source in the patient's psychodynamics. The existence of an intense relationship is not as clearly demonstrated. We expect there will be a patient-therapist relationship, but whether sufficiently intense is another matter. Unfortunately, Bateson et al. give us no idea of how intense it must be, and, in any case, there are no scales to measure this. Likewise, we cannot clearly know how compelling the therapist's injunction is. If there is a metamessage, it is not obvious. Finally, if this is a double bind, it may or may not be a repeated one. I have seen it used on a one-time basis with several therapy groups. After careful analysis of the situation, whether or not it is a double bind seems much less clear than it does at first sight. One needs to know much more about the patient's inability to say "no" to requests before it can be said whether any kind of bind is present. For example, is this inability applicable to all requests, or only to certain kinds? Another point is the artificiality of the group situation, which is not likely to be associated with the same affect as a life situation. This, too, may neutralize any bind that might otherwise exist.

Some of the classes of binds and double binds that Erickson and Rossi talk about seem to reflect merely a *superficial difference in wording and no fundamental differences.* They may be in the form of a question, as in, "Would you like to go into a trance standing or sitting?" Or, "Which one of your hands will first go up?" According to them, these are respectively typical *bind and double bind questions.* "How would you like to go into a trance, quickly or slowly?" is an example of what they call a *time bind* because time is an element in producing the response. It is obviously also a bind question. "Let me know when you begin to experience warmth in your hand" is a *time double bind.* Not only is time used to evoke the response, but there is also an implication (metacommunication) that the response will take place at an automatic level. At least, this is what Erickson and Rossi say about these communications. I question that, as it stands, the last injunction constitutes a double bind. One can more readily view it as a somewhat indirect way of suggesting that a hand will feel warm. It also has a certain degree of inherent permissiveness.

An example of a "conscious-unconscious" double bind was given earlier. Erickson was usually less subtle and more direct in his use of this kind of double bind. More typically, he would first very briefly lecture to the subject regarding differences between conscious and unconscious (automatic) behavior, then subsequently would proceed with messages and injunctions in which both the conscious and the unconscious were specifically alluded to. Thus, he might then say to a patient (1976, p. 67), "If your unconscious wants you to enter trance, your right hand will lift. Otherwise your left hand will lift." The goal is to induce hypnosis. The authors explain that this type of double bind "rests upon the fact we cannot consciously control our unconscious." They further assert that the above statement blocks any voluntary response on the patient's part and forces the mediation of a response at an unconscious level. What seems at first a rather profound observation is really a platitude, for it must follow logically *from the definition* of unconscious behavior that, indeed, if it takes place, it cannot be controlled consciously. If it could, it would cease to be unconscious! In any event, just how it follows from this that the above statement to the subject must be a double bind, or even creates a special efficacy, is anything but clear.

Many years ago, long before Rossi became Erickson's interpreter, Erickson told me, "Either way, the subject goes into a trance!" Commenting further, he explained that responding motorically at an automatic level was *ipso facto* to be in a trance. Thus, it did not make any difference *which* hand *automatically* went up. I do not agree that any automatic act, even in response to a demand, entails a trance. But supposing for a moment that this was the case; it is clear that the above contains a basic assumption on the part of Erickson—that either movement, if it takes place, will be automatic. But will this necessarily be so? Is it possible that the subject might understand the suggestion or instruction to say, "If your unconscious wants you to be in a trance, it will raise your right hand, but, if it does not do so, you will indicate this is the case by consciously raising your left hand?" This is exactly what happens in some cases. Nothing happens with the right hand, and the subject voluntarily raises the left hand to indicate his interpretation that, since his right hand does not move, his unconscious is not ready for him to go into a trance just then. In other cases, there are subjects who do nothing at all with either hand. They have, indeed, understood that either hand will go up automatically, and they wait for this to happen. It never does, because the suggestion is not effective.

There is another feature in the above example that bothers me. If it is correct that giving an automatic response is to go into a trance, then the unconscious is contradicting itself if it raises the left hand to say, "No, I am not ready to go into a trance." Obviously, by the nature of this activity, the subject will have gone into a trance! At least, this is what Erickson maintains. There is no problem, of course, if one takes the position LeCron seems to have taken in the 1950s that the unconscious can communicate through ideomotor responses with or without a trance being present. However, to take this position also means that the above maneuver is not necessarily a double bind insuring the production of a trance.

The two authors also speak of a *double-dissociation double bind.* As an example, Erickson says to the subject (p. 70), "You can as a person awaken, but you do not need to awaken as a body." Then, following a pause, he continues with, "You can awaken when your body awakes, but without a recognition of your body." It is not particularly hard to see that the above does propose by implication that two different dissociations will take place. Much less clear is what specifically constitutes the double bind in this case, and, in particular, whether the double dissociation is an essential element of this double bind, if it is one. Unfortunately, the authors do not choose to clarify the matter. Possibly the double bind is because the subject is told one moment that he *will not* awaken as a body and then, next, that he *will,* and also because awakening is not normally, if ever, a voluntary activity. But then what is the role of two different dissociations? The authors should have explained further. If pressed, Erickson might have pointed out that dissociating can only be an automatic act and that it is an additional way of satisfying the requirement that one response must be automatic. On the other hand, they go on to say that (p. 70) "double-dissociation double binds tend to confuse the subjects' conscious mind and thus depotentiate their habitual sets, biases, and learned limitations." This, they add, clears the way for greater autonomous, unconscious activity. But if the sole purpose of this double bind is to create confusion in the subject's mind, there are many other ways of doing so, including the use of other double binds, and this can hardly be a basis for considering it a special class of double bind. In this case, it would be better used as an example of something that could be called the "confusion double bind." If it seems that I am going to extremes in my analysis, it is because it seems to me that if there is a unique reason for having a double dissociation as part of a double bind, we ought to know what it is. I have come to the conclusion that there is none. The very simple answer to this puzzle lies in asking *what is the purpose of this double bind,* and Erickson tells us this a number of pages back in his book when he points out that his introduction of this double bind was for the purpose of preparing the subject for the production of dissociation and of posthypnotic responses. What this example then shows us is how a desired effect can be coupled to a double bind. I therefore no longer regard the "double-dissociation double-bind" as a legitimate category.

Next is the *reverse set double bind.* This appears to be an approach to be specifically used in dealing with resistance. It amounts to using the subject's very resistance to get the desired response, and thus is a utilization technique, too. The technique boils down to encouraging, even demanding, that the subject demonstrate his resistance in every possible way. This, of course, creates a paradoxical situation and a quandary for the subject, since resisting now becomes an act of acquiescence. This is the very thing the subject does not want to or cannot do. Perhaps more to the point, the subject forcibly has to produce the very response he started out to resist in order to continue to resist. An example reported by Haley (1958) is that of an individual who, at a demonstration, had challenged Erickson to hypnotize him. Without comment, Erickson invited him to join him on the lecture platform, asked him to sit down, and then said to him, "I want you to stay awake, wider and wider awake, wider and wider awake." Whereupon the subject entered a hypnotic state! Haley's interpretation and assumption of what happened was that the invitation to come on the platform contained the subtle metamessage of "Come up here and go into a trance," which contradicts Erickson's subsequent primary message of "stay awake." According to Haley, now speaking of the subject, "He knew that if he followed Erickson's suggestions he would go into a trance. Therefore he was determined not to follow the suggestions. Yet if he refused to follow the suggestion to stay awake he would go into a trance. Thus he was caught in a double bind." I find this explanation somewhat confusing. Superficially it seems to make sense, but when closely examined, it becomes much less clear. For example, it is not clear what suggestion is being talked about. Furthermore, is the injunction to stay awake truly a suggestion, or is it an instruction? In either case, why should going along with it bring about a hypnotic sleep? In any event, there is the possibility of other factors being involved, which Haley fails to consider. By getting the subject to come to the platform and then to sit down at his request, Erickson has begun to establish a "yes" set, which is an important step toward neutralizing the "no" set expressed by the resistance. Possibly the subject perceived a further, implied suggestion in what Erickson said to him in the form ". . . stay awake . . . but the more you try to do so the more you will tend to go into a trance . . ." Finally, one cannot exclude the strong possibility that the subject really wanted to be hypnotized, but only by the right person—in this case, Erickson.

The case of Lal described by Erickson and Rossi (1975) is another example particularly worth examining. It is reproduced below as given by the authors:

The serious question of what constitutes power and dominance and strength and reality and security had apparently been given considerable thought by Lal, approximately eight years old. At all events, shortly before the evening meal, he approached his father and remarked interrogatively, "Teachers always tell little kids what they have to do?" An interrogative "yes" was offered in reply. Lal proceeded, "And Daddys and Mammas always, always, tell their little children what they got to do?" Another interrogative affirmation was offered. Continuing, Lal said, "And they make their little children do what they say?" A questioning assent was given.

Bracing himself firmly with his feet widely apart, Lal declared through clenched teeth, "Well, you can't make me do a single thing and to show you, I won't eat dinner and you can't make me."

The reply was made that his proposition seemed to offer a reasonable opportunity to determine the facts, but that it could be tested in a manner fully as adequate if he were to declare that he could not be made to drink an extra large glass of milk. By this test, it was explained, he could enjoy his evening meal, he would not have to go hungry and he could definitely establish his point of whether or not he could be made to drink his milk.

After thinking this over, Lal agreed but declared again that he was willing to abide by his first statement if there were any doubt in the father's mind about the resoluteness of his declaration. He was airily assured that the glass of milk being extra large would be an easily adequate test.

A large glassful of milk was placed in the middle of the table where it would be most noticeably in full view, and dinner was eaten in a leisurely fashion while the father outlined the proposed contest of wills.

This exposition was made carefully and the boy was asked to approve or disapprove each statement made so that there could be no possible misunderstandings. The final agreement was that the issue would be decided by the glass of milk and that he, Lal, affirmed that his father could not make him drink the milk, *that he did not have to do a single thing his father told him to do about the milk.* In turn, the father said that he could make Lal do anything he wanted Lal to do with the milk, and that *there were some things he could make Lal do a number of times.*

When full understanding had been reached and it was agreed that the contest could begin, the father commanded, "Lal, drink your milk." With quiet determination the reply was made, "I don't have to and you can't make me."

This interplay was repeated several times. Then the father said quite simply, "Lal, spill your milk."

He looked startled, and when reminded he had to do whatever he was told to do about his milk he shook his head and declared "I don't have to." This interplay was also repeated several times with the same firm negation given.

Then Lal was told to drop the glass of milk on the floor and thus to break the glass and spill the milk. He refused grimly.

Again he was reminded that he had to do with the milk whatever he was told to do, and this was followed with the stern admonition, "Don't pick up your glass of milk." After a moment's thought, he defiantly lifted the glass. Immediately the order was given, "Don't put your glass down." A series of these two orders was given, eliciting consistently appropriate defiant action.

Stepping over to the wall blackboard the father wrote "Lift your milk" at one end and at the other he wrote, "Put your milk down." He then explained that he would keep tally of each time Lal did something he had been told to do. He was reminded that he had already been told to do both of those things repeatedly, but that tally would now be kept by making a chalk mark each time he did either one of those two things he had been previously instructed to perform.

Lal listened with desperate attention.

The father continued, "Lal, don't pick up your glass," and made a tally mark under "Lift your milk" which Lal did in defiance. Then, "Don't put your milk down" and a tally mark was placed under, "Put your milk down" when this was done. After a few repetitions of this, while Lal watched the increasing size of the score for each task, his father wrote on the blackboard, "Drink your milk" and "Don't drink your milk," explaining that a new score would be kept on these items.

Lal listened attentively but with an expression of beginning hopelessness.

Gently he was told, "Don't drink your milk now." Slowly he put the glass to his lips but before he could sip, he was told, "Drink your milk." Relievedly he put the glass down. Two tally marks were made, one under "Put your milk down," and one under "Don't drink your milk."

After a few rounds of this, Lal was told not to hold his glass of milk over his head but to spill it on the floor. Slowly, carefully he held it at arm's length over his head. He was promptly admonished not to keep it there. Then the father walked into the other room, returned with a book and another glass of milk and remarked, "I think this whole thing is silly. Don't put your milk down."

With a sigh of relief Lal put the glass on the table, looked at the scores on the blackboard, sighed again, and said, "Let's quit, Daddy."

"Certainly, Lal. It's a silly game and not real fun and the next time we get into an argument, let's make it really something important that we can both think about and talk sensibly about."

Lal nodded his head in agreement.

Picking up his book, the father drained the second glass of milk preparatory to leaving the room. Lal watched, silently picked up his glass and drained it.

That a reverse set is involved is fairly clear. But why is it so complicated to produce? Also, where does the double bind reside? Is all of the above the reverse set double bind? If not, what is the purpose of all the extra material? Rossi and Erickson give the following explanation: The father realizes at the start that the real issue is not whether to eat dinner; it is, however, a matter of principle. He therefore shifts the battle from eating an entire dinner to a single act, that of drinking a glass of milk. That is, the child's message initially being "you can't make me do anything," the reverse set is established by apparently accepting this and stating, "You do not have to do anything I request of you regarding the milk." At the primary (object) level of communication, the messages are about drinking milk, but at the metalevel, a much more general communication is being made, namely, "you will do in every situation the opposite of what I ask of you." The interchange that then follows is instigated in order to establish firmly the reverse set by repetition. The use of tallies is next introduced to demonstrate to Lal that, after all, there are things that his father can make him do. When it becomes obvious to the father than Lal realizes he is hopelessly losing the battle, the father allows him to save face by giving one last command, "Drink your milk," and then, just as Lal is about to do the opposite, proceeds to shift to a different act than drinking milk. He finally accepts the child's unstated surrender. At face value, this seems a fairly reasonable account of what has happened. But is this really what happened? What has actually happened *that is observable?* The father says to the child, "Do A," but also reminds him that he is not to do it. The child could choose to do nothing, but chooses instead to demonstrate his negativism by doing the opposite, B, whereupon the father says, "Do B," and the child proceeds to do A. This continues, with the father *always* commanding Lal to do A or B *after* it has already been initiated, or even completed, by Lal. This continues until, at some point, the father indirectly says, in essence, "See, I have told you to do A a number of times, and you have done this N times, and I told you to do B several times, and you have done it N − 1 (or N + 1) times. I rest my case." Quite true, but what the father fails to recognize overtly is that A was *never done when he said, "do A,"* and B was *never done when he said, "Do B." In other words, Lal never did what he was told to do upon being told to do it.* The best the father had done was to demonstrate that he could get Lal to do something when he commanded it, but not necessarily what he had specifically commanded at any given moment. Now, if at some point, when the father had said, "Do A," Lal had reversed himself and done A, and had done B when father said, "Do B," and then C when father said, "Do C," and so on, then we would have support for a special effectiveness of the technique in overcoming resistance. But this never happened. Possibly, the father conned Lal into believing, or at least into agreeing, that the father controlled his actions. I say "possibly," because nowhere in the account do we hear Lal admitting this overtly. Furthermore, by the time things are brought to an end, Lal or his father may have wearied of the game. I am not convinced that Lal was at all ready to concede defeat. Did Lal really save face by what his father eventually did, or did his father try to save his own face? What his father did is certainly an obvious way of arbitrarily terminating the game. That Lal eventually drank the milk when his father drank some, too, is hardly conclusive that the maneuver worked. There are a number of other equally plausible reasons for the child doing so of his own free will.

Finally, we come to the *non sequitur double bind*. As an example of this, Erickson, Rossi, and Rossi (1976) cite the following situation: To a child who does not want to go to bed, one might say, "Do you wish to take a *bath* before going to bed, or would you rather put your pajamas on in the *bathroom?*" According to the authors, the child, not being able to make any sense out of this sentence, will tend "to go along with it." One can only ask, at this point, what it is the child will go along with. There are at least three choices. We know this presumed double bind is given for the purpose of getting the child in bed, so we must assume that this is the "it" the authors have in mind.

How well does this example satisfy the criteria for being a double bind? That there is a choice of activities is agreed. However, none can be said to be contradictory of the others. There is no evidence of a metamessage. Nor is there any response involved that could only take place at an automatic level. Furthermore, does the child have another alternative besides to make one of the two choices? He certainly could have a tantrum. At best, perhaps one can then speak of a bind, but certainly not of a double bind! Is there really any question as to what the likely choice will be? I know from my experience with children, and from my own recollections as a child, that a child wanting to put off going to bed, and who does not hate baths more than going to bed, would choose to take the bath. Baths can be a lot of fun for a child, and they can be made to last! Besides, this option is face-saving, and it does postpone the undesirable and inevitable bedtime. Baths are quite relaxing, and the child, by then, is quite ready for bed anyway. On the other hand, while putting on his pajamas is getting one step closer to going to bed, it does not entail going to bed immediately. The child could still insist on playing some more in his pajamas! I take this example with a grain of salt, and I suspect that it was made up for the occasion rather than extracted from Erickson's experience, as the case of Lal mentioned earlier probably was.

There is another important flaw in this example, although it is different and from another viewpoint. Before I state what it is, let me remind the reader of what *non sequitur* means. To quote Rune (1962), a *non sequitur* "is any fallacy which has not even the deceptive appearance of valid reasoning, or in which there is a complete lack of connection between the premises advanced and the conclusions." A *fallacy* is, of course, any unsound step or process of reasoning; thus, it always involves *the supposed derivation of a seeming conclusion from some seeming premise*. Keeping this in mind, a careful examination of the above statement to the child shows that it *does not* involve a *non sequitur* statement! There is unquestionably a certain discontinuity, a lack of connection between the two choices that are offered and an adult might be led to seek a non-existing logical connection between these choices. I doubt a child would. This same example can be found in a slightly modified form in the 1975 article on the double bind with a somewhat more detailed discussion of it which provides strong evidence neither authors have a clear understanding of what *non sequitur* consists of.

This concludes our survey of Erickson's double binds. Table 7.3 (Erickson & Rossi, 1975, p. 155) on the next page, most likely drawn up by Rossi, sums up the features that they feel defines the Bateson and the Erickson double bind and indicates in what ways they differ.

Surprisingly, this table is offered by Erickson and Rossi to justify their claims to be using double binds. I say "surprisingly," because any similarity that can be found is *very* superficial and, in their effort to demonstrate a parallel between the two presumed processes, their end result was that one was shown to be the *opposite* of the other. If there are any remaining doubts about this, they are removed by the following summarizing statements of the authors (Erickson & Rossi, 1975):

> It may be noted in summary that the schizogenic double bind carries *negative injunctions that are enforced* at the metalevel or abstract level that is outside the victim's control on the primary level. Erickson's therapeutic double binds, by contrast, always emphasize *positive agreement on the metalevel and offer alternatives that can be refused at the primary level.* Erickson has stated that 'While I put the patient into a double bind they also sense, unconsciously, that I will never, never hold them to it. They know I will yield any time. I will then put them in another double bind in some other situation to see if they can put it to constructive use because it meets their needs more adequately.' For Erickson then, the double bind is a useful device that *offers* a patient possibilities for constructive change. If one double bind does not fit he will try another and another until he finds a key that fits. (p. 155)

The authors' efforts to validate their use of the double bind concept by using such additional qualifiers as "schizogenic" and "therapeutic" is pure equivocation. It is a play with words aimed at obfuscating the obvious, or at least denying that their applications of the concept are frequently questionable.

One probably comes closer to the true nature of the communications that have been reviewed if one looks upon them as creating a potential *forced choice;* one that can, at best, only be said to be *intended.* Even this proposition might be questioned because of Erickson's final statements. Erickson does, however, specify that it is the patient's unconscious that knows there is the freedom to refuse. The possible implication, then, is that the patient's conscious perception of the situation is, indeed, one of *having* to make a choice. This is, however, conjecture.

TABLE 7.3.   The Batesonian and Ericksonian Double Bind Contrasted

The Bateson Schizogenic Double Bind	The Erickson Therapeutic Double Bind
1. *Two or More Persons* The child "victim" is usually ensnared by mother or a combination of parents and siblings.	1. *Two or More Persons* Usually patient and therapist are ensconced in a positive relationship.
2. *Repeated Experience* Double bind is a repeated occurrence rather than one simple traumatic event.	2. *A Single or Series of Experiences* If one is not enough a series of double binds will be offered until one works.
3. *A Primary Negative Injunction* "Do not do so and so or I will punish you."	3. *A Primary Positive Experience* "I agree that you should continue doing such and such."
4. *A Secondary Injunction Conflicting with the First at a More Abstract (Meta) Level, and Like the First Enforced by Punishments or Signals Which Threaten Survival.*	4. *A Secondary Positive Suggestion at the Metalevel That Facilitates a Creative Interaction between the Primary (Conscious) and Metalevel (Unconscious).* Responses at both levels are permitted to resolve stalemated conflicts.
5. *A Tertiary Negative Injunction Prohibiting the Victim from Escaping the Field.*	5. *A Tertiary Positive Understanding (Rapport, Transference) That Binds the Patient to His Therapeutic Task but Leaves Him Free to Leave if He Chooses.*
6. Finally, the complete set of ingredients is no longer necessary when the victim has learned to perceive his universe in double bind patterns.	6. The patient leaves therapy when his behavior change frees him from transference and the evoked double bind.

Source: Erickson & Rossi, 1975. Reprinted with permission of *American Journal of Clinical Hypnosis*.

There is no question that one can observe situations in daily life that can be said to be "binds," or dilemmas. That is, we see individuals caught up in situations *where they are impelled or compelled to make a choice between carrying out two equally motivated actions, and they have no alternative but to make a choice,* or to develop a pathological reaction that gets them out of, or resolves, the dilemma (bind). There are situations in which individuals receive contradictory injunctions from others, and in which they have no other choice but to carry out one or the other injunction; the idea that these situations are of the above type has merit. But I would also point out that 30 years after Bateson et al. offered their ideas on the subject, the problem of schizophrenia is still unresolved with regard to etiology, nature, and treatment. As far as schizophrenia is concerned, the double bind "theory" turns out to be just an unconfirmed hypothesis. What, then, is its reality as a source of unusual behavior? If Bateson et al. and Haley had not also advanced the proposition that the double bind was applicable to hypnotic behavior, would Erickson and his co-workers have adopted it? There is no way to know, but one cannot help but wonder whether the multiplicity of double binds that Rossi has evolved does not represent a procrustean effort to deal with the various practical and conceptual difficulties that we have seen arise.

Whether or not we agree that the term "double bind" is applicable in some or all instances, I see no reason why one should stop using the procedures that have been discussed in this section, even though their nature and modes of action have most likely been misunderstood. These procedures *may be quite effective* at times, for other reasons than being double binds or binds. I do see, however, every reason for ceasing to call them double binds with or without special adjectival qualifiers. I am not sure that "intended forced choice" is the most appropriate designation, but it seems to me to be a better one until we can either confirm the validity of this label or come up with something more appropriate.

One should also listen more carefully to Erickson and Rossi's warning that double binds are maneuvers *that do not always function as such.* What works with one individual will not work with the next, and when it does work, it may or may not work because it is a double bind. So much for magical formulas.

SUGGESTION, DIRECT SUGGESTION, AND INDIRECT SUGGESTION

Is Erickson's conception of suggestion the same as that of traditional and semi-traditional hypnotism? More particularly, do his *indirect* suggestions meet the criteria of a suggestion as outlined in Volume 1? This last question is especially pertinent because much literature on Ericksonian hypnotism tends to give the impression there is a basic difference. Neither Erickson nor Rossi gave a brief, explicit, definition of what they understood a suggestion to be. Both expressions, suggestion and indirect suggestion, are frequently used in the same context, giving the impression that they are interchangeable. But are they? This is not altogether clear. There are also references to "direct" suggestions, "hypnotic" suggestions, and occasionally, to "non-hypnotic" suggestions. Do these expressions denote the same thing they denoted in Volume 1? For the most part, definitions in the Ericksonian literature are interspersed throughout the texts and must largely be derived indirectly from the many examples that are given.

Occasionally, suggestion is said by the authors to be a "process." For instance on p. 313, the authors (Erickson, Rossi, & Rossi, 1976) assert,

"So-called suggestion is actually this process of evoking and utilizing a patient's own associations, mental skills, and mental mechanisms." The "this" refers to the various procedures that were discussed in connection with the microdynamics of trance induction. However, most examples that are given by Erickson and Rossi clearly identify at least indirect suggestions (or "hypnotic forms") as *communications*. For instance, "Erickson views the separate issue of hypnotic suggestions as a problem in communication . . ." (1976, p. 20). Erickson thus seems to share with Bernheim the ambivalence the latter had regarding suggestions being a process and a communication. That a process is involved is not to be questioned. Neither is the fact that we are dealing with a communication. Perhaps what we need are two distinct designations.

There is a pretty clear message in the Ericksonian literature, particularly in the 1976 volume, that *there is some kind of basic difference between "direct" and "indirect" suggestions.* This is both implied and stated. Historically speaking, the distinction made between these two kinds of suggestions antedates Erickson. Not only have direct and indirect suggestions been contrasted, but many other kinds of suggestions have been proposed. I mentioned some of these briefly in Volume 1 and discussed them more completely elsewhere (Weitzenhoffer, 1953). Without repeating what was said previously, I will add a few pertinent comments. The action of the Trap Line Test, the Progressive Line Test, and the Progressive Weight Test, which are three well-known examples, can probably be accounted for in terms of implication and the creation of a "yes" set or of a conditioned response. The Picture Report Test seems best understood as an application of implication. Thus, in the case of the picture with the spurious spotted dog, there is an indirect suggestion of the dog being present since to speak of its spots presupposed its existence. No explanation in terms of elementary mental or neurophysiological processes has as yet been advanced to account for the observed effects. However, one can reasonably argue that an idea is subtly implanted in the subject's mind without his conscious participation and in such a way that it leads to a related non-voluntary response in each case.

I also call attention to the research of Boris Sidis (1910) because it seems to bear directly on the concept of imbedded suggestions. In his case, Sidis used non-verbal imbedding and on the basis of his results concluded that indirect suggestions could be further classified as "mediate" and "immediate." As pointed out elsewhere (Weitzenhoffer, 1953), it is possible to view the research of Sidis as experiments in perception and recall that have nothing to do with suggestions.

Having been personally acquainted with Erickson over a period of some 30 years and having carefully studied his writings, I feel comfortable in stating that in his earlier years, when Erickson spoke of using suggestions, it was always in the context of eliciting non-voluntary behavior from subjects and patients by means like those used by traditional and semi-traditional hypnotists. The non-voluntary aspects of the response to suggestions was retained by Erickson in later years. This is a theme which, for the most part, one finds still consistently carried through all three of the Erickson and Rossi books. For instance, on p. 9 we find Erickson saying of the patients (Erickson, Rossi, & Rossi, 1976), "So you build your techniques around instructions that allow their conscious mind to withdraw from the task and leave it all up to the unconscious." And a few lines further, "You don't want them to have conscious control but to allow their unconscious to function smoothly by itself." Further, on p. 20, one can read, *These hypnotic forms are communication devices that facilitate the evocation and utilization of the patient's own associations, potentials, and natural mechanisms in ways that are usually experienced as involuntary by the patient.*" On p. 309 they say, "Erickson's indirect forms of suggestion are all means of arranging such suitable conditions so that individuals can accomplish things that are within their behavioral repertory but usually not available to voluntary control . . ." Further on this same page we find, "The wonder and fascination of hypnosis is that it enables us to control these responses that are usually mediated by unconscious mechanisms outside the normal range of consciousness." The authors add that indirect suggestions are aimed at providing this control.

The above statements were made by Erickson and Rossi mainly in reference to the use of indirect (forms) of suggestions and "hypnotic forms." For the most part, they could have just as easily and correctly been made regarding direct suggestions such as were discussed in Volume 1. It would therefore seem that, insofar as the elicitation of non-voluntary behavior is concerned, there is no major difference between the Ericksonian indirect suggestion and the traditional and semi-traditional direct suggestion. However, this is not the way Erickson and Rossi view the matter, for on p. 268 they asserts, "Direct suggestion is mediated by internal processes that the subject usually has some awareness of. The subject recognizes that they made the response happen. The response is more or less under voluntary control. Indirect suggestion, by contrast, is usually mediated by internal processes that remain unknown to the subject. The response, when it is noticed, is usually acknowledged by the subject with a sense of surprise. The response appeared to occur in an involuntary and spontaneous manner. It has a curiously dissociated or autonomous aspect that is usually acknowledged as hypnotic."

This is a most puzzling assertion if we are to believe that it comes from Erickson who was well acquainted with traditional hypnotism as described in Volume 1 and many other texts. Does it mean he has a perception of direct suggestion that differs from the traditional and semi-traditional one?

It is my understanding that when the above was written Rossi's *only* experience with hypnotism was that which he had had with Erickson and that his reading of the literature had been very limited. Because of this, he was probably unaware of something that Erickson knew: that *when using the traditional methods of direct suggestion one encounters the very same kinds of reactions from subjects that have just been described as being unique to indirect suggestions!* As Erickson also knew, ideodynamic action is considered by traditional hypnotism as being responsible for suggested effects. This is an internal process that is unknown to the subject. It is also true that not all subjects experience a suggested response as having been altogether outside their voluntary control. As we have discussed in Volume 1, this is a function of their suggestibility and other determinants. It remains true, though, that there is a class of subjects in traditional and semi-traditional hypnotism who respond to and experience direct suggestions exactly as Erickson and Rossi describe the situation for indirect suggestion. Since I am certain Erickson was aware of these facts, the statement quoted in the last paragraph most likely expresses only Rossi's view and not that of Erickson.

I think it is true that when some of Erickson's rather intricate suggestion techniques are used, such as the interspersal method, the subject is least likely to know when and where the suggestion proper was given and what it was, but not because there is any intrinsically different process involved, but because it is well hidden. It is in this sense that we should understand this further statement (1976, p. 304), "Most of these approaches can be described as more or less indirect because consciousness is not entirely aware of exactly what is happening."

It is clear from the writings of Erickson and Rossi that they use the expression indirect suggestion in respect to *any* non-voluntary normal process, usually a covert action, being set in motion by the hypnotist's actions. For Erickson, hypnotism is nothing else than a utilization of the subject's repertoire of possible overt and covert responses and of all underlying and associated mental mechanisms. Certainly this model goes well beyond a traditional suggestions model which limits itself to a simple ideodynamic reflex. However, as was indicated in Volume 1, Bernheim, who originally developed the model, considered under ideodynamic action the setting in motion of the many automatisms upon which normal behavior and mental functioning depend. The more restrictive view was one that some of his successors took for lack of a clear understanding of what Bernheim had said. In any event, I believe that Volume 1 has made it clear that semi-traditional hypnotism views the response to suggestions as being a complex product and resultant of many processes that occur outside of the subject's awareness and independently of his volition. There can be no question that *communication* is as essential a feature of Erickson's indirect suggestions as it is of traditional direct ones. If any essential differences exists between the two, they will have to be found elsewhere.

One might look for differences in the neurophysiological and mental mechanisms and processes that are set into motion. The hypothesis would be that the wording of direct suggestions invokes different ones than the wording of indirect suggestions. A review of the relevant material in Volume 1 will show that for the time being there are few reasons, if any, for believing this is the case. It has been hypothesized by a number of writers, Rossi included, and by some investigators that the right cerebral hemisphere is specifically associated with hypnotic behavior. As we shall see in more detail further on, the data regarding this are quite ambiguous and support the hypothesis less and less.

Some writers, such as Bandler and Grinder, have sought the answer to what determines a suggestions in the linguistic structure of known, effective suggestions. We shall examine this in more detail in Chapter 8. Let it be said for the time being that their work sheds no light on what differentiates a direct from an indirect suggestion beyond the obvious: Erickson's indirect suggestions are convolute and often elaborate. The idea that is to be communicated is invariably conveyed in a round-about way. With direct suggestions the situation is the opposite.

In the above context, proponents of the hemispheric theory of hypnosis have gone a step further in claiming that Erickson's forms of indirect suggestion communicate with the subject in an analogic language, the latter being that which is specific to the unconscious and to the right hemisphere. Presumably, this makes these indirect suggestions particularly effective. This is all highly speculative and, in my opinion, the distinction between analogic and linear language in this context has very little to go on. I do not want to go into details here regarding the nature of this distinction beyond saying for those not familiar with it that it is partially based on the fact that most languages make use of sequences of words. Leaving out the questions of whether or not indirect suggestions are overall more effective than direct ones, and the evidence is increasingly showing this is not so, it is a fact that one can produce the same effects with direct suggestions as one can produce with indirect suggestions. This seems to indicate then that any difference that exists between the two kinds of suggestions is not be found in the dichotomy analogic/linear. Additionally, the distinction that has been made between analogic and linear languages outside of the computer sciences is anything but a clear-cut one. Most so-called analogic communications are formulated using a linear language! Typically, a metaphor, which is said to be an analogic communication, is stated in terms of everyday English, hence is also transmitted as a linear communication.

The difference between the direct form a suggestions can take and its indirect form can be very slight. For instance, in the midst of talking to a patient about other matters, Erickson once interjected casually, ". . . the unimportance of keeping your eyes open . . ." This was his way of indirectly suggesting eye closure. The direct form would simply have been, "Your eyes will close," "Your eyes are closing," or "Now your eyes can close."

An example of a much more subtle and indirect suggestion aimed at producing posthypnotic amnesia can be found on p. 261 of the 1976 book. Erickson had talked at great length to the subject about totally unrelated matters. Rather abruptly, he shifted to talking about how it is generally unnecessary for "one to remember one's dreams." He then went on to elaborate at some length on this theme by pointing out that recalling can take place very much later, can be only partial, be only as needed, that there is no need actually to remember, and so on. Then again, in a somewhat disconnected manner, Erickson said, "An illustration is when you awaken. One of the most pleasant things you have to experience is coming out of the trance . . . thinking you are ready to go into a trance . . . for the first time. And then becoming aware that you have been in a trance." As a way of insuring this last sentence did not remove the amnesia he hoped to obtain, he went on to further explain to the patient that he would infer this fact from the surroundings, possibly from changes that had occurred since the induction began. In contrast, a direct approach would have simply been to say, "After you awaken you will have no memory of anything that happened while you were hypnotized, including having been hypnotized." A simpler direct suggestion would be, "After you awaken you will have no awareness you have been hypnotized." Obviously this last direct suggestion uses implication to produce amnesia for all intra-hypnotic events and shows that even in working with direct suggestions some of the features said to be unique to Ericksonian hypnotism are used here. One should note that Erickson's way of proceeding in the above example contained some use of non sequitur, although not as a double bind.

Many of Erickson's indirect suggestions, like the one just described, are characteristically made up of two parts. One part, as Erickson himself spoke of it, is the suggestion proper. The other part constitutes a scaffold for it, so to speak, and prepares a receptive ground for the suggestion proper. It does so by causing other, non-suggested effects to occur, such as a depotentiation of consciousness. Erickson called it the preparatory part. A direct approach to depotentiating might be to suggest to the patient that he is becoming confused. To do this, Erickson preferred to make confusing statements, startle the subject, and so on. Although I do not believe Erickson ever reasoned thus, one could present the extreme argument that since getting confused is not a voluntary act, by the definition of a suggestions, any device or act that causes confusion is a suggestion. Carried far enough, this sort of reduction can lead to absurdities. Keeping these points in mind, I think it may be legitimate to refer to the entire communication used by Erickson to produce amnesia as an "indirect" suggestion. In any event, it must be understood that much of the time when "trance induction" and "indirect suggestion" is referred to in the Ericksonian literature it consists of an involved sequence of more elementary communications, and only segments of the total communication are suggestions proper.

To ask a subject or patient to recall his experiences when having received an injection of Novocaine in the past or to recall how an arm feels when it has gone "asleep" are seen by Erickson as instances of indirect suggestions of anesthesia. Whey they should not be viewed as examples of reintegration is not clear. Possibly they are both. But how far should one go along this line of action in speaking of indirect suggestion? Asking a subject to recall a time when he was on a beach on a sunny afternoon or describing to him someone's experience of doing the same, with the result the subject begins to experience warmth and may even show evidence of a dilation of his superficial blood vessels, is seen by Erickson as an indirect suggestion, too. Without saying categorically that it is not, I feel that doing so may be diluting the concept of indirect suggestion to the point where it ceases to have much meaning.

In final analysis, I believe that for Erickson one difference between direct and indirect suggestion is to be found along the following lines (Erickson, Rossi, & Rossi, 1976):

> In direct suggestion it is possible for the patient to have some conscious awareness of how the hypnotic response is mediated within and he may in consequence attempt either to inhibit or to facilitate the hypnotic response with conscious intentionality. With indirect suggestion care is taken so that the typical patient will not become aware of how the hypnotic response is mediated within; hence there is less opportunity for conscious intentionality either to facilitate or to block the response. (p. 269)

Traditional and especially semi-traditional hypnotism recognize that the subject's awareness of what is going on, especially when not hypnotized, can be an impediment. He may, as Erickson states, attempt intentionally to help or to hinder the production of the suggested effects. Furthermore conscious thinking activated by whatever he experiences may have unforeseen influences upon his responses. This is a major reason why it was recommended in Volume 1 to begin work with a subject by initially saying to him something like "Let whatever happens happen. Do not try to make anything happen or prevent it from happening. You may or may not experience what you expect." Presumably one can eliminate these instructions by using indirect suggestions because the subject does not know when and where the suggestion proper is given, nor what it is. This may be true with the more subtle forms used by Erickson, but one can wonder how well this is the case when such an indirect suggestion as "I wonder when you will go into trance" is used.

With these observations made, we are now in position to examine further Erickson's idea that a "truism" is a suggestion. In particular we can look more closely at Erickson and Rossi's (Erickson, Rossi, & Rossi, 1976, p. 21) assertion that suggestions are statements the patients cannot argue with because they are statements about obvious established facts and self-evident truths. Such a position goes against common sense, for if it were so, then a statement of fact such as "people cannot touch the moon from the earth" and "objects held aloft and released either go up or down" would be suggestions. Furthermore, since probably 90%, if not more, of everyday communications are of this type, the term suggestion is rendered meaningless. We could certainly agree to consider all truisms to be suggestions but then what would we do with those statements traditional hypnotism considers to be "suggestions"? Most are not truisms until they produce the suggested response. Also, all truisms do not produce responses that are non-voluntary, to use only this criterion, it being the only one of the three listed in Volume 1 that Erickson considers. In brief, some truisms could function as suggestions, but all do not. The reverse of the coin is that many examples of suggestion that Erickson and Rossi give are not truisms when initially given.

All of this is not to say that truisms may not influence the subject's response in other ways. Conceivably, at times they may have a synergetic action. As explained in Volume 1, pacing is based on stating truisms. For instances, if the direct suggestion of a hand movement has initiated a small movement, the next statement, "your hand has just moved," is a truism that is expected to aid the production of the desired response. This is also pacing. It is not clear how its effect comes about, if it has one. It can be viewed as a form of reinforcement and, as such, may be based on the same kinds of mechanisms that underlie other forms of reinforcement that affect learning. On the other hand, as an alternative to this truism being a suggestion, one might also offer an Ericksonian-type of explanation that "your hand has just moved" elicits an unconscious or semi-conscious "yes" set which promotes suggestibility.

Erickson and Rossi's approach to suggestion can easily lead one into seeing suggestions where, strictly speaking, there may be none. Consider the following example which, ironically, was used by Rossi (Erickson, Rossi, & Rossi, 1976, p. 267f) in a section specifically aimed at explaining the difference between the dynamics of indirect and direct suggestions. This example start out with a reference to a segment of an induction of hypnosis described in an earlier portion of the book. In this segment, Erickson embarked on a somewhat elaborate discussion of an experience both he and one of his sons had as children when learning how to multiply. He does this under the guise of giving the subject an example of what he means by certain things he has just told her regarding unconscious activities. The account he gives is an unlikely occurrence, and one cannot help but wonder if Erickson invented it for the occasion. It does exemplify to some extent what he had been talking about to the patient, but certainly not clearly. What it seems to add up to is that in arithmetical problem solving, the unconscious can provide answers to the conscious mind by using a general advanced mathematical method of solving certain types of problems without the individual having any notion of how the answers are obtained, and with the individual possessing only the most elementary knowledge of mathematics. That unconscious problem solving has led to important scientific developments is well-known. But in all cases this happened with brilliant scientists possessing advanced knowledge and training in their fields and who had long worked toward finding the solution in question. I mention this, because whether or not the event related by Erickson ever took place, it does reflect a truism.

It is clear from the account that Rossi, who was an observer, was quite puzzled by what Erickson had done and one wonders what went on in the subject's mind. Later, Erickson privately explained to Rossi that he wanted the subject to become bored. He went on to explain that her innate need to be polite would force her to listen politely with increasing boredom and this, in turn, would lead her to become fatigued because of past associations of becoming fatigued in other like situations. Summing up the whole maneuver, Erickson stated that its main purpose was to get the subject to experience feeling tired *without directly telling her to do so.*

Did the subject actually experience boredom and then fatigue? No attempt was made by Erickson to verify this and the matter must remain a surmise on his part. Was this an indirect suggestion as it is said to be in the text? Erickson never says so. It is Rossi who, in his next comment to the latter, interprets the above maneuver as Erickson using an indirect suggestion of fatigue. The latter neither acquiesces to or denies the correctness of this interpretation. However, later, he makes it clear that actually for him the significance of the maneuver is that it is one of many steps undertaken by him to depotentiate the subject's consciousness, thereby facilitating subsequent unconscious responses. Thus, for Erickson it is not the suggestion that Rossi perceived it to be. What did the subject perceive? No one knows!

Rossi goes on to state the dynamics of this presumed indirect suggestion are as follows: The boring story, *which he specifies to be the suggestion proper,* is a stimulus that arouses internal responses of acting polite that, in turn, evokes mental fatigue by association. Rossi also hints at utilization being involved, adding, in this connection, that processes already existing within the subject are also evoked.

One can agree that *if* the above maneuver did produce a feeling of tiredness, then it may qualify as being a very indirect way of doing so without ever directly bringing up the idea. But there is no evidence for this. Also, according to such a view, any stimulus, *no matter how remotely connected* it may be with the desired effect, is an indirect suggestion if it can be said to have elicited the effect, no matter how circuitous a chain of intervening processes are set into motion. Were we to follow along Rossi's line of reasoning, one could also conclude that a simpler *indirect suggestion* of tiredness would consist in physically tiring out the subject by having the latter exercise on a treadmill! Once again we are led to a use of the term suggestion which comes close to making it meaningless.

Further, let us assume for the moment that politeness really played a special part in the above situation. Was it really the cause of tiredness because, as Erickson explains at one point, being polite "can be awfully fatiguing?" If this was indeed what happened, we can stop right here. There is no need to go on and speak of associations with past experiences to account for the fatigue supposed to be present. I would be more inclined to consider that politeness created a need for the subject to remain in the situation which, possibly, might be better understood as a double bind (although I am not saying it was one). More to the point, one should ask whether it is not the case that people simply and naturally tire listening to a boring discourse and that issues of politeness and of associations with past experiences are simply extraneous and unnecessary considerations. In brief, there may never have been an indirect suggestion in the situation that has been described.

The elucidation of the difference between Erickson's conceptions of an indirect and a direct suggestion is considerably hampered by the fact that above all he was a clinician. More often than not he looks at suggestions within the context of doing psychotherapy. This becomes increasingly evident in his writings published after 1944. Most of the time Erickson fails to differentiate matters specific to psychotherapy per se, specific to suggestions per se, and specific to the use of suggestion as an adjuvant in psychotherapy. Additionally, issues specific to suggestion get confounded with issues specific to hypnosis or trance, as Erickson would put it.

This last remark brings us to the question whether or not Erickson made a meaningful distinction between hypnotic suggestions and non-hypnotic suggestions. If he did, what was it? There seems to be no question that in his early writings Erickson meant by "hypnotic suggestion" that which was called intrahypnotic suggestion in Volume 1, that is, a suggestion given to a person who is presumed to be hypnotized. Understandably, he had little to say regarding non-hypnotic suggestions because he only worked with individuals he considered to be in a hypnotic state. There are only a few brief mentions of such a distinction in the 1976 work of Erickson et al. On page 20, Erickson makes the unexpected point that *non-hypnotic suggestions are acted upon by the conscious and carried out in a voluntary manner.* What sense can we make out of this statement? For all intents and purposes, he is describing any one of the forms an injunction can take and with regard to which we expect a voluntary response, hence, which we *would not* call a suggestion in Volume 1. One expects there should be something in common between a non-hypnotic and a hypnotic suggestion and if this is not the elicitation of a non-voluntary response what is it? Possibly Erickson is attempting in the above to make the same distinction I made in Volume 1 between an intended and an effective suggestion. I say this on the basis that by 1976 Erickson was no longer distinguishing between the traditional "waking" and "hypnotic" suggestions, believing that the evocation of any non-voluntary response automatically carries a trance state with it. Obviously, from this standpoint, any intended suggestion, given in the absence of a trance, that was carried out by the subject could not, by definition, be an effective one, being carried out at a voluntary level.

Elsewhere, according to Erickson and Rossi (Erickson et al., 1976, p. 19), "Trance and hypnotic suggestion are to be viewed as distinct phenomena which, at any given instant, may or may not be associated." We are further told that Erickson views the "issue" of hypnotic suggestion as a "problem" in communication and utilization. However, at this point matters become quite confused and confusing. For we are next told that *hypnotic forms* of communication are used to facilitate suggestion. There is a problem here because throughout the work "hypnotic forms" is shown to be synonymous with forms of indirect suggestion. What we have just been told then is that forms of indirect suggestions facilitate suggestions. This is plainly circular unless we take the position a suggestion and a form of indirect suggestion denote different things. There is little basis for thinking this; what one is to make out of all this is at best confusing.

I do know from my contacts with Erickson that by 1976 he had had a long-standing position that suggestibility is not a characteristic of trance. This is possibly what he had in mind when he referred in the above to an "issue" and to a "problem." However, as we shall see in the next section, this position is not fully consistent with his attribution of "receptivity" to trance. One should probably not be too concerned about Erickson and Rossi's use of "hypnotic" as a qualifier on some occasions since I doubt that they are trying to make a major differentiation. We find them stating on p. 269 of the 1976 volume "Weitzenhoffer (1957, 1974, 1975) has emphasized that the defining feature of hypnotic suggestion is the absence of conscious volition in the production of the hypnotic response. We agree with the basic formulation."

Actually in the writings referred to I made this statement in regard to *both* hypnotic and non-hypnotic suggestions. I suspect the authors' statement is merely a reflection of Erickson's tendency to view all suggested behavior as implying the presence of a trance.

I have thus far attempted to state what Erickson's position is on the kinds of suggestions that may exist and what their nature may be. The final question I will examine is to what degree does Erickson's overall conception of suggestion coincide with the traditional and semi-traditional concept as detailed in Volume 1.

It seems reasonable to say that Erickson conceived of suggestion as being associated, either as an agent or as a mechanism (physiological or mental process), with the production, through communication from one person to another, of non-voluntary behavior. To this extent there is agreement.

However, in the traditional and semi-traditional conception there is a third defining criterion to be met. This is that the subject's eventual response must be a reflection or actualization of the ideational content of the suggestion. This is an aspect upon which neither Erickson nor Rossi have touched. They may have deliberately ignored it, they may have failed to recognize its importance as a defining feature or it may have been so obvious to them that they have taken it for granted. Whatever the case may be, this is a feature that is certainly quite evident in many of the examples of indirect suggestion they provide. But there are also examples in which this is not so. The one in which Erickson used a boring discussion about solving mathematical problems is such a case. This remains true whether we view it as a way of depotentiating the subject's conscious or of creating an experience of fatigue. We are thus led to the conclusion that Erickson apparently used the term suggestion in *two senses,* of which only one coincides with the traditional and semi-traditional definition.

Is there value in having and using his other conception? I do not think so if we are ever to have a true science of hypnotism. As I have pointed out in Volume 1, ambiguity is not consistent with good science. It also calls for concepts that are well-defined. If we agree to follow in Erickson's footsteps, we inevitably end up with ambiguities. The alternative is to choose one view of suggestion over the other. Inasmuch as Erickson offers us one way of looking at suggestion that seems also to cover all cases that satisfy the traditional and semi-traditional conditions, this would seem to be a strong argument for following this approach. The trouble with it is that, as we have seen, it leads to a conception of suggestion that is so comprehensive that it loses all meaningfulness and leaves us far worse off than we were before. It seems to me that Erickson and Rossi have pushed the process of enumerating and categorizing suggestions, especially indirect suggestion forms, too far. One can agree there are some things one is tempted to call suggestions, even though they do not meet all of the criteria for being one. Rather than force the issue, why not accept the fact they do not meet the criteria and give them a designation all of their own, if they merit one? Then let us study them in their proper context.

TRANCE AND HYPNOSIS

As with suggestion, Erickson's does not provide a good definition of "trance." Trance and non-trance phenomena are at times so completely interwoven with one another in his writings and case presentations that telling them apart is just about impossible. The material of this section will attempt to supplement earlier material about Erickson's use of the words "trance" and "hypnosis," but mostly it will highlight and summarize his position. We shall be particularly interested in what Erickson means by "trance." Does he mean something other than traditional hypnosis?

One conclusion that might be derived from previous material is that Erickson does not distinguish producing a suggestion-effect from being in a trance. Yet there are times when, in a similar context, Erickson specifically speaks of suggestion *and* specifically speaks of trance in a way that strongly intimates they are not the same.

I have come to the conclusion that this represents an issue that Erickson was never able to resolve satisfactorily and that must therefore remain an open issue where he is concerned.

In Erickson, Rossi, and Rossi (1976), it is stated that for Erickson trance is four things:

1. An inner directed state
2. A highly motivated state
3. An actual unconscious learning
4. An altered state of functioning

A more precise and correct statement would probably have been that the above four *aspects* of trance were those that were of primary interest to Erickson.

"Trance," according to Erickson and Rossi (Erickson et al., 1976, p. 138), "is actually an active process wherein the unconscious is active but not directed by the conscious mind." This, like so many others statements they make in other connections, seems too broad to be useful because it fails to differentiate between trance and processes that, from a scientific standpoint, one would probably not want to identify fully, if at all, with a trance. For example, would one really want to identify natural sleep, when dreaming, with trance? This condition does fit the above definition. Some writers, going as far back as Bernheim, have proposed a relation exists, although not an identity, between the dream state and hypnosis, or trance. There is no question that Erickson does see trance as a rather broad phenomenon embracing ordinary everyday activities, as shown when he asserts that a person who, during a lecture, absent-mindedly looks through a window, "is in a trance with wide open eyes." This is also purely conjectural.

On p. 41 we find that trance "is simply a modality wherein the patient's processes have an opportunity to interact in a more spontaneous and autonomous manner with the therapist." This, too, lacks specificity and has a certain amount of built in ambiguity. It may even contain an inherent contradiction. For how much autonomy and spontaneity can really exist when, in all of his writings, Erickson is clearly calling the shots and being very much the director, no matter how permissive and indirect he seems to be. At best, any spontaneity and autonomy is limited. "You can go into a trance when you are ready," presumably allows spontaneity and autonomy only in regard to *when* the trance will take place. According to Erickson himself, there is no question that it will occur.

The point has already been made that, for Erickson, trance and hypnosis seem to be synonymous terms. For example, Erickson, at times, speaks of "deep hypnosis." I once asked him how deep hypnosis differs from other forms of hypnosis. At that time, his answer was that "deep," "medium," and "light" are all adjectives that denote artificial demarcations. He did not elucidate further. However, in the 1976 work, Erickson specifies that deep hypnosis is that level of hypnosis that allows direct and adequate functioning (on the part of the subject) at an unconscious level without consciousness, that is, the conscious mind, interfering. But this is essentially what he also says trance is! This being the case, are we to infer that other "levels" of hypnosis are not trance? Probably not, because there is ample evidence in the remainder of his writings that, for him, trance can be said to have levels, too, depending on the extent to which unconscious processes dominate the subject's behavior.

In Erickson's earlier writings, one finds many references to the production of a very "deep," highly passive hypnosis, a lethargic condition in which the subject shows very little responsiveness, and of a somnambulic state into which deep hypnosis can be converted and in which the subject can be very active and function as if awake. The concept of a somnambulic state was retained by Erickson to the end of his life, and references to it can be found in the three volumes coauthored with Rossi, especially in the 1979 volume. Here, on p. 251, one finds the somnambulic state being defined as "a person acting as if he is awake but capable of following the therapist's hypnotic suggestions." In a later discussion (p. 393), Rossi attempts to make Erickson elucidate on this matter by voicing his impression that he has seen Erickson demonstrate three kinds of trances: a state of self-absorption in which the subject seems to be oblivious to the hypnotist; a condition in which the subject is very much in rapport with the hypnotist and responds to suggestions, but does not appear awake, and that Rossi identifies with the popular view of hypnosis; and, finally, somnambulism, in which subjects may have their eyes open and act as if they are awake. Typically, Erickson does not explicitly agree or disagree with Rossi, but comments that in practice, one observes all kinds of admixtures between the conditions just described; thus, indirectly, he is agreeing with Rossi.

The above definition does not adequately describe what Erickson really conceived the somnambulic state to be. Many hypnotized subjects who are not particularly outstanding in other ways can appear to be awake. It is clear from Erickson's earlier writings. as well as those coauthored with Rossi, that what he called somnambulic subjects were outstanding in their hypnotic performance. Whether we speak of suggestibility or not, they are the ones who are the most responsive at an automatic level to the words of the hypnotist, be they communicated directly or indirectly. Erickson's somnambulic state therefore seems to be essentially the traditional somnambulic state discussed in Volume 1. The somnambulic subject is not just capable of following suggestions, but he outstandingly does so. Furthermore, in keeping with the traditional picture of somnambulism, Erickson's somnambuls always present an amnesia for their trance experience unless told otherwise.

Although Erickson has frequently stated that there is *no* relationship between suggestibility and the presence of trance, he has also stated that the *receptivity* characteristic of trance is the basis of hypnotic suggestibility. This is an inconsistency that can be eliminated only by assuming Erickson means that, when hypnotic suggestibility is observed, such a receptivity is its basis. Since he widely spoke of suggestion, it seems reasonable to infer that suggestibility meant, for him, a responsiveness to suggestion. In fact, the consensus favoring hypersuggestibility as a sign of hypnosis is much too large to be ignored. Strictly speaking, and as explained in Volume 1, an appropriate check for hypersuggestibility calls for obtaining pre- and intrahypnotic measures of suggestibility with particular attention to the presence and absence of automatisms. There are no indications or reasons to believe that Erickson did anything of the kind with his subjects; nor did Bernheim and other investigators. However, studies in which this has been done (see Volume 1) refute Erickson's claim in a clear manner. Either Erickson and these other writers are referring to two different states, or there is a problem in communication. My best guess is that Erickson never meant to say that hypersuggestibility was *never* associated with hypnosis, but that, in many instances, he had found that this was not the case. Even so, there is still a puzzling predominance of negative assertions by Erickson.

Possibly in an effort to clarify the above, Rossi (1986, p. 50) offers his opinion that Erickson considered hypnotized subjects to be characteristically *hypersensitive* rather than *hypersuggestible*. It is this hypersensitivity, Rossi, says, that makes hypnotized individuals "amenable to accepting and carrying out suggestions." But Erickson does not appear ever to have stated this. Rossi infers it from a remark made by Erickson (1932) that is open to other interpretations. My feeling is that the above is really much less Erickson's view than that of Rossi, who tries to find support for it in the work of Ellenberger (1970, p. 115). Although this is going beyond what Erickson said, the issue is important enough to add a few comments. Ellenberger, who is merely reviewing some early historical material relevant to the origins of the concept of the unconscious, does not himself draw a conclusion such as Rossi makes. What he does is to point out that early writers such as de Puységur, Bertrand, Deleuze, and others had unanimously reported that artificial somnambulism *was characterized* by the presence of a heightening of the senses. This effect can probably be more accurately described as a lowering of sensory thresholds and an increase in the capacity to make sensory discriminations. This was presumably a psychophysiological change accompanying the development of somnambulism that had no obvious relationship with those responsible for the production of suggestion-effects, and thus of suggestibility. In fact, a person can be suggestible and even hypersuggestible without showing any increased sensitivity. The converse is also true. One might note that a decrease in sensibility, at least for pain, was also considered to be a characteristic of the somnambulistic state.

Erickson, in 1948 (p. 573f), and again in 1979, had the following to say about the role of suggestion in hypnosis:

> The next consideration concerns the general role of suggestion in hypnosis. Too often, the unwarranted and unsound assumption is made that, since a trance state is induced and maintained by suggestions, and since hypnotic manifestations can be elicited by suggestion, whatever develops from hypnosis must necessarily and completely be a result and primary expression of suggestion. Contrary to such misconceptions, the hypnotized person remains the same person. Only his behavior is altered by the trance state, but even so, that altered behavior derives from the life experience of the patient and not from the therapist. At the most, the therapist can influence only the manner of self-expression. The induction and maintenance of a trance serve to provide a special psychological state in which the patient can reassociate and reorganize his inner psychological complexities and utilize his own capacities in a manner concordant with his own experiential life. Hypnosis does not change the person, nor does it alter his past experiential life. It serves to permit him to learn more about himself and to express himself more adequately.

Direct suggestion is based primarily, if unwittingly, upon the assumption that whatever develops in hypnosis derives from the suggestions given. It implies that the therapist has a miraculous power of effecting therapeutic changes in the patient, and disregards the fact that therapy results from an inner resynthesis of the patient's behavior achieved by the patient himself. It is true that direct suggestion can effect an alteration in the patient's behavior and result in a symptomatic cure, at least temporarily. However, such a "cure" is simply a response to the suggestion and does not entail that reassociation and reorganization of ideas, understandings and memories so essential for an actual cure. It is this experience of reassociating and reorganizing his own experiential life that eventuates in a cure, not the manifestation of responsive behavior which can, at best, satisfy only the observer.

Some comments are needed regarding these two paragraphs. Overall, Erickson wants to make the point that hypnotic behavior is more than the effects of suggestions, and that hypnosis, or trance, also makes specific contributions of its own to this behavior. He also wants to make it clear that hypnotherapy entails much more than specific responses to suggestions. These are good points. His remarks regarding the tendency of many users of hypnotism to reduce everything to suggestion are also well-taken.

On the other hand, it has never come to my attention that anyone, except possibly Erickson (who seems to be doing this in the above), has claimed or argued that the reduction of all hypnotic behavior to suggestion implies a change in personality when a person becomes hypnotized. This certainly cannot be considered a logical conclusion. To my knowledge, as discussed in Volume 1, Pierre Janet is the only authority on hypnosis who has ever taken the position that a personality change affecting the self was associated with hypnosis, and more specifically, its somnambulic form. However, he did not relate this to suggestion. In fact, he did not employ suggestion to produce the hypnotic state, and he did not consider suggestibility to be a characteristic of the condition. If, indeed, Erickson saw such a connection, he has never explained what its basis is.

Actually, as mentioned in Volume 1, it is possible to argue on other grounds that the hypnotic state entails at least a superficial change in personality (but not in the self). What one can say depends a great deal upon how one defines personality. Can we really say, for example, that at a descriptive level, the individual who becomes highly suggestible or receptive to instructions after being hypnotized presents himself as the same person as he was prior to the induction and will be after dehypnotization?

When Erickson states, "Hypnosis does not change the person, nor does it alter his past experiential life," it is not clear whether he is referring to the hypnotic state only or to the state in combination with the use of suggestion.

It is also not clear what "person" denotes. Is he talking of the essence, the self of an individual, or of the outward manifestations of this self? In regard to the first of these issues, Erickson, like many other professionals, had a tendency to use the term "hypnosis" in both senses. This point is important because the validity of the above assertion is questionable if hypnosis as a combination of the state and the use of suggestions is being referred to. The very interesting clinical case Erickson and Rossi (1979) refer to on page 461 as the "February Man" may demonstrate that a person's experiential life can be altered by hypnotic interventions. In Volume 1, I have also reported a case, bearing some similarity to that of the February Man, that points in the same direction. Erickson's report (Erickson et al., 1968, p. 113) on the case of Leonard A., an age regression that got out of hand, casts some doubts on the idea that personality changes, at least, cannot be brought about when hypnotic suggestions are involved.

Why Erickson makes the remarks he does regarding the derivation of hypnotic behavior is not clear. I can see why he might make them were he writing for laymen, but this is not the case. I do not know of any professionals who have used hypnotism who conceive of suggested behavior having any other source than the subject's life experiences. If I suggest to a subject the hallucination of a duck swimming in a pond, it stands to reason that the suggested hallucination will have to be built out of the subject's past experiences with ducks and ponds. What the subject has not experienced cannot be created by hypnosis and/or suggestion. These are obvious conclusions. At the same time, one must recognize that, when successful, such a hallucination can be said to have had its source in, thus to have derived from, my actions.

Just how one should understand the first sentence of the second paragraph is also open to question. There is no basis for such a statement if Erickson is referring to the concept of a direct suggestion. Historically, it was repeatedly observed that very straightforward, "direct" statements made to a subject elicited the automatic, unconscious production by the subject of relevant behaviors and experiences. It was natural to refer to these statements as "direct suggestions." I think what Erickson really meant to say is that the use of only direct suggestion in hypnotherapy is based on the false understanding that everything that develops during the state of hypnosis, including its induction, is to be attributed to, and only to, the action of direct suggestions, and, especially, that creating effect by suggestion alone is sufficient to effect therapy. Erickson may have been very particular about what he said to his patients and subjects, but I do not think that this care was always extended to other areas of verbal intercourse. For example, how else can one account for Erickson speaking at a seminar (Erickson et al., 1961, p. 112) of a subject's retina having been anesthetized by suggestion when discussing the subject's development of a selective "blindness" for her handwriting. Erickson was far too knowledgeable regarding the physiology of vision to believe such a complex effect could thus be accounted for! I doubt that Erickson even seriously considered that suggestions could affect sensations at the receptor level. For reasons such as this, I am not hesitant in recommending that students of Erickson's work should not take everything he says at face value.

Within the framework of the use of indirect suggestion by Erickson, there is frequently no sharp demarcation between the induction of a trance and the giving of non-hypnotic and hypnotic indirect suggestions. Nonetheless, in published transcriptions, Erickson frequently seems to distinguish between a phase of an induction in which trance is not obviously there, and a phase in which it is. Furthermore, he frequently announces its appearance at specific points by calling attention to one or more of its clinical signs. The trance stare and catalepsy are among signs he uses most for this purpose. Others include decreased blinking, changes in respiration, and swallowing movements.

Traditional and semi-traditional hypnotism view hypnosis as a mental condition. Erickson sometimes gives the impression that he views trance as also being a physical condition that can involve only parts of the body or extend to the whole body. Thus, one finds him speaking of a cataleptic arm or an anesthetized hand as "being in a trance." He has also spoken of a patient's body being in trance while his mind is not. The idea that one "hypnotizes" an arm in which a rigidity has been induced is not unique to Erickson, although it is not widespread. Whether Erickson really believed that only part of an individual could be in a "trance," or whether he spoke thus for the benefit of his patients and audience, is not clear. Normally, this was said when it became obvious that there was a loss of voluntary control over some part of the body. In this context, Erickson and Rossi (Erickson et al., 1976, p. 195) speak of Erickson inducing trance "in fragments." That is, a trance is "built up" by eliciting a small automatic effect, then another one that can be associated with it, and so on. Each elicited effect constitutes a fragment of trance. This is nothing more than the chaining of suggestions that was discussed in Volume 1. However, in traditional and semi-traditional hypnotism, these effects are usually not seen as anything more than suggested effects that are conducive to an eventual mental state that appears in toto. My understanding of Erickson's position is that, because he views trance as synonymous with functioning at an automatic level, any evocation of an automatic effect means that some degree of trance, minimal as it may be, has been established. The more automatic behavior is exhibited, the more trance there is. It may seem more reasonable to Erickson to think of an analgesic hand as being in a trance, rather than the entire person being in a slight trance. For me, as it was for Erickson, trance implies the presence of directed intelligent behavior. I find it difficult to ascribe this kind of behavior to a part of the body, such as a hand. Possibly, this was said by Erickson only as a figure of speech, although I do not think so.

Looking at how Erickson perceives trance induction does not lead to further insight into what trance means for him. According to Erickson, Rossi, and Rossi (1976, p. 302), there is a threefold purpose to trance induction:

1. To reduce the foci of attention
2. To facilitate or alter habitual patterns of direction and control
3. To facilitate the subject's (or patient's) receptivity to his inner skills so that they can be integrated in the production of desire responses

But, basically, this is nothing more than what indirect suggestions aim to do! In final summary for Erickson,

1. "Trance" and "hypnosis" are synonymous. Erickson preferred the former term.
2. Trance is a state of abstraction and of inward focusing.
3. Trance is a condition of receptivity to stimuli capable of evoking inner mechanisms of automatic behaviors.
4. Trance has depth.
5. Trance and suggestion are distinct objects.

In regard to Rossi and Erickson's many references to the "therapeutic trance," does this refer to something other than what they refer to as simply "trance?" As with many other concepts that are ambiguously used in their writings, the authors go back and forth from "trance" to "therapeutic trance" as if either the difference was clear or there was no difference. From my study of the pertinent writings, I have concluded that, where the presence of a special state is concerned, it is probably the same fundamental state that is present in both situations, and that the difference, if there is one, most likely lies in the shaping and utilization of the trance. As in the case of suggestion, Erickson has considerable difficulty in separating psychotherapeutic steps and processes that *do not* specifically belong to hypnotism from those that do, and the "therapeutic trance" seems to be a mixture of the two. I shall leave the further discussion of this matter to the section on Ericksonian hypnotherapy.

ERICKSONIAN CONSCIOUS/UNCONSCIOUS DICHOTOMY

I have covered this topic earlier in this chapter. The following will, therefore, be more of a summarizing statement than a presentation of new material. Erickson's extensive use of and references to the patient's "unconscious" can be said to be a mark of his work. There can be no question that the unconscious has a central position in his writings. For Erickson, the shift from conscious to unconscious functioning is the essence of trance (hypnosis):

Nowhere in his writings, however, can one find an explicit definition of the term "unconscious," or, for that matter, of "conscious." The closest one comes to any definition of this kind is when he states (Zeig, 1980), "The unconscious mind is made up of all your learnings over a lifetime, many of which you have forgotten, but which serve you in your automatic functioning." It is clear that at the time his students began to write about and with him in the late 1970s, Erickson did not have the Freudian unconscious in mind. As Germain Lavoie, a Canadian psychologist who is very knowledgeable about both hypnotism and psychoanalysis, has aptly remarked to me, the Ericksonian "unconscious" lacks, in particular, the hostile and aggressive aspects so characteristic of Freud's system UCS. In fact it has a Jungian quality.

Many statements of Erickson regarding the unconscious, such as the one taken from Zeig's book, say little about such properties of the unconscious as being alogical and atemporal, or as being the source of drives and goal-directed action, or as possessing an intelligence of sort. Other statements by Erickson give one the distinct impression, however, that these are also characteristics of the Ericksonian unconscious. Erickson also often presented the unconscious as an entity with many features of Morton Prince's subconscious: an autonomous counterpart of a person's conscious, whose activities are unknown to the latter, except, at times, through their impact upon his consciously perceived world. Although I cannot say this with absolute certainty, it is my impression that Prince did not place all automatic actions and behavior within the province of the subconscious, whereas Erickson seems to have done so. Also, I do not believe that Prince viewed the subconscious as being alogical and atemporal. The Ericksonian unconscious appears to range in its inclusiveness from simple reflex actions to intricate intellectual activities. At times, it seems to be able to have all of the capacities of the conscious, and perhaps even more. The only superiority the Ericksonian conscious seems to have over the unconscious is that, in a normal and awake individual, the conscious holds dominance over much of an individual's behavior and holds sway over some unconscious activities. Another differentiating feature in Erickson's case seems to be that attitudes, beliefs, and acquired mental sets belong to the province of the conscious, and, in any case, influence its actions, but not those of the unconscious. As we have seen, Erickson's forms of indirect suggestion are all intended to activate unconscious activity freed of all conscious interference and control.

Erickson also makes references to "conscious awareness" and "unconscious awareness." It would have been helpful if he had clarified just what "awareness" meant to him and how it differed from consciousness. As it stands, the first expression is redundant and the second is self-contradictory, because awareness usually implies consciousness when these are not used synonymously. The above seems to express Erickson's belief that there are certain covert processes or activities that influence a person's behavior as if they were conscious processes. Just what happens when he tells a subject or patient something like, "You (or your conscious) need not know . . . but your unconscious will," or, "Your unconscious will have full awareness . . ." can only be guessed. I see very little difference between doing this and doing what Hilgard does when he creates a hidden observer. Obviously, Erickson was making use of hidden observers long before Hilgard did. Like Hilgard's hidden observers, Erickson's unconsciouses are most likely suggested artifacts. They may nevertheless be useful devices for purposes of therapy.

Much of the above material is not explicitly stated in Erickson's writings. Such a conceptualization of the conscious and unconscious leaves us with a number of questions, such as what the function of the conscious is. One sometimes gets the impression from his writings that man might be a far more effective creature had he only an unconscious. A question of a different order is whether this concept may not be too comprehensive. For example, if ideodynamic action is a reality, should it be considered to be a part of the "unconscious," or merely one of many non-conscious activities that can be and are equally used by a directing conscious and a directing unconscious? Bernheim made it fairly clear that the automatisms on which he founded hypnotic behavior were also used in the service of conscious action, and I find Erickson's concept of utilization to include the same view.

Erickson's modus operandi with respect to the unconscious has a certain paradoxical quality. We find him frequently saying to the patient, "Your unconscious will know . . . ," "As soon as your unconscious knows your hand . . ." Or he may say, "Your conscious needs not be aware . . ." or even, "You need not know . . ." with the intended implication that the unconscious, however, will be aware, or will know. The question that one must ask is just whom or what is being referred to by the words "you" and "your." Who or what is being addressed? One has the impression that two messages are being simultaneously given, one to the conscious and one to the unconscious. Indeed, Erickson does tell in his articles of doing this, and he and Rossi (1976) make the point that multilevel communication is a characteristic of Ericksonian hypnotism. But why the need to communicate in this way with the conscious when one wants to communicate with the unconscious? It is as if the former was a necessary mediator or, at least, a go-between. If so, what, then, of situations in which the patient is viewed as being in a "deep" trance? According to Erickson, in this case all conscious activities should be eliminated, or nearly so. Yet Erickson still uses "you" and "your" in these situations. Of course, this is not a new problem. We encountered it earlier, in Volume 1 when examining the nature of the hypnotic state. Apparently, it is one that was never of concern to Erickson, and he, like all other workers in this field, employed hypnotism with a very loose and vague use of the concepts of conscious and unconscious.

This matter of communication with the unconscious becomes even more complicated when one considers such maneuvers as the interspersal technique. As previously explained, with this technique, certain words, sentences, and even phrases intended for the unconscious are interwoven with other words, sentences, and phrases intended for the conscious. Somehow the unconscious knows this is the case and is able to sort out what is intended for it. But how does the unconscious know these things? One can only wildly speculate as to how the unconscious knows in general that there is material intended for it and which material it is. Regarding the issues of the unconscious knowing what in the material is intended for it, Erickson and Rossi (Erickson et al., 1976) tell us that this portion of the material is usually "underlined" in a number of ways by voice intonation, by stress on words, by other speech characteristics, and by non-verbal cues. But, similarly, the remaining material also stands out by not being thus underlined, and one cannot help but wonder why the unconscious might not act, instead, on this material. In other words, why and how does the unconscious specifically know it is the underlined and not the remaining material that it must act upon and that the underlined material is not intended instead for the conscious mind? Likewise, why and how does the conscious know this underlined material is not intended for it? Sidis, to whom I have already referred, showed that what stands out and influences people is not always what is expected.

It is easy to assert that when I say to a subject, "Your hand will rise," this is clearly heard by the unconscious as a request for it to raise the hand at an automatic level. Likewise that the statement, "I want you to do your best to stay wide awake," contains the metamessage to the unconscious, "and go into a trance," upon which the unconscious then acts. But either assertion is quite gratuitous. The only thing that can be said with any certainty is that, if the subject is carefully paying attention, his conscious mind probably hears these words. Just how he perceives or what he does with them is problematical and can be known only through his subsequent action and reports. As to what the unconscious hears or does, we can only guess.

Finally, we come to Erickson's use of story telling, allegories, and metaphors as a means of indirect suggestion. Some of Erickson's students have been so excited by this approach that they use this method to the exclusion of all others. It is not my impression that Erickson made as extensive a use of these devices as is intimated, although I think he did make more use of them in later years than earlier in his career. The idea seems to be that stories, allegories, and metaphors are ideal media of communication with the unconscious. However, there is no solid evidence that this kind of material specifically stimulates unconscious processes more than other kinds of communications, or that it is in the "language" of the unconscious. Metaphors, stories, and allegories are not unique in their ability to evoke associations that remain outside of consciousness. Any stimulus, whether it is verbal or not, has the potentiality for eliciting associations that may or may not enter consciousness. More to the point, the use of these linguistic devices may have very little to do specifically with hypnotism. They appear to be tools that can equally well be effectively used outside the context of hypnotism; it is my impression that Erickson used them as much, if not more, in a non-hypnotic therapeutic context. They may be ways of giving indirect suggestions, but this does not necessarily mean that this is the only way they function. They can be used to make a point or clarify an issue. Also as Zeig (1980) points out in connection with the use of anecdotes, they may, for example, serve to create confusion; they are non-threatening ways of communication; and they may be an aid in bypassing resistance. I have not found evidence indicating that Erickson used these devices extensively to induce hypnosis or to produce hypnotic phenomena, although he did use them to some degree for these purposes.

It needs to be added that, when used for purposes of indirect therapeutic action, anecdotes and other related forms of indirect communications must be carefully chosen and constructed. Their contents must be such that they reflect the patient, his problems, and the solution to these. In other words, there must be an isomorphism. Readers who are especially interested in pursing this subject further will find Gordon's (1978) work on therapeutic metaphors both interesting and useful. They should also keep in mind as they study it that it is largely grounded on speculation.

LEFT/RIGHT BRAIN FUNCTIONS AND HYPNOTISM

Rossi states (Erickson, Rossi, & Rossi 1976):

> From this session it is finally clear that a neurophysiological model utilizing the differences between right- and left-hemispheric functioning is also implicit in Erickson's work. (p. 277)

This is a gross misstatement of facts. More specifically, Rossi concludes that individuals in their normal state of consciousness (awake) predominantly make use of their left hemisphere, whereas when hypnotized (in trance), they predominantly use their right hemisphere. In a subsequent volume (Erickson & Rossi, 1979), the "conscious" is stated to be associated with the left hemisphere, whereas the "unconscious" is said to be associated with the right hemisphere.

The above statement is made on inferences based on the work on hemispheric functions reported by Sperry, Gazzaniga, and Bogen between 1967 and 1969. Rossi also makes reference to research of Bakan, Morgan,

McDonald, and Hilgard that touches more directly on the relationship of hemispheric functions to hypnotic behavior. Toward the end of his discussion, Rossi admits that it may be too simple to view trance as a function of only the right hemisphere, and he then recognizes the possibility that some trance inductions affect both hemispheres. Furthermore, whether intentionally or not, Rossi speaks of suggestions being given simultaneously to *both* hemispheres. However, in subsequent volumes (Erickson & Rossi, 1979 and 1981), there is no longer any hesitation on the part of the authors in taking the position that trance phenomena (which include all suggestion effects) are primarily a right hemisphere function. These works give the impression that this is now a settled matter. On the basis of this association between suggested effects and the right brain, Erickson and Rossi are now able to explain that all of their indirect methods work because they are worded in the language that the right brain specifically understands and that the left brain does not. Perhaps this is so, but I am not at all convinced that, for example, when Erickson speaks to the patient of "the unimportance of keeping your eyes open," the right brain receives the message "close your eyes," and proceeds to act upon it, whereas the left brain hears only that it is unimportant to keep the eyes open and that nothing more ensues from this. For me, this opens up a number of questions that have no answers.

One can only wish that the relationships in question were that clear and that matters were that simple. The session to which Rossi alludes in the quoted paragraph in no way clearly shows the model referred to is implicit in Erickson's work. Furthermore, today, more than ten years later, the relationship of hemispheric functions to hypnotic behavior is no better established than it was at the writing of the quote. In fact, a recent work of Gazzaniga (1985) strongly suggests that the above conclusion was highly premature. Two even more recent reports by Bower (1987) and by Kosslyn (1988) also make it clear that there is still too much controversy regarding hemispheric functions to permit one to draw conclusions regarding their relation to hypnotic effects. Kosslyn has indicated that both hemispheres are involved in mental imagery.

ERICKSONIAN HYPNOTHERAPY AND STRATEGIC THERAPY

In their 1979 book, Erickson and Rossi say:

> We view hypnotherapy as a process whereby we help people utilize their own mental associations, memories, and life potentials to achieve their own therapeutic goals. (p. 1)

It is difficult to tell whether this is intended to be a definition of what hypnotherapy is or a statement of their view of what therapy using hypnotism should be like. The above could be said of many other non-hypnotic forms of therapy, and it does not uniquely define hypnotherapy as done by Erickson. It is equally applicable to the work of a number of well-known psychotherapists and hypnotherapists, such as Wolberg, who have quite different orientations.

Speaking of Erickson, Rossi (Erickson & Rossi, 1976) says:

> He simply tries to evoke the natural processes within the patient that will enable them to be receptive to their own inner realities and experience the possibility of new creative inner work being done to resolve a problem. (p. 303)

Unless one maintains that any procedure that accomplishes the above must necessarily involve hypnosis, or at least suggestion, there is, again, nothing in the above that uniquely distinguishes what Erickson is described as doing as being hypnotherapy.

Thus far, what we have is a brief statement of Erickson's philosophy of psychotherapy. The following, also from the 1979 work, does, however, give us some idea of how hypnotism fits into the picture. According to the authors:

> suggestion can facilitate the utilization of abilities and potentials that already exist within a person but that remain unused or underdeveloped because of a lack of understanding or training. The hypnotherapist carefully explores a patient's individuality to ascertain what life learnings, experiences and mental skills are available to deal with the problem. The therapist then facilitates an approach to trance experience wherein the patient may utilize these uniquely personal and internal responses to achieve therapeutic goals. (p. 1)

Of course, such an exploration on the part of the hypnotherapist as is mentioned in the above is again not specific to doing hypnotherapy. It is only to the extent that it is done with the aid of hypnotism or in a hypnotic state that it can actually be considered to be a hypnotherapeutic element. To make this point clear, I would ask the reader to contrast exploring the patient's past by asking him questions in the normal state and exploring it, using, for example, age regressions. It is my impression that what Erickson is mainly interested in with this kind of exploration is to discover what type of responses are available at an automatic (unconscious) level, and to this end he utilizes what Erickson and Rossi refer to as the "therapeutic trance," which they say:

> . . . can be understood as a free period of psychological exploration wherein therapist and patient cooperate in the search for those hypnotic responses that will lead to therapeutic change. (p. 10)

The therapeutic trance is thus understood to be more than just the trance. It is trance *combined* with its utilization along the lines just indicated. Furthermore, as in the 1976 work:

Therapeutic trance is a special state that intensifies the patient-therapist relationship and focuses the patient's attention on a few inner realities. (p. 228)

Trance thus serves another function in Erickson's scheme of therapy. Note, however, that the effects of trance on the patient-therapist relationship is not a unique aspect of Ericksonian hypnotherapy. As pointed out in Volume 1, this effect has long been recognized by traditional and semi-traditional therapists, such as Wolberg (1948), who have also capitalized on it.

The authors add that Erickson uses the forms listed in column 3 of the microdynamics of trance induction to evoke, to mobilize, and to move the patient's associate processes and mental skills in certain directions with the hope of reaching certain therapeutic goals.

On page 311, they say that Erickson's invention and systematic use of the various hypnotic forms, discussed in the section on dynamics, was for the purpose of studying and utilizing "a patient's own associative structure and mental skills in ways that are outside his usual range of conscious ego control to effect therapeutic goals." So was Erickson's use of anecdotes, metaphors, and so forth.

Also on page 303 they state that "the approaches to clinical induction . . . are simply a convenient means by which the therapist can initiate a process of inner focus and unconscious learning." A little further on they add, "He [Erickson] simply tries to evoke the natural processes within the patient that will enable them to be receptive to their own inner realities and experience the possibility of new creative inner work being done to resolve a problem."

Finally, on page 267, it is said of Erickson, "He helps the patient to recognize the value of his unique inner experiences and provides suggestions about how it may be utilized therapeutically." Of course, the suggestions are largely indirect.

Erickson's 1948 article, to which I have already referred, contains several statements that throw a useful additional light on the above material. He says:

Another common oversight in hypnotic psychotherapy lies in the lack of appreciation of the separateness or the possible mutual exclusiveness of the conscious and the unconscious (or subconscious) levels of awareness. (p. 575)

Erickson goes on to make the point that while full knowledge regarding a specific subject matter may exist within the unconscious, it may be unavailable to the conscious mind. The point of this remark is that:

In hypnotic psychotherapy, too often, suitable therapy may be given to the unconscious but with the failure by the therapist to appreciate the tremendous need of either enabling the patient to integrate the unconscious with the conscious, or of making the new understandings of the unconscious fully accessible, upon need, to the conscious mind . . . . Properly, hypnotherapy should be oriented equally about the conscious and the unconscious, since the integration of the total personality is the desired goal in psychotherapy. . . . good unconscious understanding allowed to become conscious before a conscious readiness exists will result in conscious resistance, rejection, repression and even the loss, through repression, of unconscious gains. By working separately with the unconscious there is then the opportunity to temper and control the patient's rate of progress and thus to effect a reintegration in the manner acceptable to the conscious mind. (p. 575f)

What appears to evolve out of the above material is that, as we have seen to be the case for traditional and semi-traditional hypnotism, hypnotherapy is also for Erickson the use of hypnotism for purposes of bringing about therapeutic change. In this respect, there is not any major difference between the approaches. However, what is not made evident by the above, but largely comes out of a study of his therapy cases, is that, whereas in traditional and semi-traditional hypnotherapy the therapist generally decides early what specific effects will be produced and how they will specifically be used in support of or to affect the therapy, Erickson leaves the choice of effects and how they will be used somewhat of an open-ended issue. He does not so much choose as he gives the patient the opportunity to choose unconsciously according to the patient's own patterns of response. For him, each individual is a storehouse of past experiences that can be reinstated and of learnings that can be activated by appropriate stimuli. What he says to the patient is intended to be a stimulus for the elicitation of responses peculiar to the patient. Having elicited such responses, he then helps the patient utilize them in new, therapeutic ways, but never tells him specifically how to do this. His belief is that given these responses, the patient will find in his own way how to make use of them. The patient is the one who finds the solution to his problems; the therapist is merely instrumental in facilitating the process. The therapeutic trance is particularly useful for this. In Erickson's own words (Erickson, 1948):

The induction and maintenance of a trance serve to provide a special psychological state in which the patient can reassociate and reorganize his inner psychological complexities and utilize his own capacities in a manner concordant with his own experiential life. Hypnosis does not change the person, nor does it alter his past experiential life. It serves to permit him to learn more about himself and to express himself more adequately. (p. 514)

It is of course understood that in the above, Erickson is speaking of hypnosis induced and used in the context of therapy. However, outside of this context, Erickson's approach from at least 1960 on is not appreciably different. This can readily be seen from such transcriptions as those of Sue's (Erickson, Haley, & Weakland, 1959) and Ruth's (Erickson & Rossi, 1981, p. 155f) inductions, as well as many other later transcriptions to be found in volumes by Erickson and Rossi and one by Zeig. Erickson approaches the production of hypnotic phenomena for demonstration purposes in exactly the same way he approaches the use of hypnotic phenomenology for therapeutic ends. The study of these transcriptions can therefore be as useful for therapists as it can be for researchers. The main difference is that, in the case of demonstrations, Erickson aims at producing certain specific effects in the present or in the immediate future, whereas in the case of therapy, he can usually content himself with laying down the grounds, in an open-ended way, for a number of processes and effects that can happen at an often unspecified future time, and elsewhere than in his office. Furthermore, because of the nature of demonstrations, he is forced to direct and limit the manifestations of suggested effects along certain lines. This is not the case with therapy, where he can allow the initiated processes to go on quasi-autonomously, possibly initiating other, unspecified processes. Finally, different goals obviously guide his utilization of the effects that are elicited.

I said a moment ago that Erickson's approach to the induction of hypnosis and its utilization had a certain open-endedness, and one frequently gets the impression that it was Erickson who followed the patient wherever the patient took him, and not the other way around. I do not think this really is the case. Paraphrasing Erickson to some degree, I have heard him say on more than one occasion in reference to the subject or patient, "He has the illusion that he is in control and has choices, but he really does not have any choice." This illusory choice is well-demonstrated in many of the so-called bind and double bind maneuvers used by Erickson. The study of transcripts of Erickson at work clearly shows that he always has a goal in mind and that he very clearly guides the subject or patient in that direction. How could it be otherwise? If a patient comes in with a sexual problem, surely what Erickson is going to do, no matter how seemingly circuitously he does it, will be oriented toward bringing about a resolution of this problem. In this regard, he is no different than any other therapist. But Erickson is a patient man who is not in a hurry; he is not going to allow the patient to pressure him into premature action. It is true that he does not force the patient to produce a specific response at any precise moment. He simply waits for the patient to produce one that he can utilize, but he does not wait passively; he is constantly stimulating the patient to produce specific classes of responses. He is constantly taking calculated steps aimed at producing specific effects.

If he fails to obtain an effect that is of importance to him, he will take other steps aimed at getting it. Furthermore, it is clear that open-ended as he may be, he also adheres to a specific sequential scheme of operation detailed, for example, in Erickson and Rossi (1979, p. 1ff). There we see that, in principle, he begins with a preparatory phase and then goes on to the therapeutic trance, which itself sequentially involves four steps: fixation of attention, depotentiation of habitual frameworks and belief systems, unconscious searches, and the activation of unconscious processes. These lead to a final step: the production of hypnotic responses. In other words, there is a great deal more directing in Erickson's permissive and indirect approach than may seem or than has been admitted by adherents to his methods and views.

Erickson's approach to each patient obviously has to be highly individualized. For this reason, it is not possible to categorize his modes of treatment except in very broad, general terms. There is no such thing in Ericksonian hypnotherapy as saying, "This is the general way to treat phobias," "This is what you do with a hysterical paralysis," and so forth. Erickson was extremely creative and ingenious in his practice. But one can find some things in the writings that have been referred to that would seem to be of general applicability. One example is the idea that a symptom is often overdone and that the patient's needs can often be satisfied with a less extensive and intensive form of the symptom. This is the way that Erickson once treated a woman for a large, ugly skin lesion that was diagnosed as psoriasis: by suggesting a series of gradual reductions in its size and severity, until it was no more than a small, barely noticeable lesion. Even this remnant eventually spontaneously disappeared. He has used this method and variations of it successfully in a variety of other cases, and I have had success in doing the same.

Exacerbating first a presumably intractable symptom before starting to reduce it by suggestion is another method that appears to have some general applicability. Erickson told me of the case of a man who had come to him because of rather massive jerky movements of his hands and forearms that were thought to be organically based. As I remember it, initial efforts by Erickson to stop the movement by direct suggestion failed. Even a reduction was impossible. Erickson then directly suggested that the movement would increase and become at least double in frequency, then triple. Having succeeded with these steps, he then suggested the movement would become reduced to a half; then, having succeeded with this, he suggested a further reduction to a third. He had the patient go home with the additional posthypnotic suggestion that during the week there would be a further reduction by half, and each week thereafter there would be more reductions by one half each week, until there was no need for further reduction. Shortly thereafter, the patient reported a cessation of the movements. Erickson explained to me that he did not expect that he could directly decrease the movements, but felt certain that they could be increased. Having now added a suggested component to the movements, he could also remove the added component and thereby establish some control in the desired direction. The first reduction merely removed some of the added movement, but the second reduction not only removed the remainder of the added movement, but went further and actually reduced the original movement to a half. Having established that this could be done, he left the patient with instructions that would continue the process. As he remarked to me, whether or not the movement fully stopped, it would eventually become imperceptibly small. Erickson told me that determining early in the treatment that some form of control by suggestion could be established was important, but not just in helping him plan his strategy, but also in creating a beneficial positive attitude in the patient. He added that had this step failed, he would have tried other suggested alterations of the movement. Frequency was only one of several possibilities. This was many years before the dynamics discussed in his collaborations with Rossi were evolved. In any case, he made no allusions to them in discussing the above case with me. It is interesting, however, to look retrospectively at his procedure in such terms. There are many things possibly going on. There is the creation of a "yes" set, or of a conditioning. There are the implications inherent in the factuality of his being able to cause a change, even though it is in an undesirable direction. This can even be viewed as a use of a reverse set. There may be a use of confusion in his clever use of doubling, tripling, and then taking fractions as he does. In any event, by using the order ½, then ⅓, he is very subtly and indirectly able to suggest a half reduction of the original movement. Fragmentation is also used. Total reduction of the symptom is accomplished by doing it in small steps rather than one large step. Finally, there is a certain open-endedness in his posthypnotic suggestion. Erickson's approach was mostly direct. It is not particularly hard to do the same in more indirect ways. As an exercise, the reader might want to try reformulating the above.

Was the above case as purely organic as stated? Erickson felt it was. If so, the success of his approach raises some interesting questions as to how the results were actually accomplished. One can only speculate regarding this. On the whole, Erickson seems to have treated relatively few purely somatic problems. As I mentioned in Chapter 2 of this volume, Erickson was, to my knowledge, the first to successfully treat a case of Reynaud's disease. The physiological processes set into motion in this instance are quite clear. The treatment depended upon an understanding of the associated circulatory physiology.

One of Erickson's (Erickson, 1963) most remarkable treatments of an organic problem is probably the case of a woman who had suffered serious brain damage and had been reduced to a vegetative life filled with intractable pain.

Reading Erickson's article is highly recommended. The treatment was long and complex and presents a large number of interesting features which will be summed up. While the problem was purely organic, the treatment was strictly psychological. Yet to the extent that somatic changes toward health took place, there had to be a beneficial psychosomatic interaction. The case also clearly shows that good hypnotherapy does not necessarily mean the use of only hypnotism, and that hypnotism, in fact, can constitute only a small percentage of the total treatment, yet still be an important part of it. It also shows that its use does not necessarily mean a brief and easy treatment. Furthermore, it exemplifies how subtly and indirectly hypnotism can be induced and used. There are unfortunately a great many desirable details missing in the account regarding this use. These details would show us to what extent Erickson had made use of the various forms discussed in the section on dynamics, as well as just how hypnotism was actually employed. What we primarily know is that hypnosis was induced a number of times; we know little else about its use. The case is also a remarkable exemplification of utilization on a very wide scale going well beyond the production of hypnotic effects. Such a utilization clearly requires a detailed understanding of the patient's psychological composition.

It also needs to be emphasized that rather unique conditions seem to have existed in this case that insured the success of the treatment. Not only is the kind of necessary detailed cooperation Erickson was able to secure from members of the patient's household remarkable, but so is the fact that time after time individuals with just the right kind of personality, skills, and lack of skills were brought into the patient's household as helpers at opportune times. At least it seems so from the account, but possibly it was as much a matter of Erickson capitalizing on whatever became available at a certain time. Finally, there must have been a tremendous investment of Erickson's energy and time in this case.

Lest there be any misunderstanding, this case is not a demonstration that hypnosis per se, or specific suggestions to this effect, can bring about organic ameliorative changes. As was pointed out in Volume 1, the effectiveness of direct suggestions aimed at producing organic changes is generally very limited. What this case demonstrates is that, through a complex hypnotic intervention, one can set into motion non-hypnotic actions that can indirectly bring about organic changes or be supportive of other actions having such an effect. Erickson believed in Lashleys's theory of the equipotentiality of brain cells. He reasoned that because of this theory, any intact cluster of cells in the patient's brain could substitute for those that had been affected by disease, and that the patient thus had the potentiality to regain all lost functions. His entire strategy was one aimed at promoting such a reacquisition through life experiences. This case is therefore a good example of Erickson's application of his utilization principle.

In looking at Ericksonian hypnotherapy, it is essential to recognize that

Erickson used techniques and procedures that were not unique to his use of hypnotism, but were unique to his approach to psychotherapy per se. The study of Ericksonian hypnotherapy is confusing because in any given therapy session, Erickson frequently alternates between non-hypnotic and hypnotic therapy with little to no obvious transitions. To add to the confusion, he would often use the very same maneuver to bring about effects that were probably purely hypnotic, as well as others that were purely therapeutic and non-hypnotic. For example, he utilized resistance whether it was resistance to hypnosis or some other form of resistance. He did the same with presumed double binds. Compare, for example, the double binds, "Will you go into trance now or later?" and "Will you start on your diet today or tomorrow?" It is doubtful that a therapeutic effect will result from the first question and a trance from the second. Erickson might use both in the same session for different ends, while at the same time doing this in a integrative manner.

Since my purpose in this volume is to write about hypnotherapy rather than therapy in general, I will not discuss in detail those procedures used by Erickson that are clearly non-hypnotic. They belong largely to the domain of what has been called strategic therapies. There has been a tendency to consider these therapies as being hypnotherapies. To do so is an error. We owe the concept of strategic therapy to Haley (1973), who states (p. 17), "A therapy can be called strategic if the clinician initiates what happens during therapy and designs a particular approach for each problem." On this same page he also states, "Strategic therapy is not a particular approach or theory but a name for those types of therapy where the therapist takes responsibility for directly influencing people." *There is definitely nothing in these two definitions that implies that hypnosis or suggestion is an essential agent in the therapies.* When Haley wrote the above, and even before, there were already therapies being performed that met the requirement for being called strategic and that had no association with hypnotism. I suspect that the association of strategic therapies with hypnotism originated because the clinical work of Erickson was the starting point for Haley. There are no sharp boundaries between hypnotic and non-hypnotic therapy in Erickson's work. Haley (p. 19) has stated, "One way to see Milton Erickson's strategic therapy is as a logical extension of hypnotic techniques." I think that one could equally well make a case for the converse. Actually, it may be neither the one nor the other, since Erickson has often spoken of using his (strategic) techniques and procedures in daily situations that were neither therapy nor hypnotism.

FINAL CONSIDERATIONS

In reviewing Erickson's writings, I have noticed that his therapy articles prior to 1975 are considerably detailed regarding the dynamics of the therapies that are described. In contrast, after 1975 the emphasis in his writings is on procedures and techniques. It is also noticeable that the first group of writings were Erickson's individual work, whereas the second group represents a collaborative effort, primarily with Rossi. I cannot help but conclude that the difference may represent the influence of his co-authors, who were much more interested in looking at techniques than at dynamics. They were under the misperception that techniques alone were the answer to Erickson's success. The pressure was on Erickson to talk about techniques, not dynamics, and Erickson was obliging. Furthermore, Rossi has greatly overdone the breaking down of Erickson's procedures into his many "hypnotic forms." This has resulted in a bewildering overabundance of forms of indirect suggestion. Also, the validity of many examples must be questioned; so must the actuality of some of these forms. Broken down too finely, linguistic structures become mere combinations of words that, although they may retain some meaning, no longer reflect their original function in the total communication of which they were once a part.

One aspect that is not well-recognized in comparing Ericksonian hypnotherapy to the more traditional forms is that, as I made the point some years ago (Weitzenhoffer, 1962), a great deal can be and has been accomplished hypnotherapeutically in the framework of traditional and semi-traditional lines with limited suggestibility. The immediate production of the so-called "deeper" phenomena is no more a requirement here than it is in Ericksonian work. In many applications, neither approach to hypnotism requires that such phenomena ever be produced. A portion of Erickson's greater success is probably to be found in his early recognition of these facts (a fact not recognized by the majority of other practicing hypnotherapists of his time). The latter have been concerned about the issue of "depth" of hypnosis, whereas Erickson has concerned himself very little with it. We rarely find him talking about the extent of trance, and much of the time, one does not see him overly concerned with whether or not trance is even present.

There is a pretense of looking at dynamics in the works written with Rossi, but this always remains quite superficial. That Erickson had a much wider and deeper understanding of dynamics than is shown, and that *making effective use of these was an important key to his success,* is clearly shown in his earlier individual writings. One may counter this by pointing out that the later writings include this aspect under the umbrella notion of utilization. This may be true, but in doing so, essential details have become lost.

In spite of Rossi's emphasis that his collaborative writings with Erickson are about "approaches" as opposed to techniques, the resulting works remain primarily ones about techniques and procedures. I could possibly agree with Rossi if I knew exactly how he differentiates "approaches" from "techniques." Unfortunately, he remains silent on this matter, and he and Erickson go on to make as many references to "techniques" as they make to "approaches." If there is a difference, one can only conclude that it is not critical.

And, indeed, what is the commotion about? It seems to center around a dedicated effort to convince readers that there is a form of hypnotism— Ericksonian hypnotism—that is radically different from and far superior to traditional and semi-traditional hypnotism. *But solid documentation that this is a fact is sorely lacking.* Ericksonian hypnotism is no more nor less founded on conjecture than traditional and semi-traditional hypnotism. Conceivably, Erickson's trance state is not always the same as traditional or semi-traditional hypnosis. *This remains to be shown.* It is quite true that traditional hypnotism paid very little attention to dynamics, and it took an inflexible formula-like approach to the production of hypnotic phenomena. But this is hardly true of semi-traditional hypnotism, particularly after its incorporation in psychoanalytic therapies. Looking at Erickson's personal accounts, I am impressed that his success seems to lie not so much in whether he uses implication here, a "yes" set there, a bind over there, and so on, as it does in his greater recognition *of the importance of taking into account the general and individual dynamics of behavior* and utilizing them to bring about the desired results. Indeed, *utilization* is used to a unique extent by Erickson, as are *indirect suggestions.* My contention, however, is that this a *procedural* matter and not one having to do with the nature or essence of the phenomena that are evoked. I find it proper to speak of Ericksonian hypnotism in distinction to other forms of hypnotism, but only in that sense. I believe that it is the only scientifically applicable one. Any intimations that it is intrinsically different from traditional and semi-traditional hypnotism in other respects is unfounded and undocumented.

A great deal is said in the writings of Erickson and Rossi that seems to intimate that in Ericksonian hypnotism, the hypnotist does not control or direct the subject's or patient's behavior. I seriously question this. No matter how permissive and indirect he is, all of Erickson's maneuvers are clearly goal directed, the goal always being to bring about a definite change in the subject's or the patient's behavior. I think this is clearly indicated when, for example, we are told (Erickson, Rossi, & Rossi, 1976) that when the subject is asked, "Do you prefer to go in a trance now or later?" he has no other choice but to go into a trance, and that when a double bind fails, Erickson will try another one, again and again, until he obtains the desired behavior or change. The whole idea of depotentiating consciousness is clearly to get around conscious control. The Ericksonian hypnotist is very definitely instrumental in bringing about changes in directions of his choosing, and he is aware of this. He does differ from the traditional and the semi-traditional hypnotist in that he does not attempt to specify how the final result will be attained. Thus, for example, he is more likely to tell an obese patient, "I do not know how and your conscious mind does not know how, but your unconscious knows just what to do for you to lose the weight you need to lose," than to say, "From now on you will refrain from eating more than you should, because as soon as you have eaten just enough, you will feel completely satiated," or something even more direct. Clearly, the patient is being as much directed toward a goal set by the hypnotist in the first case as he is in the second one. There is, however, a difference that must be recognized. In the first instance, it is left up to the patient, or, rather, his unconscious, to find the path to his cure. This is the principle of utilization carried to the limit: *Let the patient find his cure from within himself and let him carry it out.* This precept and rule can be seen as increasingly constituting the foundation of what Ericksonian hypnotism is becoming.

Finally, I also see evidence in his writings of Erickson's strong overconcern to place hypnotism and hypnotherapy within a framework of normalcy. He forgets that in no way do people normally behave the way they are described to behave in any of the available transcriptions. *Each of these situations constitutes a highly artificial life situation.* That mechanisms and processes involved in normal behavior are used is not denied. This is the very point I tried to make over 30 years ago in *O.S.* There was never really that much of an issue in this regard within the scientific community. Braid's monoideism was nothing more than the result of putting to use the normal mechanisms of attention, and even animal magnetism was postulated to be based on the misperceived existence of certain natural phenomena. Where the issue of abnormality came in for a short time was when certain investigators, such as Charcot, attempted to relate hypnotic phenomena to various pathologies. Others saw a relationship between these phenomena and presumed paranormal and supernatural manifestations. It is true that the much-acclaimed "marvels" of hypnotism promoted by stage and lay hypnotists, and just plain hucksters, plus the ignorance and gullibility of a general public always seeking miracles and shortcuts to health, success, and happiness, has contributed to a public picture of hypnotism involving something well beyond the "normal." This, however, is another aspect of hypnotism that, hopefully, one should not have to be concerned with when working with professionals.

In ending this discussion, I would like briefly to contrast some of the advantages and/or disadvantages of Ericksonian hypnotherapy with those of traditional and semi-traditional hypnotherapy. One obvious problem of the Ericksonian approach is in regard to its applicability in other languages than English. Certain features, such as the utilization principle, present no problems. Some of the communication aspects of the approach may. For example, many languages do not have any satisfactory equivalents for many of the plays on words that are involved. Such a play on the words "change," "know," and "no" that I have discussed could not be replicated in French or German. Most other languages, however, may also offer opportunities for similar uses that would not be available in the English language. Metaphors probably work equally well in whatever language is used. Thus, the problem may actually not be a serious one, but it should be kept in mind by anyone wishing to use the approach in another language.

I have touched several times on the question of the claimed greater effectiveness of the Ericksonian approach. Effectiveness has a number of dimensions, each of which ought to be considered when making comparisons. For example, are we talking of duration of therapy to reach a certain end-results, or are we talking of the permanency of the end-result regardless of how long it took to get to it? Are we talking of percentages of successes versus failures? Presumably, the Ericksonian school means in all respects.

There is surprisingly little said about failure in Erickson's writings or in those of his followers. It would appear that he never failed! No matter how great a therapist he may have been, this is hard to believe. Perhaps he did fail sometimes. I have been told that some of his failures had been reported somewhere, but I have not been able to locate the material.

One also gets the impression, largely from his seminar talks, that Erickson accomplished remarkable results in relatively short single sessions. But seminar talks of the kind that Erickson gave are largely anecdotal, and are not intended to meet the rigors of formal presentations. They are often limited, by the nature of the situation, to brief statements that may be far from reflecting the true situation; they may leave many details out. One should also not confuse a unique spectacular success with a demonstration of general effectiveness. Franz Alexander tells of a cure effected in a single, short analytic session. Apparently, this was the only one in his experience. He knew this was not typical of analytical treatment in general, and he made that clear. Erickson's spectacular success in inducing breast development in a patient was, as far as I know, a unique case. So was his treatment of the brain damaged woman, which was a treatment that turned out to be quite laborious and lengthy. What generalization can one draw regarding effectiveness from these types of situations?

Most clinicians do not report the results of their therapeutic work except in special circumstances. Erickson did publish details on a number of his cases, but far more came to light under the special stimulus constituted by seminars. How many similar cases were brought to a successful conclusion with other approaches? This has not been reported because the right stimulus has not been present. I can think of any number of successes that I have had using traditional and semi-traditional approaches that compete favorably with Erickson's in regard to several aspects of effectiveness. However, I did not have the opportunity to report these.

Sometimes, one does not bother to bring up a case because, at the time, it all seemed part of the day's work, and not really unusual. I have in mind Erickson's case of a woman who, for physical reasons, could not have a vaginal orgasm. Erickson tells (1986) how he made it possible for her to experiences orgasms with other parts of her body. I can report having done something similar in a somewhat different context, but using a few very direct suggestions and nothing like the rather drawn-out method that Erickson used. I would say that my approach was actually more effective than Erickson's!

There is at least one area in which some data is available regarding the issue of comparable effectiveness. In a brief review, Hammond (1987) concludes that data now available indicate that indirect suggestions are not always superior to direct ones. They can even be inferior. One study has shown, in fact, that there is a normal distribution for the responses to indirect suggestions, just as there is one in the case of direct suggestions.

In brief, I do not believe that there are clear grounds for claiming the Ericksonian approach to therapy is generally more effective than the traditional and semi-traditional ones. With highly suggestible individuals, and even persons of medium suggestibility, there is probably a tie. Although certainly not clearly demonstrated, the Ericksonian approach may be more effective with individuals of low suggestibility. I say this, however, more on theoretical than on factual grounds.

AN ADDENDUM: MIND-BODY HEALING

Mind-body healing is the latest development in Ericksonian-type therapy. Rossi (1986) credits Erickson with being the originator. To my knowledge, Erickson did not speak of mind-body healing per se; I think that Rossi has carried such thoughts as Erickson may have had on the subject matter far beyond what Erickson would have been willing to talk about. Erickson did have a firm belief in the "wisdom of the body," an expression that I believe we owe to Walter Cannon. More specifically, in earlier years, before he and Rossi met, Erickson would frequently remark that the human body, and especially the mind, possessed the potentiality for bringing about almost any somatic, and especially physiological, change that is possible. He would point out that throughout life, for example, the body has many occasions for controlling the blood circulation in response to the need to lose or preserve body heat. The digestive system regularly controls the production of acid and enzymes as needed for proper digestion. The mechanisms are there ready to be activated. This may have been partly what Erickson had in mind when he spoke of "experiential learning," and later of the mind's potentials for naturalistic self-healing. In any event, Erickson believed, with certain good reasons, that, through hypnotism, and especially indirect suggestions, it was possible to activate these mechanisms. In later years, he came to believe that even though one did not know how specific psychosomatic effects came about, the patient's mind or body somehow knew just what to do, as, for example, in the case of the breast development that he induced in one of his patients.

In any event, as the expression "mind-body healing" suggests, the focus is on the possibility of producing profound somatic therapeutic changes in individuals through the use of their mental processes, particularly unconscious ones, acting directly and indirectly upon the soma.

This is largely based on the argument that if it is true that mental/emotional processes can produce diseased conditions in the body, then it should be possible for mental/emotional processes to reverse disease processes of purely somatic origin. Logically speaking, this conclusion does not directly follow from the premise, but it is a reasonable hypothesis. As Rossi points out, the popular and technical literature abounds in largely anecdotal material pointing to this possibility. There is also some consensus among physicians and nurses that patient attitudes and beliefs make the difference between a good and a bad prognosis in an illness or injury. Although the authentication of relevant material is on the whole very poor, there is such an abundance of it as to make one feel that there must be some basis for it. The placebo effect has been one of the few and better established and studied actions of this kind.

We do know that thoughts and emotions are associated with physiological changes. Data supporting this come from laboratories, clinics, and even everyday living. We also have good reasons to think that specific diseased somatic conditions can result in this way. One thing that is still poorly understood, in spite of the relatively long existence of this knowledge, is how and why certain organs and tissues are selected to become diseased. There also seems to be little question that psychotherapy can be quite effective in bringing about relief of such conditions, thus giving support to the idea that appropriate mental activity can reverse the process. To a large degree, such treatment tends to be of a trial-and-error nature, even when it is guided by psychodynamic principles and various theories regarding the etiology of these pathologies.

The possibility of bringing about somatic therapeutic changes through direct action by the mind naturally leads to the related question of whether or not such an action could be rendered more effective by the presence of hypnosis or through the use of hypnotic suggestions. In particular, could the production of such somatic changes be thus stimulated, and in some way specifically directed, toward the alleviation of a specific disease condition? I have already mentioned Erickson's early views on this matter. Although limited in scope, past reliable laboratory reports of specific tissue changes and organ activity changes having been brought about by means of hypnotic suggestions lend support to the idea of this being a potentiality, if not a reality. Reliable clinical reports, such as those of the successful reversal of the effects of Reynaud's disease and of induced breast development through the use of suggestions directed at bringing about specific relevant physiological changes, bring the matter much closer to the level of reality. Rossi gives the impression that Erickson did a fair amount of this kind of therapy; however, it may not have been as extensive as one is led to believe if one goes by a posthumous book by Erickson (Erickson, 1986) on hypnotic mind-body communication. It is quite disappointing in this regard. Actually, the book was not written by Erickson; it is part of a collection of Erickson's seminar talks and was edited by Rossi and Ryan.

To provide additional credence for the belief that one can alter somatic conditions by directed mind influence, Rossi has attempted, in a rather simplistic fashion, to relate psychosomatic manifestations to what he refers as "state-bound memory, learning and behavior." It has now been well established that data or information stored in memory when a person is in a given state of being cannot be retrieved, or only partially and with difficulty when the state is changed; full retrieval depends upon the person being back in the original acquisition condition. This was first shown to be the case following the ingestion of appreciable amounts of alcohol, and later of other chemicals. Since then, mood changes have been shown to have a similar action, although never as drastic. These findings have led to the hypothesis that internal cues in the form of bodily conditions of the moment are among the contextual cues that become associated with any stored memory. For full recall, all cues, external and internal, need to be present. Extending the hypothesis to the acquisition of complex learned behavior is the next logical step. One can expect the evocation of behavior to be generally subject to state-dependency effects. Rossi has done a creditable review of the relevant literature, to which readers interested in further details are referred to.

Rossi then makes the further hypothesis that stress situations are highly conducive to the formation of state-dependent behaviors that become symptoms. The idea seems to be that a severely stressed individual tends to respond in an adaptive manner to the stressing situation or stressor with a behavior that is basically maladaptive and is thus a disorder symptom under normal conditions. It is reasonable to expect that such behavior should become associated with the internal cues (changes) existing at the time and thus become state-dependent. The further expectation is that reinstating these internal cues would tend to evoke the behavior and the symptom in question. Superficially, this model of symptom formation and evocation is attractive, but it quickly breaks down when one attempts to apply it in a detailed step-by-step manner to specific instances of psychosomatic illnesses. Rossi has apparently failed to make this closer examination.

Just how "therapeutic hypnosis" brings about results is not as clear as Rossi seems to think it is. At one point, he says that it allows one to "access" the state-bound material because individuals under stress enter a spontaneous "hypnosis." Induced hypnosis presumably reinstates the same changes as those that characterize this spontaneous hypnosis. Keeping in mind that the existence of the latter is anything but well-demonstrated, the above explanation does not take into account that in the stress situation there would be equally and probably more important changes, also caused by the stressor, *added* to the changes characteristic of hypnosis. These would not be expected to be automatically reinstated when hypnosis is induced, and retrieval would therefore not follow. Perhaps recognizing this problem, Rossi also mentions the traditional and semi-traditional use of suggestion techniques aimed at getting the patient to reexperience the original trauma. This should be effective. However, Rossi offers no explanation as to how such a procedure can remove the state-boundedness of the symptom and thereby eliminate it. There are reasons to think that Rossi also sees this problem, because the therapeutic approach that he advocates calls for the addition of "reframing." Reframing is a procedure apparently borrowed from Bandler and Grinder, who introduced it around 1977. I will have more to say about it in the next chapter; for the time being, I will merely state that, properly speaking, reframing is a name given to the process of reassociating and reorganizing a problem in order to bring about its resolution. Procedures for doing this were being used by psychotherapists long before Bandler and Grinder labeled them. What they did was to recognize their existence, give them a generic name, and then proceed to develop first a three-step and later a six-step procedure, which they also called "reframing," but that certainly involved more than reframing as defined above. Rossi, who prefers a three-step approach, seems also to prefer the expression "basic accessing formula" to denote it, and, clearly, it too is more than just reframing in the above sense. It is also more than just "accessing," if this is understood to mean retrieving. The demarcation between the steps that can be conceived as accessing proper, reframing proper, and "ratifying" are quite fuzzy at times in some of the examples discussed by Rossi. The whole process is always a procedure that is aimed at contacting the patient's unconscious and setting into motion inner processes. This is done largely by giving vague, open-ended instructions (indirect suggestions) that presumably lead the patient's inner processes to develop and to apply unspecified healing solutions. They include such procedures as the patient holding a dialogue with his symptoms, just as is done in Gestalt therapy. I shall not attempt to describe in detail the different variations of the three steps that are given by Rossi. They are all mostly as follows:

The therapist begins by reviewing and discussing the problem with the patient. The idea that the patient's inner mind is capable of creative problem-solving is introduced, as well as the idea that this ability can be put to use in the present situation. Judging at some point that the patient is ready to go on with the therapy that, Rossi believes, was initiated from the start, the therapist begins by telling the patient, for example:

> When your unconscious knows how it can solve your problem, you will become more relaxed, and your eyes will close.

This constitutes what Rossi calls getting a readiness signal for inner work. The second step consists in saying something like:

> Your unconscious can continue to work out a resolution of your problem that will meet all your needs. There are all kinds of memories, past experiences, and abilities that your unconscious can use for this purpose.

This is what Rossi refers to as the accessing and transducing of state-bound resources. In the final step, something like the following is said:

> When your unconscious knows that the problem has been resolved as much as it can be at this time, and that you can deal effectively with it, you will open your eyes and be alert.

This is the stage of ratification.

Rossi, I might add, seems to prefer to use the "inner mind" and the "deep part of the inner mind" where I used the term "unconscious." Clearly, Rossi's approach is very indirect and naturalistic, and it is in the spirit of Ericksonian therapy. However, it is rather disconcerting also to find him reverting to the traditional approach by offering the reader 13 fairly structured formulas (or recipes) for doing body-mind healing. *Plus ça change, plus c'est la même chose!* Unquestionably, such formulas have a strong appeal for many readers of his work.

Rossi does not at all make clear how the procedures overcome the state-boundedness of symptoms. The procedures may work, but the theory does a poor job of explaining how or why they do.

Rossi's enthusiasms and speculations are unlimited; not only does he not hesitate to propose the production of effects at cellular levels through the mental control of immune processes, but he also quite seriously proposes a "mind-gene connection" whereby the mind can alter the genetic make-up at the cellular level! He does not, however, provide a recipe for instigating this.

Were this to become a possibility, there would theoretically be important implications for genetically based disorders.

Rossi's work is interesting and stimulating reading. It needs be kept in mind, however, that he has built a hypothetical edifice whose foundation and many of its bricks are themselves nothing more than speculations. This does not produce a sound scientific structure. The mortar also shows weaknesses. Rossi has a tendency to confuse speculation with fact. A great deal of the data he bases his speculations on come from animal studies. Some of the results most likely apply to humans, but possibly not all. The fact that humans possess languages far more complex than any other known animal, and apparently have a far more extensive ability for manipulating abstract symbols, brings in elements that animal studies cannot even begin to touch. Because Rossi presents his theories as being information-theoretical, it is surprising that he has missed this point. However, he does generally ignore any data that contradict his position, and he frequently misrepresents facts to suit his own purpose. Actually, his use of information theory is quite minimal and primitive; it amounts to not much more than the use of a few key words and concepts and a view of information theory as a source of unification of all natural phenomena that became outmoded about 30 years ago.

SELECTED BIBLIOGRAPHY ON THE ERICKSONIAN APPROACH

Erickson, M. H., Rossi, E. L., & Rossi, S. I. *Hypnotic realities.* New York: Irvington, 1976.

Erickson, M. H., & Rossi, E. L. *Hypnotherapy. An exploratory case book.* New York: Irvington, 1979.

Erickson, M. H., & Rossi, E. L. *Experiencing hypnosis.* New York: Irvington, 1981.

Haley, J. *Advanced techniques of hypnosis and therapy. Selected papers of Milton H. Erickson, M.D.* New York: Grune & Stratton, 1967.

Rossi, E. L. (Ed.). *The collected papers of Milton H. Erickson on hypnosis.* Volumes 1, 2, 3, and 4. New York: Irvington, 1980.

Zeig, J. K. *A teaching seminar with Milton H. Erickson.* New York: Brunner/Mazel, 1980.

The Haley collection and the Rossi collection of the writings of Erickson have considerable overlap. The Rossi collection is by far the more complete, including many articles never before published as well as papers of Erickson published after the publication of the Haley book. The latter does, however, give an excellent sampling of Erickson's papers. Since Erickson's death, many books and articles on Erickson, his methods, and his philosophy have been published. Many of the articles are available in edited collections.

8

Ericksonian Hypnotism: The Bandler/Grinder Interpretation

INTRODUCTION
NLP AND PSYCHOTHERAPY
NLP AND ERICKSONIAN HYPNOTISM
DISCUSSION AND CRITIQUE

INTRODUCTION

In the early 1970s, John Grinder, a linguist, and Richard Bandler, a psychologist, developed the idea that an analysis of the ways that noted psychotherapists such as Virginia Satir, Fritz Pearl, and Milton H. Erickson communicated with their patients might uncover the key to their reputed success. *Neurolinguistic programming* (NLP) was the eventual outcome of this analysis. NLP proper, as originally developed in *Structure of Magic I and II* (1975, 1976) has *nothing* to do directly with hypnotism. It is not about hypnotism, and its only relationship to it is that the Bandler/Grinder interpretation of Ericksonian hypnotism grows out of their use of the same linguistic type of analysis to elucidate the mechanism or action of communications done in the contexts of psychotherapy and hypnosis. There is no more connection between the two, as a result of this analysis, than between geometrical entities and electrical circuits as a result of using algebra to discuss and describe their respective properties.

At the time that the above analysis was attempted, Erickson was unique;

while he had acquired the reputation of being an outstanding psychotherapist, much of the therapy he did involved the use of hypnotism, and his greater reputation was as a hypnotherapist, and especially as a hypnotist.

As we have seen, it is very difficult to separate out cases of Erickson's in which one can be certain that no hypnotism, as understood and used by him, was involved from those cases in which it was clearly used. Possibly for this reason, Bandler and Grinder have had relatively little to say specifically regarding NLP as it applies to Erickson's *non-hypnotic* therapeutic work; they have focused their study on Erickson's *modus operandi* as a hypnotist.

While it is not entirely inconceivable that a linguistic analysis of non-hypnotic psychotherapeutic communications might lead to the same results as a similar analysis of hypnotic communications, the likelihood of this happening is rather low. It is therefore not surprising that Bandler and Grinder found that Ericksonian hypnotic communications involved a *reversal,* so to speak, of the way successful psychotherapists were found to apply certain linguistic principles. In brief, from a linguistic viewpoint, there seems to be no similarity between Ericksonian hypnotism and effective psychotherapy when approached from the standpoint of NLP.

The relevant material is found primarily in three works by Bandler and Grinder. Their original formulation is found in *Patterns I* (1975). *Patterns II* (1977), coauthored with Delozier, published two years later, and presumably intended to be a continuation of the first work, appears to be primarily an attempt to explain further what is happening in the person being hypnotized as a result of the kinds of communications that have been made to him by the hypnotist (and that have been analyzed in *Pattern I*). It also attempts to incorporate some of the new developments that have occurred in NLP proper during this two year interim. The first of these works is poorly written. Both suffer from ambiguities, a certain amount of disorganization within an apparent organization, and the vagueness with which the authors repeatedly use obviously basic concepts, such as those of "pattern" and "system." These defects, as well as others, are not particularly obvious until one attempts to study these works in depth. The third work, *TRANCE-formation* (1981), is based on edited and combined transcripts of ten seminars or workshops on hypnotism conducted by Bandler and Grinder. It is a later work and, again, incorporates further developments that have occurred in NLP. In contrast to the two earlier works, it combines non-hypnotic NLP procedures with Ericksonian hypnotism, and thus it cannot be said to be purely an exposition of Ericksonian hypnotism. Of the three works, it is by far the better and more readable one.

I wish to make it clear that my references to Bandler and to Grinder jointly in this order should not be regarded as indicating that I view NLP as more a product of Bandler than of Grinder. The work is so heavily based on complex linguistic considerations that, if anything, one is tempted to feel the other way around, but this is overlooking the fact that Bandler may also have had a strong minor in linguistics. Obviously, the two writers have to be listed in some order, and I have arbitrarily chosen one with no special intimations in mind.

NLP AND PSYCHOTHERAPY

According to contemporary linguistics, all utterances in natural languages (languages as spoken and written) possess a *surface structure* and a *deep structure*. The first of these structures is reflected by the arrangement of words in the language as spoken or written. It is what we see written or hear spoken. It consists of words put together according to *syntactical* rules *without regard to meaning*. The resulting sentences are said to be *well-formed* sound sequences or utterances. It is the deep structures that hold meaning, or, more technically, the corresponding semantic representions. Deep structures are not directly observable, and linguists state that they can be only "intuitively" known. Each individual who uses a language is considered to have the necessary deep structures stored in him. All well-formed sound sequences are not necessarily meaningful.

Only those sound sequences that are meaningful are said to be *well formed in meaning*. Linguists consider surface structures to be *derived* from deep structures. It is possible for one surface structure to be associated with several different deep structures, and conversely. Without explaining why this is so, linguists state that surface structures are more often than not *less complete* than deep structures.

Partly in explanation of the last statement, Bandler and Grinder go a step beyond the above formulation by stating that in every individual, there is also a *reference structure* from which all deep structures are themselves derived. They define the reference structure to be *the sum total of all the experiences an individual has and has had of the world.* This totality of organized experiences constitutes the person's internal representation of the world at any moment, and it is not usually directly accessible. Presumably, it is a somatic, and especially, a neural representation. Deep structures, they state, are the fullest *linguistic* representations, or *models,* of the world. Apparently, surface structures can also constitute fullest linguistic representations of the world, but most often they do not because various processes interfere with their accurate derivation and, as a result, they are inaccurate models of the world. Bandler and Grinder consider three classes of processes that contribute singly or in combination to inaccurate derivations: *generalizations, deletions, and distortions.* The label of distortions is somewhat peculiar, since all three processes can each be said to "distort" the derivations. Be that as it may, these are the labels used by the two writers. Although Bandler and Grinder do not specifically state it to be so, their writings give indications that they believe deep structures are also subject to the ill-effects of generalization, deletion, and distortion when they are derived from the reference structure. The consequence of this is that these fullest representations of the world are anything but accurate.

These various types of structures are viewed by Bandler and Grinder as constituting an individual's *models* of the world *at different levels of functioning.* Obviously, some of these can be very inaccurate models.

According to Bandler and Grinder, effective psychotherapists are individuals who have the ability to detect occurrences of generalizations, deletions, and distortions in the communications made by patients and to infer or intuit from their own personal deep structures what the corresponding deep structures of the patients are. Presumably, the same is true with regard to the deep structures of patients relative to their reference structures. Having done the above, the effective psychotherapist then skillfully helps the patient to recover the deep structures, correct the faulty deep structures, and derive more accurate surface structures.

Taking their cue from formal logic, the two authors define a *metamodel* to be a formal model of a model, and *in the context of NLP,* "metamodel" is now specifically used to refer to *a model of a model of the world.* Language thus becomes a source of such metamodels, and "metamodeling" denotes the construction of a linguistic metamodel. Efficient psychotherapists can be said to use metamodeling to bring about in patients new and more accurate linguistic models of the world by removing the generalizations, deletions, and distortions that these psychotherapists have detected.

This is not the whole of NLP, but it seems to represent the foundation on which it is based. Since this formulation was developed in 1975, new concepts and methods have been added to it. Some of these will be considered later in this chapter.

NLP AND ERICKSONIAN HYPNOTISM

Because the two founding works are specifically about the "patterns" of the hypnotic techniques of Erickson, one might hope to find an explicit statement of what one is to understand about this term. On the basis of the contents of the works, one minor clarification might be that it is the communication and, more specifically, the "linguistic" patterns used by Erickson. "Pattern" appears to refer to *the choice and arrangement (sequencing) of words* that Erickson uses. This, of course, is to include non-verbal elements of communication.

As we saw in the last chapter, the *depotentiation* of consciousness plays a major role in Erickson's hypnotic work. *Creating confusion* in the subject's mind is a major way in which he does this. Bandler and Grinder recognize these two observations and give them a central position, stating that *Erickson's hypnotic techniques and procedures deliberately aim to create confusion* by introducing a maximum of generalization, deletion, and distortion in the surface structures with which Erickson communicates with the patient. Thus, *whereas the efficient psychotherapist tries to eliminate these elements, the efficient hypnotist,* as exemplified by Erickson, *does just the opposite and promotes them maximally.* Hypnotism as practiced by Erickson thus involves metamodeling *in reverse.*

If I said "involves" rather than "consists of" in the last sentence, it is because Bandler and Grinder see Ericksonian hypnotism as being more than this. Again, as we saw in the last chapter, Erickson essentially views the ultimate aim of hypnotic induction techniques as one of bringing about a situation in which the elicitation of responses from the "unconscious" is maximized while, simultaneously, conscious participation is decreased and even eliminated. Consequently, many of his techniques are aimed at doing this. Bandler and Grinder agree that this is the case, although they prefer to speak of non-dominant hemispheric activity, while Erickson speaks of "unconscious" activity; they speak of dominant hemispheric activity, while Erickson speaks of "conscious" activity. They explicitly identify the conscious with the dominant hemisphere and the unconscious with the non-dominant hemisphere. Having done this, they restate the Ericksonian approach to hypnotism as involving these three "dimensions":

1. Pacing and distracting the dominant (language) hemisphere
2. Utilizing the dominant hemisphere language processing that occurs below awareness
3. Accessing the non-dominant hemisphere

From the writings of Bandler and Grinder, *pacing* is clearly a central concept in this analysis. According to them, pacing is the act, on the part of the hypnotist, of describing or reporting to the subject what the subject's ongoing observable and non-observable experiences are. As the writers say, it is a type of feedback. The importance of this process lies in the hypothesis the authors make that, once the subject has accepted such a description by the hypnotist as an accurate account of his ongoing behavior, the line of demarcation between the hypnotist's description of the patient's actual behavior and what the patient will experience next becomes blurred. Accordingly, a description of a response that has as yet to take place is likely to be experienced as occurring, and then will take place. For the hypnotist to continue and describe a future response as occurring is spoken of by Bandler and Grinder as *leading*. According to them, there are specific linguistic techniques that promote a *linking* between pacing and leading assertions and that promote the above. It is not possible to present their explanation of how this is done without making use of a number of technical linguistic terms used by Bandler and Grinder. To try to explain these terms at this point would take us too far afield. I have used them without explanation and left it up to readers interested in more details to consult the relevant works. Generally speaking, the specialized terms I have used without explanation are linguistic processes.

According to Bandler and Grinder, when observable changes are paced, *simple injunctions, implied causatives,* and *cause-effect* are used. These linguistic processes are particularly effective, the authors state, because they are the same linguistic principles that patients linguistically use to organize (model) their experiences.

The pacing of unobservable experiences is another matter. Guessing, even supported by intuition, is not reliable, because leading is effective only if pacing is accurate. The solution, according to Bandler and Grinder, lies in the hypnotist using a small amount of trickery by making vague and ambiguous pacing statements that leave it up to the patient to fill in whatever fits in terms of his unobservable experiences. This is done by the hypnotist using words *without referential indices,* and using such linguistic processes as *deletion, nominalization, selectional restriction,* and *mind-reading.* Presumably, the patient fills in the "blanks" without realizing that he is doing this, and he experiences being paced. Leading is, in turn, done indirectly by using such linguistic principles as those of *presupposition, conversational postulates, lesser included structures,* and *analogical marking.*

The third dimension of getting the patient to participate in the communication at the unconscious level is promoted by what Bandler and Grinder refer to as the *transderivational search.* This is done, they say, by the use of *generalized referential indices, selectional restriction violations, deletions,* and *nominalization.* The idea is to create sentences with a surface structure so poorly formed that the listener is forced to seek meaning for it by a search for the best deep structure built into him. Such a search requires a maximum unconscious (non-dominant hemisphere) activity. The authors further hypothesize that the selected response is the one most appropriate to the unconscious needs of the subject or patient. It is obvious from this analysis that, as stated earlier, the hypnotist deliberately uses generalization, deletion, and distortion to form the surface structure of his communication to the patients, whereas the effective psychotherapist attempts to remove these when they occur in his patient's communications! As Bandler and Grinder state, the Ericksonian hypnotist uses *reversed metamodeling.*

The above constitutes the essence of the contents of *Patterns I*. The next step is to look at the contributions of *Patterns II*. It is not clear at what point Bandler and Grinder began to talk and write about neurolinguistic programming. This expression does not appear in any of their earlier works. However, possibly for the first time, one finds references being made at the very start of this second work to "programs" and "programming." Typically, the authors do not bother to define this term. The best they offer toward a definition is their statement (p. 3) that we "develop programs within ourselves to cope effectively with the world at the *unconscious* level of behavior." In brief, programs would appear to be acquired problem-solving and goal-directed behaviors and organized sequences of behaviors. *Modeling* is now said to be the creation of these programs. Modeling can itself be at either the conscious or unconscious level. The outcome of modeling is also said to be *models*. On first examination, it would then seem that "models" and "programs" are synonymous. However, we are soon told that these models are also models of our world of experience. Without trying to make any more sense out of this for the moment, let us go on to the author's statement of what the new volume is about. It is concerned, they say, with the presentation of a model for effective hypnotic communication, based on Erickson's work, that consists of "the minimum number of patterns or distinctions necessary for a hypnotist to communicate effectively in the context of hypnotic communication." It is clear what "distinctions" refers to. As for "patterns," we can still take this to refer to distinct arrangements and choices of words. The intimation is that the previous work had extraneous material and that the present work will offer a condensation and more of the essence of Erickson's approach. Interestingly enough, "metamodeling," which is a central idea in the earlier work, has been dropped out of the present one. I am not sure what this signifies. As for "model" as used in the above, it would seem that it is synonymous with a way of behaving, or more specifically, of communicating.

Using a symbolic notation borrowed from mathematics and logic, which is of dubious value and significance in this context, Bandler and Grinder start developing the new model by introducing the concept of a "4-tuple," an idea also borrowed from mathematics and logic. The basic point they make is that a person's experience of the moment can be decomposed into *visual, kinesthetic, tonal auditory,* and *olfactory* experiences. These four types of experiences are said by them to form a specific 4-tuple. They use the term "kinesthetic" incorrectly by including the experience of pressure, of temperature, and other unspecified sensations that possibly include pain, touch, and vestibular sensations, but of which they, surprisingly, make no specific mention as components of experience. Their specification of the auditory experience being "tonal" is due to their desire to distinguish between the "digital" auditory experience of hearing linguistic utterance and other auditory sensations. One wonders about their failure to make a similar breakdown for visual experiences. However, this may be because, quite obviously, auditory communication is the main channel of communication in hypnotic work. One can also wonder why gustatory experiences have been left out. True, some have an olfactory origin, but not all. In any case, they make the important observation that of the many sensory experiences an individual may have or may have had at some specific time, only some of these may enter his consciousness. These conscious experiences, they add, can have an external or an internal origin, and an individual may experience a mixture of both. Language, in particular, as a representation of experiences, can itself serve as an external generator of experiences for a person receiving a communication. The possibility of one individual (the hypnotist) evoking specific experiences in another individual (the subject/patient) by a proper choice of words follows from this observation.

Let us now return to the observation that a person will often have a conscious representation of an experience that is *limited* to only some of the sensory components that make up the total experience. According to Bandler and Grinder, most individuals favor one or two sense modalities. These preferred modalities constitute what the authors refer to as this person's *most highly valued representational system.* In most cases, they remark, this most valued system coincides with that portion of the world that the individual is aware of. Effective hypnotic communication, they assert, depends partly upon taking this into account. However, as an aside, this point, if valid, has broad applicability to any communication situation and to therapeutic interactions in general, as NLP proper makes clear. For the edification of readers who might read the above mentioned text, or who may already have read it, I will add the following: the two authors make a number of references to "operators." More specifically, they speak of an "R-operator." This concept, also borrowed from mathematics and logic, is misused by the authors when they assert that (Grinder et al., 1977, p. 21) " . . . the application of the operator to the 4-tuple which represents the organism's total experience yields the portion of the experience available in the organism's consciousness." By this they mean that, by an arbitrary convention, anytime the letter R is placed in written discussions in front of the symbolic representation of a 4-tuple that denotes what is totally sensed by an individual, this indicates that the corresponding content of his consciousness is now being denoted. However, this content really has to be either directly provided by the individual or inferred from his behavior. This content will presumably be an explicit representation in the individual's most highly valued representational system. Similarly, Bandler and Grinder's subsequent reference to "the use of the R-operator and the 4-tuple" in hypnotic inductions is nothing more than a discussion of the possible importance, when pacing and leading, of taking into consideration that individuals have favored representational systems, and also that shifting an individual from a system using one sense modality to one using another modality is a useful procedure. They ascribe part of Erickson's effectiveness to his recognition and application of this observation. Furthermore, leading can be from an externally to an internally generated experience. More specifically, they conclude from their analysis of Erickson's work that he begins pacing by using words and expressions that refer to experiences specific to the sense modality in question. This amounts to talking to the patient in terms that he best understands. Since Erickson views inducing an internalization of experience as a step toward the production of a trance state, the next step follows. However, according to Bandler and Grinder, a further effect exists: shifting from a preferential representational system to one that is not. This is associated with the appearance of a trance state. This effect, however, remains to be clearly demonstrated.

In regard to the above, NLP makes a specific contribution of its own to the practice of Ericksonian hypnotism. However, pacing and leading are not procedures unique to Ericksonian hypnotism, but they are also a part of effective non-hypnotic psychotherapy where they are used, presumably, to produce other effects.

In the development of NLP proper, Bandler and Grinder evolved two ways of detecting the representational systems used by individuals. One is eye scanning movements, which they also refer to as *accessing cues* and which they claim can be elicited by asking or setting certain mental tasks to an individual. These are specific to the kind of preferred representational system the individual uses. The other method consists of noticing the kinds of words, especially predicates (verbs, adjectives, and adverbs), that an individual uses in communicating with others. *There is no evidence that Erickson consciously made use of either of these methods;* however, if he did, it was most likely the second one.

Two other NLP concepts (besides representational systems and accessing cues) that we will look at briefly are those of *anchoring* and *reframing.*

An anchor can be said to be any stimulus that consistently evokes the same response from an individual. The specific process of anchoring is the deliberate association by an operator of a stimulus with a particular experience the subject is having for the purpose of eliciting it on subsequent occasions using this stimulus. For example, the patient is asked to think back to a situation when he was experiencing certain feelings that the therapist wants to use. When the patient indicates that he is reliving the feelings, the therapist touches a part of his body in a specific way. According to Bandler and Grinder, any time the therapist again touches the patient in exactly the same way, the feelings will be reinstated. Anchoring is clearly nothing more than making use of the process that Erickson referred to as redingretation.

We have already seen how Erickson made use of it, particularly for reinducing hypnosis. NLP has interesting ways of using anchoring outside of the context of hypnotism, but to discuss them would be a digression.

Considering that Grinder and Bandler view reframing as one of the most important concepts of NLP and have devoted an entire book to it, there is something remarkable in their failure to provide a concise definition of the concept. Reframing appears to be a technique that aims to substitute a more acceptable form of behavior for one that is a source of problems for the patient. It is *partly* founded upon the hypothesis that behavior, even if it is undesirable, is generally associated with an *intention.* According to Bandler and Grinder (1979), reframing seeks to substitute a new and more acceptable behavior that can equally well satisfy the intention that is now satisfied by the behavior that is a problem. In most cases, the intention is not known to the patient or the therapist, and it is the beauty of reframing that neither ever needs to know what it is; the basic idea is to change the behavior, *not the intention.* In Bandler and Grinder's (1979) own words, reframing "is a specific way of contacting the portion or part—for lack of a better word—of the person that is causing a certain behavior to occur, or that is preventing a certain other behavior from occurring." And, they could have added, getting this part to accept a substitution. Thus, reframing is also founded upon the hypothesis that there is a hidden part of ourselves that, besides our conscious minds, controls our behavior for its own ends.

There is a parallelism between "intention" and needs, "part of the person" and the Freudian unconscious, and reframing and planned symptom substitution. There are also important differences, because what is referred to as a "part" is clearly given all of the features of a second personality that at a subconscious level effectively wills behavior.

Actually, reframing involves at least *two* parts of the patient. One is usually addressed as "that part that is responsible" for the target behavior, and the other is referred to as the "creative" part of the individual. The technique of reframing calls upon these two parts to communicate and work with each other. As suggested by the writings of Bandler and Grinder, still *other* parts may exist in an individual and need to be involved in any therapeutic reframing. Although these parts are clearly all subconscious entities, Bandler and Grinder clearly distinguish them from what they refer to as the patient's "unconscious."

In NLP proper, reframing is accomplished by having the person make the necessary contact at a conscious level. The hypnotic counterpart is getting the subject or patient to use his unconscious to make this contact. The induction of hypnosis is viewed as a way of facilitating this. The resemblance of this procedure to the use of ideomotor signaling and some of Erickson's indirect utilizations techniques is obvious. To my knowledge, Erickson never used the term "reframing," and he did not use anything comparable to the "six steps" reframing evolved by Bandler and Grinder. However, as we saw, Rossi (1986) has adopted the idea and technique.

The term "reframing" seems to have recently gathered a fair amount of popularity among therapists not identified with NLP. They mostly use it to designate any intervention aimed at changing the internal responses of an individual to a situation or to his behavior, either by modifying the meaning the person gives to the situation or behavior, or by finding a context in which the behavior becomes acceptable. A new perspective is thus created that is said to "reframe" the events and that, presumably, eventually enables the patient to produce different responses. There is, of course, nothing new in this; therapists were doing this long before NLP came into existence.

DISCUSSION AND CRITIQUE

More than 10 years after its birth, NLP does not appear to have made an appreciable impact upon the behavioral sciences, and its success seems to have been primarily that of a therapeutic fad. Despite its creators' constant direct and indirect infantile references and allusions to magic, wizards, enchantments, and so on (possibly in a metaphorical way), there is little evidence that it has lived up to the many promises it has made of providing magical solutions for ailing mankind. There is also something incongruous in speaking on the one hand of "programming" and "reprogramming" people, and on the other hand of insisting that the approach is a highly permissive one that is totally unlike that of the traditional hypnotherapist (which it is).

The major weakness of Bandler and Grinder's linguistic analysis is that so much of it is built upon untested hypotheses and is supported by totally inadequate data. Additionally, because—by Chomsky's (1972) own admission—the concept of deep structure he originated remains a reasonable but untested hypotheses, we end up with a situation in which assumptions are built upon assumptions. This is a poor, unscientific practice. Furthermore, not only do many assertions made by linguists remain indefinite in the absence of supporting evidence for making them, but Bandler and Grinder appear to have introduced terms and ideas of their own that are not a part of the accepted body of modern linguistics. I will exemplify the general kind of problem that exists in terms of their treatment of nominalization. According to Bandler and Grinder, a nominalization is a grammatical transformation whereby a process word, or verb, is converted into an event word, or noun. They give the two sentences, "I regret my decision to return home," and "I regret that I am deciding to return home" as exemplifying the "decision" as the nominalization of "deciding." Linguistically speaking, nominalization is actually a more complex matter, but the above is a fair approximation. However, according to Bandler and Grinder, nominalization also constitutes a linguistic "distortion." There is no evidence that any kind of "distortion" is present, but quite apart from this, the idea of a distortion seems to be particular to the two authors. Standard works on linguistics make no mention of a distortion resulting. In fact, the position usually held is that both of the above sentences are acceptable equivalent surface structures representing a common deep structure. Bandler and Grinder's idea of a distortion seems to be connected with their claim that much information is deleted when nominalization takes place. Again, this is not claimed by other writings on linguistics, and, in any case, it is difficult to see just what information has been deleted in the above example. The problem may be that although one of them has a degree in linguistics, the authors seem to have a confused understanding of what nominalization entails; we find them asserting that such words as "resources" and "hypnosis" are nominalizations! But of what verb is "resource" a nominalization? As for "hypnosis," it is quite clear from the historic facts that it was first introduced as a noun, and only subsequently was the verb "to hypnotize" derived! Finally, while it is true, as they point out, that "has much knowledge" is rather vague (is deficient in information) and also involves a nominalization, it is no more vague than "knows a lot of things," which is not associated with a nominalization. But why make such an issue about an incorrect association between vagueness and nominalization? Simply because it is a contention of Bandler and Grinder that Erickson effectively used planned nominalization in his work because of this associated vagueness. Now it is quite true that vagueness and ambiguity can arise out of nominalizations, but obviously this is not a universal consequence. There is a great deal more to its use for this purpose than Bandler and Grinder reveal. I have chosen nominalization to explain what some of the problems are in Bandler and Grinder's linguistic approach to Ericksonian hypnotism. Almost any other linguistic concept used by these authors could have served equally well for the purpose of showing some of the inherent weaknesses in their treatment.

Has NLP really abstracted and explicated the essence of successful therapy and provided everyone with the means to be another Whittaker, Virginia Satir, or Erickson? Quite apart from the above remarks, its failure to do this is evident because today there is no multitude of their equals, not even another Whittaker, Virginia Satir, or Erickson. Ten years should have been sufficient time for this to happen. In this light, I cannot take NLP very seriously.

Its contributions to our understanding and use of Ericksonian techniques are equally dubious. *Patterns I* and *II* are poorly written works that were an overambitious, pretentious effort to reduce hypnotism to a magic of words. This clearly has not paid off. The best testimony to this is that in all of the

NLP seminars and workshops on hypnotism that I have attended, none of this material has been used or has even been mentioned; nor is it even mentioned in *TRANCE-Formation,* written six years later. This work, incidentally, contains some glaring misstatements of facts. For example, Freud and Mesmer were depicted as contemporaries! The main conclusion drawn from the two early volumes is that Erickson's success as a hypnotist lies in his ability to confuse his subjects! There is no question that confusion is an important tool used by Erickson, but we did not need Bandler and Grinder's complex analysis to tell us that. This had been clearly stated by Erickson. Furthermore, it is clear that confusion is only one of the tools he uses so effectively. One contribution I would credit to NLP is its explication of matching, pacing, and leading, as well as providing us with these terms. It has provided a methodical approach to reframing, but can hardly be said to have originated the idea. In any case, it is not specific to Ericksonian hypnotism. Another contribution made by NLP is its calling attention to the possible importance of communicating with subjects and patients in their preferred representational mode, and to the possible value in shifting from it to other modes. Unfortunately, as with almost everything else proposed by NLP, no hard data exist in support of these propositions.

One of the most striking features of the Bandler/Grinder interpretation is that it somehow ignores the issue of the existence and function of suggestion, which, even in Erickson's own writings and those done with Rossi, is a central idea. And even though Erickson frequently fails to distinguish between extrahypnotic and intrahypnotic suggestions, he does speak of suggestion and trance as separate phenomena, even if the one leads into the other. Now Bandler and Grinder may have reasons for ignoring the concept of suggestion, but if they do, they fail to mention these reasons or even to state they have concluded that one can dispense with the concept of suggestion. Their doing so is rather surprising because their detailed analysis of some of Erickson's inductions (Grinder et al., 1977) offers possibilities for some clear answers to the question of where "suggestion" fits into their interpretation. Even the term "trance" is barely used by them, and this to the extent it sinks into insignificance. Is it that they believe "trance" is an unnecessary concept? Their extensive discussion of Erickson's experiments with Aldous Huxley suggests quite the contrary. It seems rather reasonable that in their model, "trance" or "hypnosis" would coincide with the normally non-dominant hemisphere attaining dominance or quasi-dominance as a consequence of the two steps listed earlier. On the other hand, they also make the point in their seminars (e.g., Grinder and Bandler, 1981) that (a) there is no hypnosis and (b) all communications are hypnosis. However, if everything is "hypnosis" then "hypnosis" denotes nothing in particular and (b) says nothing different than (a). Furthermore their books clearly refute this position or they are being dishonest, for if there is no hypnosis, how can they in good faith write at length on how to hypnotize and use hypnosis? To be fair they are not unique in doing this for T. X. Barber, Sarbin, their associates and their students have also continued to talk and write about "hypnosis" over the years in spite of denying its existence.

As I have mentioned in the last chapter, any references made to left and right brain functions in relation to hypnotic phenomena must be considered as poorly founded. They do not add to our understanding of nor our ability to utilize hypnotic phenomena in the style of Erickson. Indeed, references such as Bandler and Grinder make to these functions give their subject matter a false appearance of having a more scientific status than it has. Their emphasis on the use of eye movements and positions as a way of determining what representational mode the subject or patient is using is intriguing, as is the idea that changes in eye position reflect the nature of some of the mental processes that are going on. However, none of their assertions in these respects appear to have been properly documented, and one must look upon them mainly as hypotheses. In my experience with these indicators, I have often found the results to be ambiguous. Furthermore, Coe and Scharcoff (1985) have been unable to find any consistency in the use of indicators of preferred representational systems by individuals. On the other hand Yapko (1981) found that instructions and suggestions aimed at producing a relaxed state were most effective when worded in terms characteristic of the subject's preferred representational system as indicated by their verbalizations. This perhaps shows that verbal content is the more accurate indicator of those proposed by Bandler and Grinder. According to Coe and Scharcoff the limited research data in this area leads to mixed conclusions.

Anchoring, which clearly is not specific to the use of hypnotism, has had great appeal because of its apparent simplicity and because of the quasi-magical therapeutic effects that Bandler and Grinder claim can be obtained with it. In standard psychological terms, it amounts to one-trial learning or conditioning through contiguity successfully taking place in a far wider variety of circumstances and with remarkably far greater effectivity than would be expected from available laboratory data. Aside from the beliefs of Bandler, Grinder, and their students that anchoring techniques work, there are little supporting data. It must be admitted that, when viewed superficially, demonstrations of anchoring given by Bandler and Grinder at their workshops have been at times quite impressive. However, when closely examined, they have shown themselves to be far less impressive, and at times to be questionable, demonstrations. In any event, as far as Erickson's work is concerned, he did not speak of anchoring *per se,* and, to the extent he may have used it, he did not do so in the ways detailed by Bandler and Grinder. They, it seems, can be given credit for having been innovative in its uses.

With reframing, its multiplicity of subconscious entities (with which the therapist and the patient's "conscious" and "unconscious" communicate and which communicate with each other in a quasi-social cooperative manner) raises some serious questions regarding what is actually going on. One can strongly suspect that all these "parts" are artifacts created by the therapist's communications and manipulations. They are highly reminiscent of Watkin's (Watkins & Watkins, 1979) concept of "ego states" and "ego state therapy" that he claims are derived from some earlier psychoanalytic concepts of Ferdern. Either one may have had an influence on the development of the other. Watkins was very familiar with Erickson's work, had considerable contact with him, and shows a great deal of Erickson's influence in his own approach to therapy. Whatever the case may be, reframing, like anchoring, is not specific to the use of hypnotism; also Erickson did not do anything quite like Bandler and Grinder.

Finally, one might consider Jose Silva's use of "guides" mentioned in Volume 1 as a forerunner of Bandler and Grinder's "parts."

In concluding this material, I will briefly discuss the concept that a detailed linguistic study of the communications going on between individuals would not only throw light upon the nature of hypnotic phenomena, but would lead to more effective, even quasi-magical, procedures. The idea that certain signs, words, and sentences are imbued with special powers is very old and culturally widespread. Incantations and magical words, even words that make no sense and are just meaningless noises, abound in the lore of every culture. Furthermore, there is no question that traditional hypnotism generally has a strong dependence upon the process of communication. One could even say that it is a manifestation of communication. From our study of techniques in Volume 1, it is reasonable to think that the way one says things can make an appreciable difference in the results that are attained. However, the specific words that are used, including their intonation and accompanying non-verbal signs, seem to be only one aspect of the communications in question. The context in which the communication is made and the way it is received and perceived seem also to be essential determining factors. As we saw in the last chapter, even Erickson and Rossi admit that, for example, what is intended to be a double bind may not function as such because of how the subject perceives it. Other determining factors may include such elements as the personal qualities possessed by the human source of the communication and the kind of relationship that exists between this source and the recipient. For at least these reasons, it seems rather doubtful that the key to effective hypnotic communications would be found in purely linguistic considerations, and particularly in those relating to the transformational grammar of English.

I would not want the reader to leave this discussion with the idea that NLP, and particularly its view of Ericksonian hypnotism, should be altogether disregarded, or that linguistics has nothing to contribute. There may be some golden nuggets to be found among the dross. Some of the anchoring techniques and reframing procedures that are described are quite interesting and worth further examination. There is certainly something to be said for a possible special role in hypnotic work of the conjunctions "or" and "and," as well as of presupposition, implication, analogical marking, and other linguistic processes listed by Bandler and Grinder. The point is to extract what is useful and to disregard the rest.

9

Clinical Hypnotism:
The State of the Art and
Thoughts for the Future

There have been two periods during which hypnotism has been looked upon favorably by professionals and used by accredited health providers. The first period consisted roughly of the last quarter of the last century. The second period began in 1950 and continues today. Between these two periods, professionals looked askance at hypnotism, and if they had an interest in it, they did not talk much about it. Just a few were brave or foolhardy enough to be open about it. This attitude seems to have been more prevalent among clinicians than researchers, who were openly investigating hypnotic phenomena as early as 1930, and even earlier.

Whether or not the increasing acceptance and use of clinical hypnotism by health providers in the second period is really due to the large amount of laboratory work during the last 30 years or so, as Baker (1987) maintains, or should be attributed to other factors, is not entirely clear. Surely the pressure felt by clinicians, especially psychotherapists, to find briefer methods of treatment was an important element. Likewise, the *Zeitgeist* that was developing around that period may have been a determinant. Clinical hypnotism might have evolved to the same extent whether or not much research went on. I say this because those clinicians I came into contact with during that period did not appear to be particularly knowledgeable about or interested in laboratory findings, although I am sure the research activity helped to raise the status of clinical hypnotism. As far as contributing data that could be applied to clinical work, research still has to do this.

Perhaps the biggest contribution to the growth of interest in and acceptance of hypnotism by professionals came from the efforts of a group of respected and dedicated clinicians who, starting around 1950 and going from city to city, began to offer workshops in hypnotism for the professions. This group was led by Irving I. Secter, Seymour Hershman, and Milton H. Erickson. Erickson was especially dedicated to this task, and perhaps more than anyone else, was instrumental in the flourishing of clinical hypnotism during a period when research was just beginning to acquire some momentum. Erickson had been one of the charter members of the Society for Clinical and Experimental Hypnosis, which was then the only professional organization of its kind. It was also a very select one. He was in favor of widely disseminating clinical hypnotism among the professions. Strongly opposed in this by the majority of the small number of members of the society, he elected to break away and to found the American Society of Clinical Hypnotism, which he opened to any professional interested in hypnotism.

The workshops began by teaching mostly traditional techniques and then gradually shifted more and more toward semi-traditional hypnotism. So-called Ericksonian hypnotism as such never was taught, although many of the principles and techniques upon which it is based were introduced in the workshops. In later years, Erickson began to give seminars in increasing numbers. But it was not until after Erickson's death that Ericksonian hypnotism workshops fully evolved; mainly as a product of later students and followers.

I disagree with Erika Fromm (1987) who asserts that clinical hypnotism has ceased to be an art and is now a science. This seems to be a direct contradiction of the claim of many modern hypnotherapists that clinical hypnotism was successful because it finally moved away from its reliance on laboratory findings. In any case, I find very little in it that qualifies it as a true science. We simply *do not* have an understanding of the nature of either hypnotic phenomena or its clinical uses. As Baker (1987) has aptly pointed out, what has blossomed in the last 30 years is a clinical *technology* utilizing hypnotism, not a science.

One important issue that is rarely considered by clinicians using hypnotism is how effective hypnotic interventions really are. A second and even more important question, usually ignored, is how much of the observed or believed effectiveness *is attributable to hypnosis or to the specific effects of suggestions, and how much to other factors.* As we have seen, these are particularly vexing problems with the Ericksonian approach. The second question is unquestionably the harder of the two to answer, and, essentially, nothing has been done in regard to it. On the other hand, Frankel (1987) has recently shown evidence that a start has been made with regard to the first issue, but there is still far to go.

There is a continuing tendency among some clinicians to promote questionable practices. One physician who was treating female patients for obesity became convinced that all his obese patients were overweight because they had secondary malignant personalities. His treatment approach, I might add, was guaranteed to create such personalities! Regressions to past lives may be a useful therapeutic device, but I have serious questions regarding clinicians whose practice is centered in the production of such regressions to the exclusion of other approaches. One fairly well-known psychiatrist goes a step further in this specialization. It would appear that all of his patients have been priests and priestesses or have served in some other capacity in ancient temples!

The concept of the "unconscious" is being used much too loosely and indiscriminately by clinicians. Therapeutic practices center around it that are *based entirely on conjectures*. Can one really talk in such a way that the "unconscious" will know it is specifically being addressed? Does the unconscious really possess a type of mentality as seems to be implied? Furthermore, if so, why should it be as compliant as it appears to be? Why should it be so much wiser than the therapist with regard to the changes that need to be made, particularly when it belongs to a person with no clinical knowledge? To make matters worse, we have seen a proliferation of "unconsciouses" with some clinicians who maintain we all have many unconscious "parts" capable of interacting with each other and even with our "conscious." With some therapists, these "parts" pass under the more technical sounding label of *ego states*. Are these parts or ego states merely suggested artifacts appearing as secondary personalities? Do they produce the observed therapeutic changes, or are these brought about through some totally different mechanism? Even though therapeutic changes may take place in this context, I must admit that I feel rather uncomfortable about the matter. It sounds too much like mumbo jumbo, and therapeutic sessions done in this context are too reminiscent of spirit seances and exorcisms. There is a dangerous over-reliance on benign unconsciouses affecting cures with an accompanying disregard of psychodynamics.

Looking to the future, one would hope to see clinicians begin to tackle the many questions that have been raised throughout this volume and above. Closer ties to relevant laboratory work and findings are needed, not lesser ties, and one might hope to see more clinically oriented research take place.

There is a need for better training. A major deficiency of most workshops is the inadequate amount of supervised practice that is offered and the lack of available follow-up supervision. The ideal situation would be a one-semester graduate/post graduate university course combining lectures, demonstrations, and a practicum. It would be primarily open to approved graduate students in their last year of clinical training, senior medical students, residents, and, of course, qualified health providers in the community or from outside. It has been my experience that it is nearly impossible to accomplish this. The demands on the time of residents and medical students is particularly bad. The next best alternative may be to offer at intervals a sequence of short courses, limited to small groups (20 maximum), such as those I have given in the French-speaking part of Canada. These courses are four days in length (Thursday through Sunday) and consist of lectures, extensive demonstrations, and short, supervised practicums each day. They total 24 hours each of intensive training and consist of an introductory and an intermediate-level course given at six-months intervals. Each participant gets a total of one hour of closely supervised practice in each course with one supervisor allocated to small groups of three to four participants. These practice sessions are as important as, if not more than, the didactic portions. One hour of practice is by no means adequate, but under the circumstances, supplemented by appropriate demonstrations, this seems to do a reasonably good job.

Who shall be trained and allowed to use hypnotism professionally is a heated topic. In the early days of the Society for Clinical and Experimental Hypnosis, there were members who advocated that only psychiatrists should be trained and use hypnotism. Some were even in favor of restricting the sale of books on hypnotism to the professions. This organization and the American Society of Clinical Hypnosis are still adamant about only individuals with doctoral degrees in psychology, medicine, and dentistry being allowed to take part in professional level workshops. I believe it is only a matter of time before these restrictions must break down. In the meantime, for a number of years fully accredited members of the two societies have been openly giving workshops that have been open to professionals who do not have doctoral degrees, even though such an activity is expressedly forbidden by at least the Society for Clinical and Experimental Hypnosis. In any case, anyone who really wants to learn how to hypnotize and utilize hypnosis and suggestions can readily do so by reading the many books now available and by taking unaccredited courses. Personally, I would much rather see individuals who are professional licensed health providers at a masters degree level or the equivalent (registered nurses, psychiatric social workers, marital and family therapists, among others) get their training under the auspices of the above-named societies than on their own, and, especially, from questionable sources. I doubt there is more likelihood of their misusing it than there is of individuals with doctoral degrees doing so. If they have been properly selected and trained in their specialties, they will be aware of their limitations and will not go beyond what they are qualified or instructed to do. I have yet to see a registered nurse seriously exceeding her qualifications. I can see many advantages, for example, in registered nurses and dental assistants being able to prepare patients for hypnotic therapy in clinics, offices, and hospitals. Properly trained nurses who work with surgery and obstetric patients, and especially those on oncology units, are among those who could use hypnotism very effectively. Hypnotism can be a very useful pre-operative and post-operative adjunct; it could be very useful with patients undergoing chemo- and radiation therapy. Nurses thus trained could relieve physicians of a time-consuming activity, and hypnotism could be made more available on a routine basis to patients. There is, however, a need to offer specialized courses for these people, possibly following a short basic course. In fact, the ideal situation would be to be able to offer further specialized "advanced" courses to all professionals on a continuing education basis.

Glossary

The definitions given for the terms that follow are not necessarily those that will be found in dictionaries, but pertain to my particular use. For the most part, they will be found to agree with accepted uses. Where important, more than one use is listed; the first listed is the one I prefer. Words used in the definitions that are in capitals will be found in this glossary.

Age Regression: A re-experiencing of earlier events in life, usually limited to a specific time or time period.

Amnesia: Normally refers to a pathological form of extensive forgetting. In the context of HYPNOSIS it is always a *reversible* forgetting. It may occur spontaneously or be suggested. It may be *partial* or *total* according to how much material is forgotten or not retrievable.

Approach: A general, overall, characteristic *modus operandi.*

Arousal: Level of excitation of the nervous system, especially of the reticular system, associated with a state of vigilance or readiness of the cortex. Reticular activation is frequently viewed as the physiological counterpart of CONSCIOUSNESS. More properly it should probably be said to be associated with and necessary for its occurrence.

Authoritarian: Commanding, forceful, injunctive. Said of SUGGESTIONS and APPROACHES. Particularly used in connection with DIRECT SUGGESTIONS.

Autohypnosis: See SELF-HYPNOSIS.

Automatic: Said of actions that are not being voluntarily controlled. All AUTOMATISMS are of this kind.

Automatism: Synonymous with INVOLUNTARY and NON-VOLUNTARY behaviors and actions. Automatisms comprise *both* and range from simple reflex acts to complex activities.

Autosuggestion: A SUGGESTION given by an individual to himself.

Awareness: See CONSCIOUSNESS.

Braid Effect: The hypnotic state James Braid elicited by means of visual fixation only.

Chaining: Synergetically relating the effects of one SUGGESTION to another SUGGESTION or the response to it. Sometime spoken of as LINKING.

Coconscious: See SUBCONSCIOUS.

Component Response: Each distinct response in a sequence of SUGGESTION STEPS.

Conscious: That which is known and experienced. Also, the knowing, experiencing, intelligently controlling aspect of the psyche. As such, it is the reservoir and embodiment of the totality of all that is known and experienced at a given time. Used as an adjective to denote activities controlled by the conscious.

Consciousness: Frequently synonymous with CONSCIOUS. Also a quality or aspect of being defying proper definition and best considered one of the fundamental givens of the psychological universe of discourse.

Consciousness, Altered State of: A poorly defined concept which hypothesizes the possibility of occurrence of a multiplicity of "consciousnesses" differing in various ways from the "normal" or modal "consciousness" of an individual and partaking of its main features.

Consciousness, Depotentialization of: Preventing CONSCIOUS action from taking place. There is usually an implication in the use of this expression that the CONSCIOUS is put out of commission.

Consciousness, Primary: The normal, that is, usual CONSCIOUSNESS of an individual. Synonymous with "normal" CONSCIOUSNESS.

Consciousness, Secondary: Any more or less temporary *other* CONSCIOUSNESS substituted for a PRIMARY CONSCIOUSNESS.

Deautomatization: Making AUTOMATISMS accessible to voluntary control; transformation of AUTOMATISMS into voluntary acts.

Depth, Hypnotic: Extension ascribed to HYPNOSIS. Frequently measured by the degree of SUGGESTIBILITY possessed by a presumably hypnotized individual.

Dissociation: A term with several meanings. It is used as a broad term referring to hypothesized separations of mental processes normally considered to be bound together. Has also been more specifically used to denote conditions in which some overt and covert activities of an individual normally in his consciousness occur outside of it. When the scope of the activities involved is limited one speaks of a PARTIAL DISSOCIATION. When all activities are affected one then speaks of a TOTAL DISSOCIATION. In the latter case the overall effect has the appearance of a person's normal CONSCIOUSNESS having been displaced or replaced by another one.

Dissociation, Hypnotic: DISSOCIATION taking place in the context of hypnotic manifestations and, more particularly, in the course of an induction of HYPNOSIS.

Dissociation, Partial: See DISSOCIATION.

Dissociation, Total: See DISSOCIATION.

Dissociative Effect: The occurrence of any dissociation.

Elaborations: Refers to ongoing modifications of the manifestations of SUGGESTION EFFECTS brought about by these manifestations acting as stimuli. As such they are capable of setting other mental processes into motion that alter the overall response. These extraneous processes include the subject's natural reactions to what is going on at the time.

End Response: The ultimate response or goal aimed for by a PROCEDURE.

Feedback, Negative: Use of a part of or of the whole of a system's output or response to decrement the input giving rise to this output.

Feedback, Positive: Use of a part of or of the whole of a system's output or response to increment the input giving rise to this output.

Heterohypnosis: HYPNOSIS induced by one person in another person.

Hypersuggestibility: Refers to SUGGESTIBILITY above a norm or above an individual's base line.

Hypnopsychotherapy: Use of HYPNOTISM in doing psychotherapy. With few exceptions it consists of HYPNOTHERAPEUTIC INTERVENTIONS.

Hypnosis: An inferred psychophysiological state characterized by HYPERSUGGESTIBILITY, i.e., increased SUGGESTIBILITY, and/or one or more of a widely accepted set of other clinical signs. Often hypothesized to be an ALTERED STATE OF CONSCIOUSNESS. It may occur in a number of forms each constituting a state of its own. Some authorities do not recognize HYPERSUGGESTIBILITY to be one of its characteristics. Others deny the existence of such a state.

Hypnosis, Clinical: The prophylactic and therapeutic uses of HYPNOTISM.

Hypnosis, Common: See HYPNOTISM, TRADITIONAL.

Hypnosis, Conventional: TRADITIONAL OR SEMI-TRADITIONAL HYPNOSIS which is not SOMNAMBULIC.

Hypnosis, Dissociative: A proposed form of hypnosis associated with a TOTAL DISSOCIATION.

Hypnosis, Non-Somnambulic: See HYPNOSIS, CONVENTIONAL.

Hypnosis, Semi-Traditional: HYPNOSIS produced and used in the context of a SEMI-TRADITIONAL APPROACH. Does not imply any "special" form of HYPNOSIS.

Hypnosis, Sleep: A form of HYPNOSIS showing the EEG characteristics of drowsiness or very light sleep.

Hypnosis, Somnambulic: HYPNOSIS characteristically associated with spontaneously occurring AMNESIA and HYPERSUGGESTIBILITY. Frequently inappropriately used to denote an arbitrarily defined high degree of SUGGESTIBILITY. See also SOMNAMBULISM.

Hypnosis, Traditional: HYPNOSIS used in the context of a TRADITIONAL APPROACH. Does not imply any "special" form of HYPNOSIS.

Hypnosomatotherapy: Use of HYPNOTISM as the primary agent in the treatment of somatic problems.

Hypnosuggestive: Said of an effect or action originating from a SUGGESTION given in the presence of HYPNOSIS. Synonymous with HYPNOTIC.

Hypnosuggestive Intervention: See next entry.

Hypnotherapeutic Intervention: Use of HYPNOTIC SUGGESTION to produce a therapeutic effect which is only a part of an overall therapy.

Hypnotherapy: Any therapy in which the use of HYPNOTISM constitutes the core of the treatment.

Hypnotic: Pertaining or belonging to the domain of hypnotism. More specifically, associated with HYPNOSIS.

Hypnotism: The study and use of SUGGESTION with or without the presence of HYPNOSIS. Frequently employed as a short form and synonym for TRADITIONAL AND SEMI-TRADITIONAL HYPNOTISM when greater specificity is not required. In a more restricted, infrequently used sense refers to the study and use of HYPNOSIS *per se.*

Hypnotism, Classical: Production and use of the BRAID EFFECT.

Hypnotism, Ericksonian: An approach to the production of hypnotic phenomena, particularly in a clinical setting, originated by Milton H. Erickson, and characterized by PERMISSIVENESS and the extensive use of INDIRECT SUGGESTION and UTILIZATION techniques. Also, school and movement centered around the teachings of Milton H. Erickson.

Hypnotism, Non-Traditional: ERICKSONIAN HYPNOTISM and its derivatives. Any use of hypnotism that does not come under the headings of CLASSICAL, TRADITIONAL or SEMI-TRADITIONAL.

Hypnotism, Semi-Traditional: TRADITIONAL HYPNOTISM modified by the use of such devices as PACING, LEADING, MATCHING, CHAINING, and the UTILIZATION of a subject's responses. It resembles ERICKSONIAN HYPNOTISM in these regards but historically antedates it and represents a transition phase.

Hypnotism, Traditional: Early forms of HYPNOTISM based entirely on the use of DIRECT, AUTHORITARIAN SUGGESTIONS.

Hypnotizability: The DEPTH OF HYPNOSIS attained at any given moment by a presumably HYPNOTIZED individual. It is usually incorrectly identified with the person's HYPNOTIC SUGGESTIBILITY. Has often been used as a synonym for HYPNOTIC SUSCEPTIBILITY.

Hypnotize, to: To bring about a state of HYPNOSIS in an individual.

Hypnotized: Said of a person in a state of HYPNOSIS.

Ideational Content: The essential idea or ideas contained in, or conveyed by, a communication, by an event, or a situation.

Ideoaffective Action: IDEODYNAMIC ACTION which is affective in nature.

Ideodynamic Action: A hypothesized cortical reflex whereby an idea evokes an action without mediation by the higher cortical centers. The action is therefore considered always to be NON-VOLUNTARY or to be INVOLUNTARY, hence an AUTOMATISM.

Ideodynamic Capacity: The capacity for IDEODYNAMIC ACTION. Distinguished from SUGGESTIBILITY which refers to the capacity to produce a response based on IDEODYNAMIC ACTION usually modified by various co-existing factors.

Ideomotor Action: IDEODYNAMIC ACTION which is motoric in nature.

Ideomotor Signaling: A technique used in HYPNOTISM in which NON-VOLUNTARY movements on the subject's part are used to communicate presumably with his UNCONSCIOUS.

Ideosensory Action: IDEODYNAMIC ACTION which is sensory in nature.

Induction (of Hypnosis):   Any intended production of HYPNOSIS.

Induction, Formal: In a TRADITIONAL APPROACH it is the production of HYPNOSIS by the use of precised, preestablished set rules and patterns of stepwise procedures with a clearcut beginning and end, and a set wording to be used without modifications. In a SEMI-TRADITIONAL APPROACH there is a like situation with a limited flexibility allowing some changes to be made in the steps and words used on an ongoing basis as deemed indicated by the situation. In both instances all concerned know that an INDUCTION is being performed.

Induction, Informal: Any INDUCTION OF HYPNOSIS that does not follow a preestablished, set pattern of steps and words and is largely *ad libbed.* It frequently is done on an impromptu basis and may not have a clearcut beginning or end.

Intervention, Hypnotic: Use of HYPNOTISM to produce an effect in an adjunctive manner. Most often used in the context of therapy.

Involuntary: Inborn or acquired behavior that at no time has been or can be under volitional control. Includes all spinal and autonomic and conditioned reflexes.

Leading: Communicating about an imminent event as if it was already taking place. More specifically used in reference to imminently anticipated behavior on the part of a subject.

Linking: See CHAINING.

Matching: Said of an individual deliberately reflecting in his own behavior features present in the behavior of another person. Synonymous with "mirroring."

Neurolinguistic Programming: A method of influencing others through forms of communication developed by John Grinder and Richard Bandler. Includes hypnotism but is broader in scope.

Non-Voluntary: Behavior that can be VOLUNTARY but which, at the time of observation, is deemed to be taking place without VOLUNTARY participation by the person doing it and which may even be outside his consciousness. More specifically it was neither voluntarily initiated or is being voluntarily directed.

Operator: Synonymous with hypnotist and suggestor.

Pacing: Communicating to a subject, FEEDBACK-wise, factual data regarding his current overt and covert behavior.

Permissive: The opposite of AUTHORITARIAN. Said of SUGGESTIONS and APPROACHES.

Personality, Primary: Synonymous with "normal, that is, usual personality." It is the personality usually associated with an individual's PRIMARY CONSCIOUSNESS.

Personality, Secondary: Any personality other than the PRIMARY PERSONALITY. It is always associated with a SECONDARY CONSCIOUSNESS.

Presuggestion: See SUGGESTION, PREHYPNOTIC.

Procedures: A specific sequence of steps leading to a desired response.

Ratification: A term used by Milton H. Erickson to denote the act of providing a subject or patient with evidence he has been hypnotized or has experienced hypnotic effects.

Revivification: A condition said to be present with an AGE REGRESSION when the latter is accompanied by a return to a physiological state believed to have existed at the time to which the subject has returned.

Self-Hypnosis: HYPNOSIS induced by an individual in himself.

Self-Suggestion: See AUTOSUGGESTION.

Semi-Traditional: Pertaining to SEMI-TRADITIONAL HYPNOTISM.

Semi-Voluntary: Said of behaviors that are partially but not altogether VOLUNTARY. Volition may initiate, modify or terminate these behaviors but is not in constant control. The behaviors therefore go on partially automatically. Most daily activities are of this nature.

Somnambulism: A term used to denote a number of hypothesized mental states. May denote a sleep abnormality also referred to as "natural somnambulism." It has been used to denote a pathological condition occurring in the waking state once associated with major hysteria. It has also been used to denote an artificially induced condition often qualified as being "artificial" and later called HYPNOSIS. It has been considered to be one of several forms under which HYPNOSIS manifests itself, its chief feature being spontaneous AMNESIA usually associated with HYPERSUGGESTIBILITY. As such it is synonymous with SOMNAMBULIC HYPNOSIS. In contemporary HYPNOTISM it is merely an arbitrary designation given to hypnosis associated with very high values of SUGGESTIBILITY.

Somnambulism, Hypnotic: Expression used for the purpose of making it clear that the term "somnambulism" is being employed in the context of HYPNOSIS. Synonymous with SOMNAMBULIC HYPNOSIS.

Step Response: Response to a STEP SUGGESTION.

Strategy: Choosing between available PROCEDURES to optimize the production of a result.

Subconscious: Psychic processes of which an individual is not CONSCIOUS but which otherwise appear to be like the processes involved in CONSCIOUS experience and action. One may speak of "*the* subconscious" as the embodiment of the totality of such processes going on at a given time. SUBCONSCIOUS activities differ from UNCONSCIOUS ones in that they are always integrated, goal directed activities, exhibiting "intelligence." All SUBCONSCIOUS activities are also UNCONSCIOUS ones, but the converse does not hold.

Subject: Term used traditionally to denote any individual submitting to the use of SUGGESTIONS or to an INDUCTION OF HYPNOSIS. Is frequently applied to patients with whom hypnotism is used.

Suggestibility: The capacity to respond to SUGGESTIONS. Distinguished from the capacity to produce SUGGESTION EFFECTS, and more specifically from IDEODYNAMIC CAPACITY. SUGGESTIBILITY usually differs from the capacity for SUGGESTION EFFECTS because it reflects the influence of factors influencing the final expression of the latter.

Suggestibility, Hypnotic: SUGGESTIBILITY associated with a hypnotic state. May or may not be of the same nature as that associated with the normal state of an individual.

Suggestibility, Waking: Often used to designate SUGGESTIBILITY associated with the normal awake state of an individual. Same as "non-hypnotic" SUGGESTIBILITY.

Suggestion: A communication which evokes a NON-VOLUNTARY response which reflects the IDEATIONAL CONTENT of the communication. See also SUGGESTION, TRADITIONAL.

Suggestion, Component: Any suggestion combined with other suggestions to form a COMPOUND SUGGESTION. COMPONENT SUGGESTIONS can be UNIT or COMPOUND SUGGESTIONS.

Suggestion, Compound: The result of combining several suggestions into a more complex one. Usually done by means of the conjunctions "and" and "or."

Suggestion, Direct: A SUGGESTION whose IDEATIONAL CONTENT is explicitly stated.

Suggestion Effect: The conversion of an idea into an action that satisfies the two defining criteria of a TRADITIONAL SUGGESTION. As such it is often identified with activated IDEODYNAMIC ACTION. The SUGGESTION EFFECT is not the response itself.

Suggestion, Effective: A communication planned to serve as a SUGGESTION which has been demonstrated to have acted as one, hence to have produced a SUGGESTION EFFECT.

Suggestion, Elementary: See UNIT SUGGESTION.

Suggestion, Extrahypnotic: A SUGGESTION given in the absence of HYPNOSIS.

Suggestion, Indirect: A SUGGESTION whose IDEATIONAL CONTENT is not explicitly stated. This content may be implied, contained in an association, or hidden within the communication.

Suggestion, Intended: A communication which is intended to function as a SUGGESTION but which has not yet been shown to have thus acted.

Suggestion, Intrahypnotic: A SUGGESTION given in the presence of HYPNOSIS.

Suggestion, Posthypnotic: A SUGGESTION given in HYPNOSIS, which is to become effective only in the future after the HYPNOSIS has been removed.

Suggestion, Prehypnotic: A SUGGESTION given prior to an induction of HYPNOSIS which becomes effective following or during such an induction.

Suggestion, Step: Any SUGGESTION given as part of a sequence in which each suggestion produces a distinct response which, in combination with other responses, contributes to the END RESPONSE. STEP SUGGESTIONS usually are UNIT SUGGESTIONS. See also CHAINING, PROCEDURE, and COMPOUND SUGGESTIONS.

Suggestion, Traditional: A communication made by one person to another that, (1) evokes an AUTOMATISM in the second person that, (2) reflects, that is, is a realization of the IDEATIONAL CONTENT of the communication. *This is the only sense in which the term "suggestion" is used in this work,* that is, unless otherwise stated.

Suggestion, Unit: A smallest communication capable of acting as a SUGGESTION.

Susceptibility, Hypnotic: The potentiality, capacity, or ability a person has for developing a state of hypnosis. It is usually employed in a predictive sense and is usually based on estimates of a person's HYPNOZABILITY. Commonly incorrectly associated with a person's predicted HYPNOTIC SUGGESTIBILITY. Frequently used interchangeably with HYPNOTIZABILITY.

System UCS: The specific Freudian (conception of the) UNCONSCIOUS.

Technique: Plan or method of doing something. A technique can be a PROCEDURE but, more generally, consists of a number of these. Frequently used as a synonym for PROCEDURE.

Traditional: Pertaining to TRADITIONAL HYPNOTISM, or to tradition.

Trance: Often used synonymously for HYPNOSIS. It is more reasonable to speak of a class of TRANCES of which HYPNOSIS is only one member. That is, HYPNOSIS is a special case of TRANCE. The converse, that all TRANCES are HYPNOSIS does not hold.

Unconscious: Said of psychic activities and processes going on in an individual and of overt activities on his part of which he is not CONSCIOUS. The embodiment of the totality of such activities and processes is referred to as "*the* unconscious." Frequently this last expression is used as a synonym for SUBCONSCIOUS. Many writers speak of a plurality of "unconsciouses" in this latter sense. The above mentioned activities can be viewed as inclusive of those ascribed to the Freudian "unconscious."

Unconsciousness, Clinical: Clinical state of unresponsiveness accompanied by a seeming amnesia on recovery. Often accompanied by mild to severely depressed physiological functions. The "amnesia" may actually be a reflection that stimuli are unable to make any impression.

Utilization: Making use of the subject's responses, potentials for specific behaviors, and dynamisms in the production of a suggested effect. Also making use of specific observed or sensed ongoing responses and spontaneous actions on the part of the subject when giving SUGGESTIONS. See PACING.

Voluntary: Any act experienced by an individual as having been consciously initiated or terminated by him. Such an act may be consciously directed from beginning to end or may largely go on at a NON-VOLUNTARY level in between. It may be self-terminating.

Will: The function or functions involved in (delayed) conscious action.

References

Baker, E. L. (1987). The state of the art of clinical hypnosis. *International Journal of Clinical and Experimental Hypnosis, 35*, 203–214.

Bandler, R., & Grinder, J. (1975a). *The structure of magic, I.* Palo Alto, CA: Science and Behavior Books.

—— (1975b). *Patterns of the hypnotic techniques of Milton H. Erickson, M.D., Volume 1.* Cupertino, CA: Meta Publications.

—— (1979). *Frogs into princes.* Moab, UT: Real People Press.

—— (1982). *ReFraming.* Moab, UT: Real People Press.

Bateson, G., Jackson, D. D., Haley, J., & Weakland, J. (1956). Toward a theory of schizophrenia. *Behavioral Science, 41*, 251–264.

Berger, M. M. (Ed.). (1978). *Beyond the double bind.* New York: Brunner/Mazel.

Bower, B. (1987). The language of the brain. *Science News, 132*, 40–41.

Charny, E. J. (1966). Psychosomatic manifestations of rapport in psychotherapy. *Psychosomatic Medicine, 28*, 305–315.

Chevreul, M. (1854). *De la baguette divinatoire, du pendul dit explorateur et des tables tournantes, au point de vue de l'histoire, de la critique et de la méthode expérimentale.* Paris: Mallet-Richelieu.

Chomsky, N. (1972). *Language and mind.* New York: Harcourt Brace Jovanovich.

Coe, W. C., & Scharcoff, J. A. (1985). An empirical evaluation of the neurolinguistic programming model. *International Journal of Clinical Hypnosis, 33*, 310–318.

Coons, P. M. (1988). Misuse of forensic hypnosis: A hypnotically elicited false confession with the apparent creation of a multiple personality. *American Journal of Clinical Hypnosis, 36*, 1–11.

Crassilneck, H. B., & Hall, J. A. (1975). *Clinical hypnosis: Principles and applications.* New York: Grune & Stratton.

Ellenberger, H. F. (1970). *The discovery of the unconscious.* New York: Basic Books.

English, H. B., & English, A. C. (1958). *A comprehensive dictionary of psychological and psychoanalytical terms.* New York: Longmans, Green.

Erickson, M. H. (1935). A study of an experimental neurosis hypnotically induced in a case of ejaculation praecox. *British Journal of Medical Psychology, 15,* 34–50.

———— (1939). Experimental demonstration of the psychopathology of everyday life. *Psychoanalytic Quarterly, 8,* 338–353.

———— (1944). The method employed to formulate a complex story for the induction of an experimental neurosis. *Journal of General Psychology, 31,* 67–84.

———— (1948). Hypnotic psychotherapy. *The Medical Clinics of North America,* 571–583.

———— (1958). Naturalistic techniques of hypnosis. *American Journal of Clinical Hypnosis, 1,* 3–8.

———— (1959). Historical note on the hand levitation and other ideomotor techniques. *American Journal of Clinical Hypnosis, 2,* 3–21.

———— (1963). Hypnotically oriented psychotherapy in organic disease. *American Journal of Clinical Hypnosis, 5,* 92–112.

———— (1986). *Mind-body communication in hypnosis.* E. L. Rossi & M. O'Ryan (Eds.), New York: Irvington Publishers.

————, Haley, J., & Weakland, J. H. (1959). A transcript of a trance induction with commentary. *American Journal of Clinical Hypnosis, 11,* 49–84.

————, & Rossi, E. L. (1975). Varieties of double bind. *American Journal of Clinical Hypnosis, 17,* 143–157.

————, & Rossi, E. L. (1976). Two level communication and the microdynamic of trance induction. *American Journal of Clinical Hypnosis, 18,* 153–171.

————, Rossi, E. L., & Rossi, S. I. (1976). *Hypnotic realities.* New York: Irvington Publishers.

———— (1979). *Hypnotherapy. An exploratory case book.* New York: Irvington Publishers.

———— (1981). *Experiencing hypnosis: Therapeutic approaches to altered states.* New York: Irvington Publishers.

————, Hershman, S., & Secter, I. (1961). *The practical applications of medical and dental hypnosis.* New York: Julian Press.

Frankel, F. H. (1987). Significant developments in medical hypnosis during the past 25 years. *The International Journal of Clinical and Experimental Hypnosis, 35,* 231–247.

Fromm, E. (1987). Significant developments in clinical hypnosis during the past 25 years. *The International Journal of Clinical and Experimental Hypnosis, 35,* 215–230.

Gazzaniga, M. S. (1985). *The social brain.* New York: Basic Books.

Gordon, D. (1978). *Therapeutic metaphors.* Cupertino, CA: Meta Publications.

Grinder, J., & Bandler, R. (1976). *The structure of magic, II.* Palo Alto, CA: Science and Behavior Books.

———— (1981). *TRANCE-formation.* Moab, UT: Real People Press.

————, Delozier, J., & Bandler, R. (1977). *Patterns of the hypnotic techniques of Milton H. Erickson, M.D.* Cupertino, CA: Meta Publications.

Haley, J. (1958). An interactional explanation of hypnosis. *American Journal of Clinical Hypnosis, 1*, 41–57.

———— (1969). *Advanced techniques of hypnosis and therapy. Selected papers of Milton H. Erickson, M.D.* New York: Grune & Stratton.

———— (1973). *Uncommon therapy.* New York: Norton.

Hammond, D. C. (1985). The security place. *American Society of Clinical Hypnosis Newsletter, 26*, 4.

———— (1987). Are indirect suggestions superior to direct suggestions? *American Society of Clinical Hypnosis Newsletter, 28*, 3.

Hartland, J. (1971). *Medical and dental hypnosis and its clinical applications.* London: Bailliere Tindall.

Janet, P. (1889). *L'automatisme psychologique. Essai de psychologie expérimentale sur les formes inférieures de l'activité humaine.* Paris: Alcan.

Kosslyn, S. M. (1988). Aspects of a cognitive neuroscience of mental imagery. *Science, 240*, 1621–1626.

Kroger, W. S. (1963). *Clinical and experimental hypnosis in medicine, dentistry and psychology.* Philadelphia: Lippincott.

Lyons, J. (1977). *Semantics. Volumes 1 and 2.* Cambridge: Cambridge University Press.

O'Hanlon, W. H. (1985). A study guide of frameworks of Milton H. Erickson's hypnosis and therapy. J. K. Zeig (Ed.), *A teaching seminar with Milton H. Erickson.* New York: Brunner/Mazel, 33–51.

O'Hanlon, W. H. (1987). *Taproots.* New York: Norton.

Orne, M. T. (1979). The use and misuse of hypnosis in court. *International Journal of Clinical and Experimental Hypnosis, 27*, 311–341.

Reichenbach, H. (1947). *Elements of symbolic logic.* New York: Macmillan.

Rossi, E. L. (Ed.). (1980). *The collected papers of Milton H. Erickson on hypnosis. Volumes 1, 2, 3, 4.* New York: Irvington Publishers.

Rossi, E. L. (1986). *The Psychobiology of mind-body healing.* New York: Norton.

Runes, D. D. (1962). *Dictionary of philosophy.* New York: The Philosophical Library.

Seitz, P. F. (1953). Experiments in substitution of symptoms by hypnosis: II. *Psychosomatic Medicine, 5*, 405–424.

Sidis, B. (1910). *The psychology of suggestion.* New York: Appleton-Century.

Spiegel, H. (1970). A single-treatment method to stop smoking using ancillary self-hypnosis. *International Journal of Clinical and Experimental Hypnosis, 18*, 235–250.

Stein, C. (1963). The clenched fist technique as a hypnotic procedure in clinical psychotherapy. *American Journal of Clinical Hypnosis, 6*, 113–119.

Taber's medical cyclopedic dictionary. (1981). Philadelphia: Davis.

von Dedenroth, T. E. A. (1964a). The use of hypnosis with "tobaccomania." *American Journal of Clinical Hypnosis, 6,* 326–331.

———— (1964b). Further help for the "tobaccomaniacs." *American Journal of Clinical Hypnosis, 6,* 332–336.

Watkins, J. G., & Watkins, H. H. (1979). Theory and practice of ego state therapy: a short-term therapeutic approach. In P. Olsen, & H. Grayson (Eds.), *Short term approaches to psychotherapy.* New York: Human Science Press.

Watzlawick, P., Beavin, J. H., & Jackson, D. D. (1967). *Pragmatics of human communication.* New York: Norton.

Weitzenhoffer, A. M. (1960a). Unconscious or co-conscious? *American Journal of Clinical Hypnosis, 2,* 177–196.

———— (1960b). Reflections upon certain specific and current uses of the "unconscious" in clinical hypnosis. *Journal of Clinical and Experimental Hypnosis, 8,* 165–177.

———— (1962). The significance of hypnotic depth for therapy. *International Journal of Clinical and Experimental Hypnosis, 10,* 75–78.

———— (1972a). Behavior therapeutic techniques and hypnotherapeutic methods. *American Journal of Clinical Hypnosis, 15,* 71–82.

———— (1972b). Open-ended distance hypnotherapy. *American Journal of Clinical Hypnosis, 14,* 236–248.

———— (1974). Limited hypnotherapy of a case of diaphragmatic clonus. *American Journal of Clinical Hypnosis, 16,* 147–154.

————, & Hilgard, E. R. (1959). *Stanford hypnotic susceptibility scale, forms A and B.* Stanford, CA: Consulting Psychologists Press.

Wolberg, L. R. (1945). *Hypnoanalysis.* New York: Grune & Stratton.

———— (1948). *Medical hypnosis. Volumes I and II.* New York: Grune & Stratton.

———— (1967). *The technique of psychotherapy, part one.* New York: Grune & Stratton.

Wolpe, J. (1969). *The practice of behavior therapy.* New York: Pergammon.

Yapko, M. D. (1981). The effect of matching primary representational system predicated on hypnotic relaxation. *American Journal of Clinical Hypnosis, 23,* 169–175.

Zeig, J. K. (1980). *A teaching seminar with Milton H. Erikson.* New York: Brunner/Mazel.

Author Index

Subject Index